MEDICAL TESTS
SOURCEBOOK

SEVENTH EDITION

Table of Contents

Part 2. Laboratory Tests

Part 3. Imaging Tests

Part 4. Endoscopic, Catheterization, and Electrical Tests and Assessments

Part 5. Screening and Assessments for Specific Conditions and Diseases

Part 6. Home and Self-Ordered Tests

Preface

ABOUT THIS BOOK

Regular medical tests can help find problems before they start. They also can help find problems early, when one's chances for treatment and cure are better. Screening tests identify risk factors for specific disorders, while diagnostic tests find markers of disease or dysfunction. Medical tests assist in diagnosing the causes of symptoms, making treatment decisions, and assessing treatment effectiveness. When faced with decisions about health, consumers need to understand the benefits and limitations of medical tests and how the test results guide treatment and lifestyle choices.

Medical Tests Sourcebook, Seventh Edition provides updated information about exams, tests, and other screening, diagnostic, and disease monitoring procedures. It discusses preventive care guidelines and the screening tests used for specific conditions such as allergies, cancer, celiac disease, diabetes, thyroid dysfunction, COVID-19, etc. Details about laboratory blood tests, biopsies, urine tests, and genetic tests are also presented. Imaging tests, such as x-ray, ultrasound, computed tomography (CT), magnetic resonance, nuclear, and optical imaging are described, and facts are offered about electrical, endoscopic, and home-use tests. The book concludes with a glossary of related terms and a directory of organizations related to medical tests.

HOW TO USE THIS BOOK

This book is divided into parts and chapters. Parts focus on broad areas of interest. Chapters are devoted to single topics within a part.

Part 1: Screening and Preventive Care Tests are used to identify individuals with specific risk factors for which the timely provision of medical care or other interventions can help avoid or reduce health consequences. These include high blood pressure (HBP), high cholesterol, and certain genetic characteristics. Information is included about regular health exams, newborn screening tests, and preventive screening recommendations for all ages.

Part 2: Laboratory Tests begins with an overview of lab tests. Information about commonly used diagnostic and preventive care tests, such as blood tests, urine tests, and stool tests are provided. Specific types of biopsies are also explained.

Part 3: Imaging Tests describes many types of imaging available and the accompanying risks associated with exposure to radiation emissions. Imaging tests include x-rays, contrast radiography, ultrasound exams, computed tomography (CT) scans, magnetic resonance imaging (MRI), nuclear imaging, neurological imaging, and optical imaging.

Part 4: Endoscopic, Catheterization, and Electrical Tests and Assessments describes tests that use scopes, cameras, and electrical assessments such as endoscopy, laparoscopy, cardiac catheterization, electrocardiogram, electroencephalogram, electromyography, and electronystagmography.

Part 5: Screening and Assessments for Specific Conditions and Diseases explains tests used to identify and monitor conditions such as allergy, cancer, celiac disease, cystic fibrosis, diabetes, heart disease, lung disease, sleep disorders, and thyroid disorders. Information is also provided about vision tests, prenatal tests, and infertility tests.

Part 6: Home and Self-Ordered Tests discusses products that offer consumers a private option for the initial screening of cholesterol, diabetes, drug abuse, human immunodeficiency virus (HIV), COVID-19, and other health concerns.

Part 7: Additional Help and Information provides a glossary of terms and a directory of organizations related to medical tests.

BIBLIOGRAPHIC NOTE

This volume contains documents and excerpts from publications issued by the following U.S. government agencies: Agency for Healthcare Research and Quality (AHRQ); Cancer Imaging Program (CIP); Centers for Disease Control and Prevention (CDC); *Eunice Kennedy Shriver* National Institute of Child Health and Human Development (NICHD); MedlinePlus; National Cancer Institute (NCI); National Digestive Diseases Information Clearinghouse (NDDIC); National Eye Institute (NEI); National Heart, Lung, and Blood Institute (NHLBI); National Institute of Biomedical Imaging and Bioengineering (NIBIB); National Institute of Diabetes and

Digestive and Kidney Diseases (NIDDK); National Institute of Neurological Disorders and Stroke (NINDS); Office of Disease Prevention and Health Promotion (ODPHP); Office on Women's Health (OWH); Surveillance, Epidemiology, and End Results (SEER) Program; U.S. Department of Veterans Affairs (VA); and U.S. Food and Drug Administration (FDA).

It also contains original material produced by Omnigraphics and reviewed by medical consultants.

ABOUT THE *HEALTH REFERENCE SERIES*

The *Health Reference Series* is designed to provide basic medical information for patients, families, caregivers, and the general public. Each volume provides comprehensive coverage on a particular topic. This is especially important for people who may be dealing with a newly diagnosed disease or a chronic disorder in themselves or in a family member. People looking for preventive guidance, information about disease warning signs, medical statistics, and risk factors for health problems will also find answers to their questions in the *Health Reference Series*. The *Series*, however, is not intended to serve as a tool for diagnosing illness, in prescribing treatments, or as a substitute for the physician–patient relationship. All people concerned about medical symptoms or the possibility of disease are encouraged to seek professional care from an appropriate healthcare provider.

A NOTE ABOUT SPELLING AND STYLE

Health Reference Series editors use *Stedman's Medical Dictionary* as an authority for questions related to the spelling of medical terms and *The Chicago Manual of Style* for questions related to grammatical structures, punctuation, and other editorial concerns. Consistent adherence is not always possible, however, because the individual volumes within the *Series* include many documents from a wide variety of different producers, and the editor's primary goal is to present material from each source as accurately as is possible. This sometimes means that information in different chapters or sections may follow other guidelines and alternate spelling authorities. For example, occasionally a copyright holder may require that eponymous terms be shown in possessive forms (Crohn's disease vs. Crohn disease) or that British spelling norms be retained (leukaemia vs. leukemia).

MEDICAL REVIEW

Omnigraphics contracts with a team of qualified, senior medical professionals who serve as medical consultants for the *Health Reference Series*. As necessary, medical consultants review reprinted and originally written material for currency and accuracy. Citations including the phrase "Reviewed (month, year)" indicate material reviewed by this team. Medical consultation services are provided to the *Health Reference Series* editors by:

Dr. Vijayalakshmi, MBBS, DGO, MD
Dr. Senthil Selvan, MBBS, DCH, MD
Dr. K. Sivanandham, MBBS, DCH, MS (Research), PhD

HEALTH REFERENCE SERIES UPDATE POLICY

The inaugural book in the *Health Reference Series* was the first edition of *Cancer Sourcebook* published in 1989. Since then, the *Series* has been enthusiastically received by librarians and in the medical community. In order to maintain the standard of providing high-quality health information for the layperson the editorial staff at Omnigraphics felt it was necessary to implement a policy of updating volumes when warranted.

Medical researchers have been making tremendous strides, and it is the purpose of the *Health Reference Series* to stay current with the most recent advances. Each decision to update a volume is made on an individual basis. Some of the considerations include how much new information is available and the feedback we receive from people who use the books. If there is a topic you would like to see added to the update list, or an area of medical concern you feel has not been adequately addressed, please write to: custserv@infobaselearning.com.

Part 1 | Screening and Preventive Care Tests

Chapter 1 | **Regular Health Exams**

Chapter Contents

Section 1.1 | **Why Regular Health Exams Are Important**

This section contains text excerpted from the following sources: Text in this section begins with excerpts from "Health Checkup," MedlinePlus, National Institutes of Health (NIH), July 15, 2019; Text beginning with the heading "Choosing a Doctor: Quick Tips" is excerpted from "Regular Checkups," Office of Disease Prevention and Health Promotion (ODPHP), U.S. Department of Health and Human Services (HHS), October 21, 2021.

Regular health exams and tests can help find problems before they start. They also can help find problems early, when your chances for treatment and cure are better. Which exams and screenings you need depends on your age, health and family history, and lifestyle choices such as what you eat, how active you are, and whether you smoke.

To make the most of your next checkup, here are some things to do before you go:

- Review your family medical history.
- Find out if you are due for any general screenings or vaccinations.
- Write down a list of issues and questions to take with you.

CHOOSING A DOCTOR: QUICK TIPS

When looking for a primary care doctor for yourself or a loved one, it is important to choose someone you can trust. A primary care doctor can:

- Help you stay healthy by recommending preventive services, such as screening tests and vaccines (shots)
- Treat many health problems – including physical and mental-health issues
- Refer you to a specialist when you need more help with a specific health issue

When you and your doctor work together as a team, you get better healthcare. Look for a doctor who:

- Treats you with respect
- Listens to your opinions and concerns

- Encourages you to ask questions
- Explains things in ways you understand

Try the following tips to find a doctor who is right for you.

Ask for Recommendations from People You Know

Getting a reference from someone you know and trust is a great way to find a doctor:

- Ask friends, family members, neighbors, or coworkers if they have a doctor they like.
- If you are looking for a new doctor because yours is retiring or moving, ask your current doctor for a recommendation.

Check with Your Insurance Company

If you have health insurance, you may need to choose from a list of doctors in your plan's network (doctors that take your insurance plan). Some insurance plans may let you choose a doctor outside your network if you pay more of the cost.

To find a doctor who takes your insurance:

- Call your insurance company and ask for a list of doctors near you who take your insurance plan – or use the insurance company's website to search for a doctor.
- Then call the doctor's office and ask them to confirm that they take your plan – have your insurance card handy in case they need to know your plan details.

Learn More about Your Top Choices

Make a list of the doctors you are interested in. Be sure to think about how easy or difficult it will be to travel to an appointment. Then call their offices to learn more about them. The answers to the following questions may help you make the best decision.

Questions about the doctor:

- Is the doctor taking new patients?
- Is the doctor part of a group practice? If so, who are the other doctors that might help care for me?

- Who will see me if my doctor is not available?
- Which hospital does the doctor use?
- Does the doctor have experience treating my medical conditions?
- Does the doctor have special training or certifications?

Questions about the office:

- Are evening or weekend appointments available? What about virtual appointments over the phone or on a computer (telemedicine)?
- What is the cancellation policy?
- How long will it take to get an appointment?
- How long do appointments usually last?
- Can I get lab work and x-rays done in the office?
- Is there a doctor or nurse who speaks my preferred language?

Think about Your Experience after the First Visit

Did the doctor and office staff:

- Make me feel comfortable during my appointment?
- Explain things in a way that was easy to understand?
- Listen carefully to me?
- Show respect for what I had to say?
- Know important information about my medical history?
- Spend enough time with me?
- Give me a chance to ask questions?

If you answer "no" to any of these questions, you may want to keep looking.

GET YOUR MEDICARE WELLNESS VISIT EVERY YEAR

If you have Medicare, be sure to schedule a yearly wellness visit with your doctor. A yearly wellness visit is a great way to help you stay healthy.

What Happens during a Yearly Wellness Visit

The doctor or nurse will first ask you to fill out a questionnaire called a "health risk assessment." Answering these questions will help you get the most from your yearly wellness visit.

During your visit, the doctor or nurse will:

- Go over your health risk assessment with you
- Measure your height and weight
- Check your blood pressure
- Ask about your medical and family history
- Ask about other doctors you see and any medicines you take
- Give advice to help you prevent disease, improve your health, and stay well
- Look for any changes in your ability to think, learn, or remember

The doctor or nurse will give you a short, written plan – like a checklist – to take home with you. This plan will include any screening tests and other preventive services that you will need over the next 5 to 10 years. Preventive services are health-care services that keep you from getting sick.

Plan Your Visit

WHEN CAN YOU GO FOR A YEARLY WELLNESS VISIT

You can get a wellness visit when:

- You have had Medicare Part B for more than 12 months.
- It has been at least 12 months since your last wellness visit.

DO YOU NEED TO HAVE A "WELCOME TO MEDICARE" VISIT FIRST

You do not need to have a "Welcome to Medicare" preventive visit before getting a yearly wellness visit.

If you choose to get the "Welcome to Medicare" visit during the first 12 months you have Medicare Part B, you will have to wait 12 months before you can get your first yearly wellness visit.

WHAT ABOUT COST

With Medicare Part B, you can get a wellness visit once a year at no cost to you. Check to make sure the doctor or nurse accepts Medicare when you schedule your appointment.

If you get any tests or services that are not included in the yearly wellness visit (like an extra blood test), you may have to pay some of those costs.

Who Can Get Medicare Coverage

Medicare is a federal health insurance program. You may be able to get Medicare if you:

- Are age 65 or older
- Are under age 65 and have a disability
- Have amyotrophic lateral sclerosis (ALS), also called "Lou Gehrig disease"
- Have end-stage renal disease (permanent kidney failure)

You must be living in the United States legally for at least 5 years to qualify for Medicare.

Make an Appointment

Take these steps to help you get the most out of your Medicare yearly wellness visit.

SCHEDULE YOUR MEDICARE YEARLY WELLNESS VISIT

Call your doctor's office and ask to schedule your Medicare yearly wellness visit. Make sure it has been at least 12 months since your last wellness visit.

Get Ready

GATHER IMPORTANT INFORMATION

Take any medical records or information you have to the appointment. Include important information such as:

- Your name and birth date

- The name and phone number of a friend or relative to call if there is an emergency
- Dates and results of checkups and screening tests
- A list of shots (vaccines) you have received – and the dates you got them
- Medicines you take, how much you take, and why you take them (including over-the-counter (OTC) medicines and vitamins)
- Phone numbers and addresses of other places you go for healthcare, including your pharmacy
- Any health conditions you have, including allergies

MAKE A LIST OF ANY IMPORTANT CHANGES IN YOUR LIFE OR HEALTH

Your doctor or nurse will want to know about any big changes since your last visit. For example, write down things such as:

- Losing your job
- A death in the family
- A serious illness or injury
- Surgery
- A change in your living situation

KNOW YOUR FAMILY HEALTH HISTORY

Your family's health history is an important part of your personal health record.

Ask Questions

MAKE A LIST OF QUESTIONS YOU WANT TO ASK THE DOCTOR

This visit is a great time to ask the doctor or nurse any questions about:

- A health condition
- Changes in sleeping or eating habits
- Pain or discomfort
- Prescription medicines, OTC medicines, or supplements

Some important questions include:

- Do you need to get any shots to protect your health?

- How can I get more physical activity?
- Are you at a healthy weight?
- Do you need to make any changes to your eating habits?

What to Expect

KNOW WHAT TO EXPECT AT YOUR VISIT

The doctor or nurse will ask you questions about your health and safety, such as:

- Do you have stairs in your home?
- What do you do to stay active?
- Have you lost interest in doing things you usually enjoy?
- Do you have a hard time hearing people on the phone?
- What medicines, vitamins, or supplements do you take regularly?

The doctor or nurse will also:

- Measure your height and weight
- Check your blood pressure
- Ask about your medical and family history
- Look for any changes in your ability to think, learn, or remember

Follow Up

MAKE A WELLNESS PLAN WITH YOUR DOCTOR

During the yearly wellness visit, the doctor or nurse will give you a short, written plan – like a checklist – to take home with you. This written plan will include a list of preventive services you will need over the next 5 to 10 years.

Your plan may include:

- Getting important screenings for cancer or other diseases
- Making healthy changes, like getting more physical activity

FOLLOW UP AFTER YOUR VISIT

During your yearly wellness visit, the doctor or nurse may recommend that you see a specialist or get certain tests. Try to schedule these follow-up appointments before you leave your wellness visit.

If that is not possible, put a reminder note on your calendar to schedule your follow-up appointments.

ADD ANY NEW HEALTH INFORMATION TO YOUR RECORDS

Make your next wellness visit easier by updating your medical information right away. Write down any shots you got and the results of any screening tests.

Medicare offers an online tool called "MyMedicare" to help you track your personal health information and Medicare claims. If you have your Medicare number, you can sign up for your MyMedicare account now.

Healthy Habits

TAKE CARE OF YOURSELF ALL YEAR LONG

After your visit, follow the plan you made with your doctor or nurse to stay healthy. Your plan may include:

- Getting active
- Eating healthy
- Watching your weight
- Keeping your heart healthy
- Preventing type 2 diabetes
- Quitting smoking
- Lowering your risk of falling
- Getting shots for older adults

TAKE CHARGE OF YOUR HEALTHCARE

When you play an active role in your healthcare, you can improve the quality of the care that you and your family get. Start by speaking up and asking questions at the doctor's office.

Healthcare is a team effort, and you are the most important member of the team! Your team also includes doctors, nurses, pharmacists, and insurance providers.

To take charge of your healthcare:

- Keep track of important health information.
- Know your family's health history.
- See a doctor regularly for checkups.
- Be prepared for medical appointments.
- Ask your doctor, nurse, or pharmacist questions.
- Follow up after your appointment.

Get Checkups

SEE A DOCTOR REGULARLY FOR CHECKUPS

Getting regular checkups with your doctor or nurse can help you stay healthy.

Regular checkups can help find problems early, when they may be easier to treat.

Cost and Insurance

WHAT ABOUT COST

Under the ACA, insurance plans must cover many preventive services, such as screenings and shots. Plans must also cover well-child visits through age 21 and well-woman visits.

Depending on your insurance plan, you may be able to get preventive services at no cost to you. Check with your insurance company for more information.

- Find out which services are covered under the ACA.
- Find out which services are covered by Medicare.

If you do not have insurance, check out these resources to help you get healthcare:

- Visit HealthCare.gov to find insurance options for your family.
- For low-cost or free services, find a health center near you and make an appointment.

Be Prepared

WRITE DOWN YOUR QUESTIONS AHEAD OF TIME

Write down any questions you have about your health. Take the list with you to your doctor, nurse, or pharmacist.

MAKE THE MOST OF DOCTOR VISITS

Take your list of questions and personal health record with you to the appointment. You may also want to ask a family member or friend to go with you to help take notes.

Be sure to talk about any changes since your last visit, such as:

- New medicines you are taking, including OTC medicines
- Herbs, home remedies, and vitamins you are taking
- Recent illnesses or surgeries
- Important changes in your life, like becoming unemployed or a death in the family
- Health concerns or issues
- Health information you have found online or heard from others

Section 1.2 | Women: Stay Healthy at Any Age

This section includes text excerpted from "Women: Stay Healthy at Any Age," Agency for Healthcare Research and Quality (AHRQ), U.S. Department of Health and Human Services (HHS), May 2014. Reviewed October 2021.

GET THE SCREENINGS YOU NEED

Screenings are tests that look for diseases before you have symptoms. Blood pressure checks and mammograms are examples of screenings.

You can get some screenings, such as blood pressure readings, in your doctor's office. Others, such as mammograms, need special equipment, so you may need to go to a different office.

After a screening test, ask when you will see the results and who to talk to about them.

Breast cancer. Talk with your health-care team about whether you need a mammogram.

***BRCA 1* and *BRCA 2* genes.** If you have a family member with breast, ovarian, or peritoneal cancer, talk with your doctor or nurse about your family history. Women with a strong family history of certain cancers may benefit from genetic counseling and BRCA genetic testing.

Cervical cancer. Starting at age 21, get a Pap smear every 3 years until you are 65 years old. Women 30 years of age or older can choose to switch to a combination Pap smear and human papillomavirus (HPV) test every 5 years until the age of 65. If you are older than 65 or have had a hysterectomy, talk with your doctor or nurse about whether you still need to be screened.

Colon cancer. Between the ages of 50 and 75, get a screening test for colorectal cancer. Several tests – for example, a stool test or a colonoscopy – can detect this cancer. Your health-care team can help you decide which is best for you. If you are between the ages of 76 and 85, talk with your doctor or nurse about whether you should continue to be screened.

Depression. Your emotional health is as important as your physical health. Talk to your health-care team about being screened for depression, especially if during the last 2 weeks:

- You have felt down, sad, or hopeless
- You have felt little interest or pleasure in doing things

Diabetes. Get screened for diabetes (high blood sugar) if you have high blood pressure (HBP) or if you take medication for HBP.

Diabetes can cause problems with your heart, brain, eyes, feet, kidneys, nerves, and other body parts.

Hepatitis C virus (HCV). Get screened one time for HCV infection if:

- You were born between 1945 and 1965.
- You have ever injected drugs.
- You received a blood transfusion before 1992.

If you currently are an injection drug user, you should be screened regularly.

High blood cholesterol. Have your blood cholesterol checked regularly with a blood test if:

- You use tobacco
- You are overweight or obese
- You have a personal history of heart disease or blocked arteries

- A male relative in your family had a heart attack before age 50 or a female relative, before age 60

High blood pressure. Have your blood pressure checked at least every 2 years. HBP can cause strokes, heart attacks, kidney and eye problems, and heart failure.

HIV. If you are 65 or younger, get screened for HIV. If you are older than 65, talk to your doctor or nurse about whether you should be screened.

Lung cancer. Talk to your doctor or nurse about getting screened for lung cancer if you are between the ages of 55 and 80, have a 30 pack-year smoking history, and smoke now or have quit within the past 15 years. (Your pack-year history is the number of packs of cigarettes smoked per day times the number of years you have smoked.) Know that quitting smoking is the best thing you can do for your health.

Overweight and obesity. The best way to learn if you are overweight or obese is to find your body mass index (BMI). You can find your BMI by entering your height and weight into a BMI calculator, such as the one available at the website: (www.nhlbi.nih.gov/guidelines/obesity/BMI/bmicalc.htm).

A BMI between 18.5 and 25 indicates a normal weight. Persons with a BMI of 30 or higher may be obese. If you are obese, talk to your doctor or nurse about getting intensive counseling and help with changing your behaviors to lose weight. Overweight and obesity can lead to diabetes and cardiovascular disease (CVD).

Osteoporosis (bone thinning). Have a screening test at age 65 to make sure your bones are strong. The most common test is a dual-energy x-ray absorptiometry (DEXA) scan – a low-dose x-ray of the spine and hip. If you are younger than 65 and at high risk for bone fractures, you should also be screened. Talk with your health-care team about your risk for bone fractures.

Sexually transmitted infections. STIs can make it hard to get pregnant, may affect your baby, and can cause other health problems.

- Get screened for chlamydia and gonorrhea infections if you are 24 years or younger and sexually active. If you

are older than 24 years, talk to your doctor or nurse about whether you should be screened.
- Ask your doctor or nurse whether you should be screened for other sexually transmitted infection.

GET PREVENTIVE MEDICINES IF YOU NEED THEM

Aspirin. If you are 55 or older, ask your health-care team if you should take aspirin to prevent strokes. Your health-care team can help you decide whether taking aspirin to prevent stroke is right for you.

Breast cancer drugs. Talk to your doctor about your risks for breast cancer and whether you should take medicines that may reduce those risks. Medications to reduce breast cancer have some potentially serious harms, so think through both the potential benefits and harms.

Folic acid. If you are of an age at which you can get pregnant, you should take a daily supplement containing 0.4 to 0.8 mg of folic acid.

Vitamin D to avoid falls. If you are 65 or older and have a history of falls, mobility problems, or other risks for falling, ask your doctor about taking a vitamin D supplement to help reduce your chances of falling. Exercise and physical therapy may also help.

Immunizations.

- Get a flu shot every year.
- Get shots for tetanus, diphtheria, and whooping cough. Get tetanus booster if it has been more than 10 years since your last shot.
- If you are 60 or older, get a shot to prevent shingles.
- If you are 65 or older, get a pneumonia shot.
- Talk with your health-care team about whether you need other vaccinations.

TAKE STEPS TO GOOD HEALTH

- Be physically active and make healthy food choices.
- Get to a healthy weight and stay there.
- Be tobacco free.
- If you drink alcohol, have no more than one drink per day.

Section 1.3 | Men: Take Charge of Your Health

This section contains text excerpted from the following sources: Text beginning with the heading "Need for Screening" is excerpted from "Get Screened," Office of Disease Prevention and Health Promotion (ODPHP), U.S. Department of Health and Human Services (HHS), March 24, 2021; Text beginning with the heading "Get the Screenings You Need" is excerpted from "Men: Stay Healthy at Any Age," Agency for Healthcare Research and Quality (AHRQ), U.S. Department of Health and Human Services (HHS), March 2014. Reviewed October 2021.

NEED FOR SCREENING

Screenings are medical tests that doctors use to check for diseases and health conditions before there are any signs or symptoms. Screenings help find problems early on, when they may be easier to treat.

Getting recommended screenings is one of the most important things you can do for your health. Depending on your age, sex, and medical history, you may need to be screened (tested) for things such as:

- Certain types of cancer
- High blood pressure (HBP) or high cholesterol
- Diabetes
- Osteoporosis or weak bones
- Sexually transmitted diseases (STDs)
- Mental-health conditions, such as depression

What Happens during a Screening

That depends on what problem the doctor is checking for. For example, a screening could be a blood test, a physical exam, or a list of questions your doctor asks you.

COST AND INSURANCE

The Affordable Care Act (ACA) requires most insurance plans to cover many screening tests. This means you may be able to get screening tests at no cost to you. Check with your insurance company to find out what is included in your plan.

If you do not have insurance, you can still get important screening tests.

GET THE SCREENINGS YOU NEED

Screenings are tests that look for diseases before you have symptoms. Blood pressure checks and tests for high blood cholesterol are examples of screenings.

You can get some screenings, such as blood pressure readings, in your doctor's office. Others, such as colonoscopy, a test for colon cancer, need special equipment, so you may need to go to a different office.

After a screening test, ask when you will see the results and who you should talk to about them.

Abdominal aortic aneurysm. If you are between the ages of 65 and 75 and have ever been a smoker (smoked 100 or more cigarettes in your lifetime) get screened once for abdominal aortic aneurysm (AAA). AAA is a bulging in your abdominal aorta, your largest artery. An AAA may burst, which can cause dangerous bleeding and death.

An ultrasound, a painless procedure in which you lie on a table while a technician slides a medical device over your abdomen, will show whether an aneurysm is present.

Colon cancer. If you are between the ages of 50 and 75, get a screening test for colorectal cancer. Several different tests – for example, a stool test or a colonoscopy – can detect this cancer. Your health-care team can help you decide which is best for you. If you are between the ages of 76 and 85, talk with your doctor or nurse about whether you should continue to be screened.

Depression. Your emotional health is as important as your physical health. Talk to your doctor or nurse about being screened for depression, especially if during the last two weeks:

- You have felt down, sad, or hopeless.
- You have felt little interest or pleasure in doing things.

Diabetes. Get screened for diabetes (high blood sugar) if you have high blood pressure (HBP) or if you take medication for high blood pressure.

Diabetes can cause problems with your heart, brain, eyes, feet, kidneys, nerves, and other body parts.

Hepatitis C virus (HCV). Get screened one time for HCV infection if:

- You were born between 1945 and 1965.
- You have ever injected drugs.
- You received a blood transfusion before 1992.

If you currently are an injection drug user, you should be screened regularly.

High blood cholesterol. If you are 35 or older, have your blood cholesterol checked regularly with a blood test. High cholesterol increases your chance of heart disease, stroke, and poor circulation. Talk to your doctor or nurse about having your cholesterol checked starting at age 20 if:

- You use tobacco
- You are overweight or obese
- You have diabetes or HBP
- You have a history of heart disease or blocked arteries
- A man in your family had a heart attack before age 50 or a woman, before age 60

High blood pressure. Have your blood pressure checked at least every 2 years. HBP can cause strokes, heart attacks, kidney and eye problems, and heart failure.

Human immunodeficiency virus (HIV). If you are 65 or younger, get screened for HIV. If you are older than 65, ask your doctor or nurse whether you should be screened.

Lung cancer. Talk to your doctor or nurse about getting screened for lung cancer if you are between the ages of 55 and 80, have a 30 pack-year smoking history, and smoke now or have quit within the past 15 years. (Your pack-year history is the number of packs of cigarettes smoked per day times the number of years you have smoked.) Know that quitting smoking is the best thing you can do for your health.

Overweight and obesity. The best way to learn if you are overweight or obese is to find your body mass index (BMI). You can find your BMI by entering your height and weight into a BMI calculator, such as the one available at website: (www.nhlbi.nih.gov/guidelines/obesity/BMI/bmicalc.htm)

A BMI between 18.5 and 25 indicates a normal weight. Persons with a BMI of 30 or higher may be obese. If you are obese, talk to your doctor or nurse about getting intensive counseling and help with changing your behaviors to lose weight. Overweight and obesity can lead to diabetes and cardiovascular disease (CVD).

GET PREVENTIVE MEDICINES IF YOU NEED THEM

Aspirin. If you are 45 or older, your doctor or nurse can help you decide whether taking aspirin to prevent a heart attack is right for you.

Vitamin D to avoid falls. If you are 65 or older and have a history of falls, mobility problems, or other risks for falling, ask your doctor about taking a vitamin D supplement to help reduce your chances of falling. Exercise and physical therapy may also help.

Immunizations.

- Get a flu shot every year.
- If you are 60 or older, get a shot to prevent shingles.
- If you are 65 or older, get a pneumonia shot.
- Get a shot for tetanus, diphtheria, and whooping cough. Get a tetanus booster if it has been more than 10 years since your last shot.
- Talk with your health-care team about whether you need other vaccinations.

TAKE STEPS TO GOOD HEALTH

- Be physically active and make healthy food choices.
- Get to a healthy weight and stay there.
- Be tobacco free.
- If you drink alcohol, have no more than two drinks per day if you are 65 or younger.

Chapter 2 | Family History

WHAT IS FAMILY HEALTH HISTORY?

Family health history is a record of the diseases and health conditions in your family. You and your family members share genes. You may also have behaviors in common, such as exercise habits, and what you like to eat. You may live in the same area and come into contact with similar things in the environment. Family history includes all of these factors, any of which can affect your health.

HOW CAN YOU COLLECT YOUR FAMILY HEALTH HISTORY?

You may know a lot about your family health history or only a little. To get the complete picture, use family gatherings as a time to talk about health history. If possible, look at death certificates and family medical records. Collect information about your parents, sisters, brothers, half-sisters, half-brothers, children, grandparents, aunts, uncles, nieces, and nephews. Include information on major medical conditions, causes of death, age at disease diagnosis, age at death, and ethnic background. Be sure to update the information regularly and share what you have learned with your family and with your doctor. You can use the Surgeon General's web-based tool called "My Family Health Portrait" website: (phgkb.cdc.gov/FHH/html/index.html) to keep track of the information.

This chapter contains text excerpted from the following sources: Text beginning with the heading "What Is Family Health History?" is excerpted from "Family Health History: The Basics," Centers for Disease Control and Prevention (CDC), November 25, 2020; Text under the heading "Why Is It Important to Know Your Family Health History?" is excerpted from "Why Is It Important to Know My Family Health History?" MedlinePlus, National Institutes of Health (NIH), May 12, 2021.

WHY IS FAMILY HEALTH HISTORY IMPORTANT FOR YOUR HEALTH?

Most people have a family health history of at least one chronic disease, such as cancer, heart disease, and diabetes. If you have a close family member with a chronic disease, you may be more likely to develop that disease yourself, especially if more than one close relative has (or had) the disease or a family member got the disease at a younger age than usual.

Collect your family health history information before visiting the doctor, and take it with you. Even if you do not know all of your family health history information, share what you do know. Family health history information, even if incomplete, can help your doctor decide which screening tests you need and when those tests should start.

HOW CAN YOU USE YOUR FAMILY HEALTH HISTORY TO IMPROVE YOUR HEALTH?

You cannot change your genes, but you can change unhealthy behaviors, such as smoking, not exercising or being active, and poor eating habits. If you have a family health history of disease, you may have the most to gain from lifestyle changes and screening tests. In many cases, healthy living habits can reduce your risk for diseases that run in your family. Screening tests, such as blood sugar testing, mammograms, and colorectal cancer screening, help find early signs of disease. Finding disease early can often mean better health in the long run.

WHY IS IT IMPORTANT TO KNOW YOUR FAMILY HEALTH HISTORY?

A family health history is a record of health information about a person and her or his close relatives. A complete record includes information from three generations of relatives, including children, brothers and sisters, parents, aunts and uncles, nieces and nephews, grandparents, and cousins.

Families have similar genetic backgrounds, and often similar environments and lifestyles. Together, these factors can give clues to conditions that may run in a family. By noticing patterns of disorders among relatives, health-care professionals can determine whether an individual, family members, or future generations may be at an increased risk of developing a particular condition.

A family health history can identify people with a higher-than-usual chance of having common disorders, such as heart disease, high blood pressure (HBP), stroke, certain cancers, and type 2 diabetes. These complex disorders are influenced by a combination of genetic factors, environmental conditions, and lifestyle choices. A family history also can provide information about the risk of rarer conditions caused by variants (mutations) in a single gene, such as cystic fibrosis and sickle cell disease.

While a family health history provides information about the risk of specific health concerns, having relatives with a condition does not mean that an individual will definitely develop that condition. On the other hand, a person with no family history of a disorder may still be at risk of developing the disorder.

Knowing one's family health history allows a person to take steps to reduce her or his risk. For people at an increased risk of certain cancers, health-care professionals may recommend more frequent screening (such as mammography or colonoscopy) starting at an earlier age. Health-care providers may also encourage regular checkups or testing for people with a condition that runs in their family. Additionally, lifestyle changes such as adopting a healthier diet, getting regular exercise, and quitting smoking help many people lower their chances of developing heart disease and other common illnesses.

The easiest way to get information about family health history is to talk to relatives about their health. Have they had any health problems, and when did they occur? A family gathering could be a good time to discuss these issues. Additionally, obtaining medical records and other documents (such as obituaries and death certificates) can help complete a family health history. It is important to keep this information up-to-date and to share it with a health-care professional regularly.

Chapter 3 | Newborn Screening Tests

Newborn screening programs across the United States currently screen four million infants each year. This public-health program detects treatable disorders in newborns, allowing treatment to begin often before symptoms or permanent problems occur. Newborn screening not only saves lives, but can also improve the health and quality of life (QOL) for children and their families.

Within the first 24 to 48 hours after birth, babies undergo a simple heel stick and a few drops of blood are collected on a special paper card. Health-care providers then test those blood spots for a number of congenital disorders (conditions that are present at birth). Infants are also screened for hearing disorders and for other serious heart problems using methods other than dried blood spots.

When a screen is positive for any condition, the newborn's parents are informed that their infant has an "out-of-range" test result for one of the conditions. But, a positive screening test does not mean the infant has a disorder. Additional testing is needed to confirm and diagnose the condition.

Only about one out of 300 newborns is later diagnosed with a treatable condition. Once the condition is confirmed, the infant is referred to an appropriate specialist so that treatment can begin as early as possible.

This chapter contains text excerpted from the following sources: Text in this chapter begins with excerpts from "About Newborn Screening," *Eunice Kennedy Shriver* National Institute of Child Health and Human Development (NICHD), September 1, 2017. Reviewed October 2021; Text beginning with the heading "Talk with Your Doctor about Newborn Screening" is excerpted from "Talk with Your Doctor about Newborn Screening," Office of Disease Prevention and Health Promotion (ODPHP), U.S. Department of Health and Human Services (HHS), October 15, 2020.

TALK WITH YOUR DOCTOR ABOUT NEWBORN SCREENING

Talk about newborn screening with your doctor or midwife before your baby is born. Newborn screening includes tests that check for certain diseases and conditions in newborn babies.

Newborn screening lets doctors find these diseases and conditions early – before your baby shows any signs of a problem. Early treatment is important to keep your baby healthy and developing normally.

Your baby will get most tests before leaving the hospital. They do not cause any harm or risk to your baby.

BLOOD TESTS

What Tests Will Your Baby Need?

All states require newborn screening, but the number and types of tests are not the same from state to state. Depending on your family health history, you may want to ask the doctor for extra tests.

Most newborn screening tests use a few drops of blood taken from the heel of your baby's foot. The same sample of blood can be used to test for many different diseases, including:

- **Hypothyroidism.** The thyroid is a gland in the neck that makes the thyroid hormone. Hypothyroidism (low thyroid hormone) can cause problems with growth and development, but it can be treated if it is found early.
- **Phenylketonuria (PKU).** People with PKU cannot process certain foods. To make up for the foods they cannot eat, they have to drink a special formula. PKU can also cause intellectual disability (mental skills that are below average) if it is not treated early.
- **Sickle cell disease (SCD).** This is a blood disorder that can cause serious pain, infections, or stroke. If it is found early, sickle cell disease can be treated.

OTHER TESTS

Heart Defects

Screening for heart defects can help find some problems with the way the heart develops before your baby goes home from the hospital. Finding and treating these defects early can help prevent serious problems or death.

Doctors test for heart defects by placing a small sensor on your baby's hand or foot. This test is painless and only takes a few minutes.

Hearing

A hearing screening checks how your baby responds to sounds using a tiny sensor or earphone. If your baby has hearing loss, finding out early can help prevent problems with speech, language, and social development.

If your hospital does not screen for hearing loss, ask your baby's doctor to check your child's hearing in the first month.

Some hearing loss starts later on, so have your child's hearing checked if you notice any problems.

If your child has hearing loss, it is important to get help early on. Getting help early helps children with hearing loss develop communication and social skills. Some children may also be able to use devices that help them hear, like a hearing aid, or get medicine or surgery.

MAKE A PLAN

If you are pregnant, talk with your doctor or midwife about newborn screening before your baby is born.

Find Out Which Tests Your Hospital Offers

Ask your doctor or midwife which newborn screening tests are offered at the hospital where your baby will be born. You can also call the hospital to ask about screening tests.

If you are not planning to give birth at a hospital, your baby still needs to get screened. Ask your midwife if she can screen your baby for you. You can also take your baby to a hospital or clinic to get screened a few days after birth.

- See which screening tests are offered in your state.
- Contact your state health department to ask about required newborn screening.

Follow Up

Ask the doctor when you will get your baby's test results. Your baby may need to get some tests again after leaving the hospital, especially if you go home less than 24 hours after giving birth.

Make a plan with your doctor about how you will follow up. And be sure to follow the instructions for any additional tests your baby needs.

COST AND INSURANCE

What about Cost

Some newborn screening tests are covered under the Affordable Care Act (ACA), the health-care reform law passed in 2010. Depending on your insurance plan, you may be able to get your baby screened at no cost to you.

Check with your insurance provider to find out what is included in your plan.

If you do not have insurance, you can still get medical care for yourself and your baby. Call the toll-free phone number below to connect with the health department in your area. Be sure to ask about free care.

For information, call toll-free at: 800-311-BABY (800-311-2229).

SCHEDULE A CHECKUP

Schedule Well-Baby Checkups

A well-baby checkup is a full checkup from your baby's doctor that you schedule ahead of time. This is different from other visits for sickness or injury. Most babies have their first well-baby checkup 2 to 3 days after coming home from the hospital.

Start Building Your Child's Health Record Now

Keep track of your baby's test results and shots. Put medical information in a safe place – you will need it for child care, school, and other activities.

Your family's health history is another important part of your baby's health record. Use the family health history tool (phgkb.cdc.gov/FHH/html/index.html) to keep track of your family's health. Keep a copy with your baby's other health information.

Chapter 4 | **Preventive Care Screening Tests for Children and Adolescents**

Chapter Contents

Section 4.1 | Checkup for Babies – Ages 0 to 11 Months

This section includes text excerpted from "Make the Most of Your Baby's Visit to the Doctor (Ages 0 to 11 Months)," Office of Disease Prevention and Health Promotion (ODPHP), U.S. Department of Health and Human Services (HHS), September 2, 2021.

Babies need to go to the doctor or nurse for a "well-baby visit" 6 times before their first birthday.

A well-baby visit is when you take your baby to the doctor to make sure they are healthy and developing normally. This is different from other visits for sickness or injury.

At a well-baby visit, the doctor or nurse can help catch any problems early, when they may be easier to treat. You will also have a chance to ask any questions you have about caring for your baby.

Learn what to expect so you can make the most of each well-baby visit.

WELL-BABY VISITS

How Often Do You Need to Take Your Baby for Well-Baby Visits?

Babies need to see the doctor or nurse 6 times before their first birthday. Your baby is growing and changing quickly, so regular visits are important.

The first well-baby visit is 2 to 3 days after coming home from the hospital, when the baby is about 3 to 5 days old. After that first visit, babies need to see the doctor or nurse when they are:

- 1 month old
- 2 months old
- 4 months old
- 6 months old
- 9 months old

If you are worried about your baby's health, do not wait until the next scheduled visit – call the doctor or nurse right away.

CHILD DEVELOPMENT

How Do You Know If Your Baby Is Growing and Developing on Schedule?

Your baby's doctor or nurse can help you understand how your baby is developing and learning to do new things – like smile or turn their head to hear your voice. These are sometimes called "developmental milestones."

At each visit, the doctor or nurse will ask you how you are doing as a parent and what new things your baby is learning to do.

1 TO 2 MONTHS

By age 1 month, most babies:

- Are gaining weight and growing
- React to sounds

By age 2 months, most babies:

- Lift their head when lying on their stomach
- Pay attention to faces and try to look at their parents
- Bring their hands to their mouth
- Make cooing sounds
- Smile at people

4 TO 6 MONTHS

By age 4 months, most babies:

- Roll over from their stomach to their back
- Reach for, grab, and hold toys
- Have different cries for different feelings (like hungry, cranky, or uncomfortable)
- Start babbling
- Recognize a parent's voice or touch
- Copy some facial expressions and sounds

By age 6 months, most babies:

- Begin to sit without support
- Roll over in both directions (from stomach to back and from back to stomach)
- Sleep for 6 to 8 hours a night without waking up

- Respond to their name
- Show interest in and reach for objects
- Begin to recognize familiar faces
- Like to look at themselves in a mirror

9 MONTHS

By age 9 months, most babies:

- Make sounds like "bababa"
- Play peek-a-boo
- Sit without support
- Stand by holding on to something
- Crawl

What If You Are Worried about Your Baby's Development

Remember, every baby develops a little differently. But, if you are concerned about your child's growth and development, talk to your baby's doctor or nurse.

GET READY

Take these steps to help you and your baby get the most out of well-baby visits.

Gather Important Information

Take any medical records you have to the appointment, including a record of vaccines (shots) your baby has received and results from newborn screenings.

Make a list of any important changes in your baby's life since the last doctor's visit, such as:

- Being sick
- Falling or getting injured
- Starting daycare or getting a new caregiver

ASK QUESTIONS

Make a List of Questions to Ask the Doctor

Before the well-baby visit, write down 3 to 5 questions you have. Each well-baby visit is a great time to ask the doctor or nurse any questions about:

- How your baby is growing and developing
- How your baby is sleeping
- Breastfeeding your baby
- When and how to start giving your baby solid foods
- What changes and behaviors to expect in the coming months
- How to make sure your home is safe for a growing baby

Here are some questions you may want to ask:

- Is your baby up-to-date on vaccines?
- How can you make sure your baby is getting enough to eat?
- Is your baby at a healthy weight?
- How can you make sure your baby is sleeping safely – and getting enough sleep?
- How can you help your baby develop speech and language skills?
- Is it okay for your baby to have screen time?
- How do you clean your baby's teeth?

Take a notepad, smartphone, or tablet and write down the answers so you can remember them later.

Ask What to Do If Your Baby Gets Sick

Make sure you know how to get in touch with a doctor or nurse when the office is closed. Ask how to reach the doctor on call, or if there is a nurse information service you can call at night or on the weekend.

WHAT TO EXPECT

Know What to Expect

During each well-baby visit, the doctor or nurse will ask you about your baby and do a physical exam. The doctor or nurse will then update your baby's medical history with all of this information.

The Doctor or Nurse Will Ask Questions about Your Baby

The doctor or nurse may ask about:

- **Behavior.** Does your baby copy your movements and sounds?
- **Health.** How many diapers does your baby wet each day? Does your baby spend time around people who are smoking or using e-cigarettes (vaping)?
- **Safety.** If you live in an older home, has it been inspected for lead? Do you have a safe car seat for your baby?
- **Activities.** Does your baby try to roll over? How often do you read to your baby?
- **Eating habits.** How often does your baby eat each day? How are you feeding your baby?
- **Family.** Do you have any worries about being a parent? Who can you count on to help you take care of your baby?

Your answers to questions like these will help the doctor or nurse make sure your baby is healthy, safe, and developing normally.

PHYSICAL EXAM

The Doctor or Nurse Will Also Check Your Baby's Body

To check your baby's body, the doctor or nurse will:

- Measure height, weight, and the size of your baby's head
- Take your baby's temperature
- Check your baby's eyes and hearing
- Check your baby's body parts (this is called a "physical exam")
- Give your baby shots they need

Section 4.2 | **Checkup for Children – Ages 1 to 4**

This section includes text excerpted from "Make the Most of Your Baby's Visit to the Doctor (Ages 1 to 4)," Office of Disease Prevention and Health Promotion (ODPHP), U.S. Department of Health and Human Services (HHS), September 2, 2021.

Young children need to go to the doctor or nurse for a "well-child visit" 7 times between ages 1 and 4.

A well-child visit is when you take your child to the doctor to make sure they are healthy and developing normally. This is different from other visits for sickness or injury.

At a well-child visit, the doctor or nurse can help catch any problems early, when they may be easier to treat. You will also have a chance to ask questions about things such as your child's behavior, eating habits, and sleeping habits.

Learn what to expect so you can make the most of each visit.

WELL-CHILD VISITS

How Often Do You Need to Take Your Child for Well-Child Visits?

Young children grow quickly, so they need to visit the doctor or nurse regularly to make sure they are healthy and developing normally.

Children ages 1 to 4 need to see the doctor or nurse when they are:

- 12 months old
- 15 months old (1 year and 3 months)
- 18 months old (1 year and 6 months)
- 24 months old (2 years)
- 30 months old (2 years and 6 months)
- 3 years old
- 4 years old

If you are worried about your child's health, do not wait until the next scheduled visit – call the doctor or nurse right away.

CHILD DEVELOPMENT
How Do You Know If Your Child Is Growing and Developing on Schedule?

Your child's doctor or nurse can help you understand how your child is developing and learning to do new things – like walk and talk. These are sometimes called "developmental milestones."

Every child grows and develops differently. For example, some children will take longer to start talking than others.

At each visit, the doctor or nurse will ask you how you are doing as a parent and what new things your child is learning to do.

AGES 12 TO 18 MONTHS

By age 12 months, most kids:

- Have at least 1 tooth
- Stand up by pulling on a table or chair
- Walk (either with help or on their own)
- Try to copy animal sounds
- Say "mama" and "dada," plus 1 or 2 other words
- Follow simple directions, like "Pick up the toy"

By age 15 months, most kids:

- Bend to reach the floor without falling
- Put things in a cup
- Make scribbles with crayons
- Take toys over to show a parent
- Listen to a story and look at pictures

By age 18 months, most kids:

- Say several single words
- Point to 1 body part (like their nose) when asked
- Point to show someone what they want
- Walk on their own
- Use a spoon to eat

AGES 24 TO 30 MONTHS

By age 24 months (2 years), most kids:

- Stand on their tiptoes
- Kick a ball without losing their balance
- Have at least 16 teeth
- Can tell someone when they are hungry, thirsty, or need to use the bathroom
- Understand instructions with 2 steps, like "Put on your shoes and then get your ball"
- Copy others, especially adults and older children
- Can name items in a picture book (like a cat or dog)

By age 30 months, most kids:

- Play simple games with other kids, like tag
- Brush their teeth with help
- Jump up and down in place
- Put on their clothes with help

AGES 3 TO 4 YEARS

By age 3 years, most kids:

- Have all 20 "baby" teeth
- Use the toilet during the day (may still need a diaper overnight)
- Copy a circle when drawing
- Put 1 foot on each step when walking up and down stairs
- Speak in sentences of 3 to 4 words
- Ask questions
- Know their first name, age, and sex

By age 4 years, most kids:

- Hop on 1 foot and balance on 1 foot for a short time
- Use child-safe scissors
- Count to at least 4
- Ask lots of questions
- Play with imaginary (pretend) friends
- Can name some colors and numbers
- Play simple board games and card games

GET READY

Take these steps to help you and your child get the most out of well-child visits.

Gather Important Information

Bring any medical records you have to the appointment, including a record of vaccines (shots) your child has received.

Make a list of any important changes in your child's life since the last doctor's visit, such as a:

- New brother or sister
- Serious illness or death in the family
- Separation or divorce
- Change in child care

Ask Other Caregivers about Your Child

Before you visit the doctor, talk with others who care for your child, like a grandparent, daycare provider, or babysitter. They may be able to help you think of questions to ask the doctor or nurse.

ASK QUESTIONS

Make a List of Questions You Want to Ask the Doctor

Before the well-child visit, write down 3 to 5 questions you have. This visit is a great time to ask the doctor or nurse any questions about:

- A health condition your child has (such as asthma or an allergy)
- Changes in sleeping or eating habits
- How to help kids in the family get along

Here are some questions you may want to ask:

- Is your child up-to-date on vaccines?
- How can you make sure your child is getting enough physical activity?
- Is your child at a healthy weight?
- How can you help your child try different foods?

- What are appropriate ways to discipline your child?
- How much screen time is okay for young children?

Take a notepad, smartphone, or tablet and write down the answers so you remember them later.

WHAT TO EXPECT

Know What to Expect

During each well-child visit, the doctor or nurse will ask you questions about your child, do a physical exam, and update your child's medical history. You will also be able to ask your questions and discuss any problems you may be having.

The Doctor or Nurse Will Ask Questions about Your Child

The doctor or nurse may ask about:

- **Behavior.** Does your child have trouble following directions?
- **Health.** Does your child often complain of stomachaches or other kinds of pain?
- **Activities.** What types of pretend play does your child like?
- **Eating habits.** What does your child eat on a normal day?
- **Family.** Have there been any changes in your family since your last visit?

They may also ask questions about safety, such as:

- Does your child always ride in a car seat in the back seat of the car?
- Does anyone in your home have a gun? If so, is it unloaded and locked in a place where your child cannot get it?
- Is there a swimming pool or other water around your home?
- What steps have you taken to childproof your home? Do you have gates on stairs and latches on cabinets?

Your answers to questions like these will help the doctor or nurse make sure your child is healthy, safe, and developing normally.

PHYSICAL EXAM

To check your child's body, the doctor or nurse will:

- Measure your child's height and weight
- Check your child's blood pressure
- Check your child's vision
- Check your child's body parts (this is called a "physical exam")
- Give your child shots they need

Section 4.3 | **Checkup for Children – Ages 5 to 10**

This section includes text excerpted from "Make the Most of Your Baby's Visit to the Doctor (Ages 5 to 10)," Office of Disease Prevention and Health Promotion (ODPHP), U.S. Department of Health and Human Services (HHS), September 2, 2021.

Children ages 5 to 10 need to go to the doctor or nurse for a "well-child visit" once a year.

At a well-child visit, the doctor or nurse can help catch any problems early, when they may be easier to treat. You will also have a chance to ask any questions you may have about your child's behavior or development.

CHILD DEVELOPMENT

How Do You Know If Your Child Is Growing and Developing on Schedule?

Developmental milestones for children ages 5 to 10 include physical, learning, and social skills – things like:

- Developing skills for success in school (such as listening, paying attention, reading, and math)
- Taking care of their bodies without help (such as bathing, brushing teeth, and getting dressed)

- Learning from mistakes or failures and trying again
- Helping with simple chores
- Following family rules
- Developing friendships and getting along with other children
- Participating in activities like school clubs, sports teams, or music lessons

GET READY

Take these steps to help you and your child get the most out of well-child visits.

Gather Important Information

Take any medical records you have to the appointment, including a record of vaccines (shots) your child has received. If your child gets special services at school because of a health condition or disability, bring that paperwork, too.

Make a list of any important changes in your child's life since the last doctor's visit, such as a:

- New brother or sister
- Separation or divorce – or a parent spending time in jail or prison
- New school or a move to a new neighborhood
- Serious illness or death of a friend or family member

Help Your Child Get More Involved in Doctor Visits

You can help your child get involved by letting them know what to expect.

ASK QUESTIONS

Make a List of Questions You Want to Ask the Doctor

- A health condition your child has (such as asthma, allergies, or a speech problem)
- Changes in behavior or mood
- Problems in school – with learning or with other children

Here are some important questions to ask:

- Is your child up-to-date on vaccines?
- How can you make sure your child is getting enough physical activity?
- How can you help your child eat healthy?
- Is your child at a healthy weight?
- How can you teach your child to use the Internet safely?
- How can you talk with your child about bullying?
- How can you help your child know what to expect during puberty?

Ask What to Do If Your Child Gets Sick

Make sure you know how to get in touch with a doctor or nurse when the office is closed. Ask how to get hold of the doctor on call, or if there is a nurse information service you can call at night or on the weekend.

WHAT TO EXPECT

Know What to Expect

During each well-child visit, the doctor or nurse will ask you questions about your child, do a physical exam, and update your child's medical history. You will also be able to ask your questions and discuss any problems.

The Doctor or Nurse Will Ask You and Your Child Questions

The doctor or nurse may ask about:

- **Behavior.** Does your child have trouble following directions at home or at school?
- **Health.** Does your child often complain of headaches or other pain?
- **School.** Does your child look forward to going to school?
- **Activities.** What does your child like to do after school and on weekends?

- **Eating habits.** What does your child eat on a normal day?
- **Family.** Have there been any changes in your family since your last visit?

They may also ask questions about safety, such as:

- Does your child always ride in the back seat of the car?
- Does anyone in your home have a gun? If so, is it unloaded and locked in a place where your child cannot get it?
- Is there a swimming pool or other water around your home?

Your answers to questions like these will help the doctor or nurse make sure your child is healthy, safe, and developing normally.

PHYSICAL EXAM

To check your child's body, the doctor or nurse will:

- Measure your child's height and weight
- Check your child's blood pressure
- Check your child's vision and hearing
- Check your child's body parts (this is called a "physical exam")
- Give your child shots they need

Section 4.4 | Checkup for Children – Ages 11 to 14

This section includes text excerpted from "Make the Most of Your Baby's Visit to the Doctor (Ages 11 to 14)," Office of Disease Prevention and Health Promotion (ODPHP), U.S. Department of Health and Human Services (HHS), September 2, 2021.

Kids ages 11 to 14 need to go to the doctor or nurse for a "well-child visit" once a year.

CHILD DEVELOPMENT

How Do You Know If Your Child Is Growing and Developing on Schedule?

Your child's doctor or nurse can help you identify "developmental milestones," or signs to look for that show your child is developing normally. This is an important part of the well-child visit.

Some developmental milestones are related to your child's behavior and learning, and others are about physical changes in your child's body.

BEHAVIOR CHANGES

What Are Some Changes You Might See in Your Child's Feelings, Relationships, and Behavior?

Developmental milestones for preteens and teens ages 11 to 14 include:

- Wanting more independence and privacy
- Having mood swings (going quickly from happy to sad or sad to happy)
- Showing more concern about what their friends and classmates think
- Developing stronger problem-solving skills
- Developing a clearer sense of right and wrong
- Challenging rules and resisting advice from parents

This is also a time when some kids may start showing signs of depression or eating disorders (EDs). Bullying and social media use may also become issues at this age. It is important to:

- Make sure the doctor screens your teen for depression

- Know the signs of ED
- Teach your kids to use social media safely
- Watch for signs of bullying

PHYSICAL CHANGES

What Physical Changes Will Your Child Go Through?

Many kids ages 11 to 14 are going through puberty. Puberty is when a child's body develops into an adult's body.

- For girls, puberty usually starts between ages 9 and 13.
- For boys, it usually starts between ages 10 and 13.

You can help by giving your child information about what changes to expect during puberty. You can also encourage your child to talk about puberty with the doctor or another trusted adult, like a teacher or school nurse.

Puberty can be a difficult time for gender-diverse children – kids who feel that they are a different gender than the sex that is listed on their birth certificate. Encourage your child to talk with you or their doctor if they have questions about their gender.

GET READY

Take these steps to help you and your child get the most out of well-child visits.

Gather Important Information

Take any medical records you have to the appointment, including a record of vaccines (shots) your child has received.

Make a list of any important changes in your child's life since the last visit, such as a:

- New brother or sister
- Separation or divorce – or a parent spending time in jail or prison
- New school or a move to a new neighborhood
- Serious illness or death of a friend or family member

Help Your Child Get More Involved in Visits to the Doctor

Once your child starts puberty, the doctor will usually ask you to leave the room for a few minutes so your child can ask questions about their health. This lets your child develop a relationship with the doctor or nurse, and it is an important step in helping your child learn about their healthcare.

Your child can also:

- Call to schedule appointments (if the doctor's office allows it)
- Help you fill out medical forms
- Write down questions for the doctor or nurse

ASK QUESTIONS

Make a List of Questions You Want to Ask the Doctor

Before the well-child visit, write down 3 to 5 questions you have – and ask your child if they have any questions to add. This visit is a great time to ask the doctor or nurse any questions about:

- A health condition your child has (such as an allergy, asthma, or acne)
- Changes in behavior or mood
- Loss of interest in favorite activities
- Problems at school (such as learning challenges or not wanting to go to school)

Here are some questions you may want to ask:

- How can you make sure your child is getting enough physical activity?
- How can you help your child eat healthy?
- Is your child at a healthy weight?
- Is your child's body developing normally?
- Is your child up-to-date on shots?
- How can you help your child succeed at school?

You may also want to ask:

- How can you talk with your child about sex?
- How can you talk with your child about tobacco, alcohol, and drugs?

- How can you teach your child to use the Internet safely?
- How can you talk with your child about bullying?

Ask What to Do If Your Child Gets Sick

Make sure you know how to get in touch with a doctor or nurse when the office is closed. Ask how to get hold of the doctor on call, or if there is a nurse information service you can call at night or on the weekend.

WHAT TO EXPECT

Know What to Expect

During each well-child visit, the doctor or nurse will ask you questions about your child, do a physical exam, and update your child's medical history. You will also be able to ask your questions and discuss any problems.

The Doctor or Nurse Will Ask You and Your Child Questions

The doctor or nurse may ask about:

- **Behavior.** Does your child have trouble following directions at home or at school?
- **Health.** Does your child often complain of headaches or other pain? How much sleep does your child get? When was their last visit to the dentist?
- **Safety.** Does anyone in your home have a gun? If so, is it unloaded and locked in a place where your child cannot get it?
- **School and activities.** Does your child look forward to going to school? What does your child like to do outside of school?
- **Eating habits.** What does your child eat on a normal day?
- **Family and friends.** Have there been any recent changes in your family? How many close friends does your child have? Has your child been bullied at school or online?

- **Emotions.** Does your child often seem sad, stressed, or bored? Does your child have someone to talk to about problems?
- **Sexuality.** Have you talked with your child about puberty? Is your child dating?

The answers to questions like these will help the doctor or nurse make sure your child is healthy, safe, and developing normally.

PHYSICAL EXAM

The Doctor or Nurse Will Also Check Your Child's Body

To check your child's body, the doctor or nurse will:

- Measure height and weight and figure out your child's body mass index (BMI)
- Check your child's blood pressure (BP)
- Check your child's vision and hearing
- Check your child's body parts (this is called a "physical exam")
- Decide if your child needs any lab tests, like a blood test
- Give your child shots they need

BEHAVIOR AND EMOTIONS

The Doctor or Nurse Will Pay Special Attention to Signs of Certain Issues

The doctor or nurse will offer additional help if your child may be:

- Depressed
- Struggling with an ED
- Using tobacco, alcohol, or drugs
- Experiencing any kind of violence

And if your child may be having sex, the doctor or nurse will talk to your child about preventing sexually transmitted diseases (STDs) and pregnancy.

The Doctor or Nurse Will Make Sure You and Your Child Have the Resources You Need

This may include telling you and your child about:

- Websites or apps that have helpful health information
- Organizations in your community where you can go for help

If needed, the doctor or nurse may also refer your child to a specialist.

Section 4.5 | Checkup for Children – Ages 15 to 17

This section includes text excerpted from "Make the Most of Your Baby's Visit to the Doctor (Ages 15 to 17)," Office of Disease Prevention and Health Promotion (ODPHP), U.S. Department of Health and Human Services (HHS), April 5, 2021.

Teens ages 15 to 17 need to go to the doctor or nurse for a "well-child visit" once a year.

A well-child visit is when you take your teen to the doctor for a full checkup to make sure they are healthy and developing normally. This is different from other visits for sickness or injury.

At a well-child visit, the doctor or nurse can help catch any problems early, when they may be easier to treat.

CHILD DEVELOPMENT

How Do You Know If Your Teen Is Growing and Developing on Schedule?

Your teen's doctor or nurse can help you identify "developmental milestones," or signs to look for that show your teen is developing normally. This is an important part of the well-child visit.

Some developmental milestones are related to your teen's behavior and learning, and others are about physical changes in your teen's body.

BEHAVIOR CHANGES

What Are Some Changes You Might See in Your Teen's Behavior?

Developmental milestones for teens ages 15 to 17 include:

- Spending less time with family and more time with friends
- Fighting with parents less than ages 13 and 14
- Worrying more about the future (such as going to college or finding a job)
- Thinking more about romantic relationships and sex
- Trying new things, including experimenting with tobacco, alcohol, or drugs

This is also a time when some teens may start showing signs of depression, anxiety, or EDs. That is why it is important to make sure the doctor screens your teen for depression.

PHYSICAL CHANGES

What Are Some Physical Changes Your Teen Is Going Through?

Teens ages 15 to 17 are usually either finished with puberty or close to finishing puberty. Puberty is when a child's body develops into an adult's body.

- Most girls finish puberty by age 15.
- Most boys finish puberty by age 16.

Teens might not ask you questions about sex, their bodies, or relationships. That is why it is a good idea for you to start the conversation. You can also encourage your teen to ask the doctor or nurse any questions they have about body changes or other health concerns.

GET READY

Take these steps to help you and your teen get the most out of well-child visits.

Gather Important Information

Take any medical records you have to the appointment, including a record of vaccines (shots) your teen has received.

Make a list of any important changes in your teen's life since the last visit, such as a:

- New brother or sister
- Separation or divorce
- New school or a move to a new neighborhood
- Serious illness or death of a friend or family member

Help Your Teen Get More Involved in Visits to the Doctor

The doctor will probably ask you to leave the room during part of the visit, usually the physical exam. This lets your teen develop a relationship with the doctor or nurse and ask questions in private. It is an important step in teaching your teen to take control of their healthcare.

Your teen can also:

- Call to schedule appointments
- Help you fill out medical forms
- Write down questions for the doctor or nurse

ASK QUESTIONS

Make a List of Questions You Want to Ask the Doctor

Before the well-child visit, write down 3 to 5 questions you have. This visit is a great time to ask the doctor or nurse any questions about:

- A health condition your teen has (such as acne or asthma)
- Changes in your teen's behavior or mood
- Loss of interest in favorite activities
- Your teen's sexual development
- Tobacco, alcohol, or drug use
- Problems at school (such as learning challenges or not wanting to go to school)

Here are some questions you may want to ask:

- Is your teen up-to-date on vaccines?

- How can you make sure your teen is getting enough physical activity?
- How can you help your teen eat healthy?
- Is your teen at a healthy weight?
- How can your family set rules more effectively?
- How can you help your teen become a safe driver?
- How can you talk with your teen about tobacco, alcohol, and drugs?

Take a notepad, smartphone, or tablet and write down the answers so you can remember them later.

Ask What to Do If Your Teen Gets Sick

Make sure you know how to get in touch with a doctor or nurse when the office is closed. Ask how to get hold of the doctor on call, or if there is a nurse information service you can call at night or on the weekend.

WHAT TO EXPECT

The Doctor or Nurse Will Ask Your Teen Questions

The doctor or nurse may ask about:

- **Behavior.** Do you have trouble following directions at home or at school?
- **Health.** Do you often get headaches or have other kinds of pain?
- **Safety.** Do you always wear a seatbelt in the car? Do you and your friends use tobacco, alcohol, or drugs?
- **School and activities.** Do you look forward to going to school? What do you like to do after school?
- **Eating habits.** What do you eat on a regular day?
- **Family and friends.** Have there been any changes in your family recently? Do you have close friends?
- **Emotions.** Do you often feel sad or bored? Is there someone you trust who you can talk to about problems?

- **Sexuality.** Do you have any questions about your body? Do you have a boyfriend or girlfriend?
- **The future.** Have you started to think about what you want to do after high school?

The answers to questions like these will help the doctor or nurse make sure your teen is healthy, safe, and developing normally.

PHYSICAL EXAM

To check your teen's body, the doctor or nurse will:

- Measure height and weight and figure out your teen's body mass index (BMI)
- Check your teen's blood pressure (BP)
- Check your teen's vision and hearing
- Check your teen's body parts (called a "physical exam")
- Decide if your teen needs any lab tests, like a blood test
- Give your teen vaccines they need

BEHAVIOR AND EMOTIONS

The Doctor or Nurse Will Pay Special Attention to Signs of Certain Issues

The doctor or nurse will offer additional help if your teen may be:

- Depressed
- Struggling with an ED
- Using tobacco, alcohol, or other drugs
- Experiencing any kind of violence

And if your teen may be having sex, the doctor or nurse will talk about preventing STDs and pregnancy.

The Doctor or Nurse Will Make Sure You and Your Teen Have the Resources You Need

This may include telling you and your teen about:

- Websites or apps that have helpful health information
- Organizations in your community where you can go for help

If needed, the doctor or nurse may also refer your teen to a specialist.

Section 4.6 | **Body Mass Index Screening for Weight Problems**

This section includes text excerpted from "About Child and Teen BMI," Centers for Disease Control and Prevention (CDC), March 17, 2021.

Body mass index (BMI) is a person's weight in kilograms (kg) divided by the square of height in meters. It is an inexpensive and easy-to-perform method of screening for weight categories that may lead to health problems.

For children and teens, BMI is age- and sex-specific and is often referred to as BMI-for-age. In children, a high amount of body fat can lead to weight-related diseases and other health issues. Being underweight can also put one at risk for health issues.

A high BMI can indicate high body fatness. BMI does not measure body fat directly, but BMI is correlated with more direct measures of body fat.

HOW IS BMI CALCULATED FOR CHILDREN AND TEENS?

Calculating BMI using the BMI Percentile Calculator involves the following steps:

- Measure height and weight.
- Use the Child and Teen BMI Calculator (www.cdc.gov/healthyweight/bmi/calculator.html) to calculate BMI. The BMI number is calculated using standard formulas.

WHAT IS A BMI PERCENTILE AND HOW IS IT INTERPRETED?

After BMI is calculated for children and teens, it is expressed as a percentile obtained from either a graph or a percentile calculator linked below. These percentiles express a child's BMI relative to U.S. children who participated in national surveys from 1963–65 to 1988–94. Weight and height change during growth and

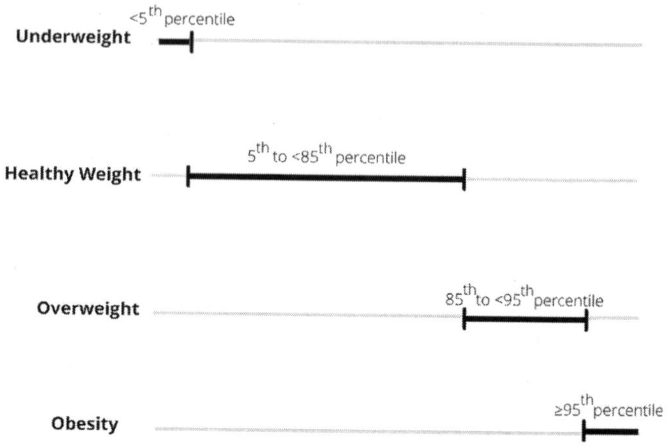

Figure 4.1. Body Mass Index-for-Age Weight Status Categories and the Corresponding Percentiles

development, as does their relation to body fatness. Consequently, a child's BMI must be interpreted relative to other children of the same sex and age.

The BMI-for-age percentile growth charts are the most commonly used indicator to measure the size and growth patterns of children and teens in the United States.

HOW IS BMI USED WITH CHILDREN AND TEENS?

For children and teens, BMI is not a diagnostic tool. Instead it is used to screen for potential weight and health-related issues. If children have a high BMI for their age and sex, a health-care provider may perform further assessments to determine if excess fat is a problem. These assessments might include skinfold thickness measurements, evaluations of diet, physical activity, family history, and other appropriate health screenings. The American Academy of Pediatrics (AAP) recommends using BMI to screen for overweight and obesity in children beginning at 2 years old. For children under the age of 2 years old, consult the World Health Organization (WHO) standards.

IS BMI INTERPRETED THE SAME WAY FOR CHILDREN AND TEENS AS IT IS FOR ADULTS?

Body mass index is interpreted differently for children and teens even though it is calculated with the same formula. Due to changes in weight and height with age, as well as their relation to body fatness, BMI levels among children and teens are expressed relative to other children of the same sex and age. These percentiles are calculated from the Centers for Disease Control and Prevention (CDC) growth charts, which were based on national survey data collected from 1963–65 to 1988–94.

Obesity is defined as a BMI at or above the 95th percentile for children and teens of the same age and sex. For example, a 10-year-old boy of average height (56 inches) who weighs 102 pounds would have a BMI of 22.9 kg/m^2. This would place the boy in the 95th percentile for BMI, and he would be considered to have obesity. This means that the child's BMI is greater than the BMI of 95 percent of 10-year-old boys in the reference population.

WHY CANNOT HEALTHY WEIGHT RANGES BE PROVIDED FOR CHILDREN AND TEENS?

Healthy weight status is based on BMI between the 5th and 85th percentile on the CDC growth chart. It is difficult to provide healthy weight ranges for children and teens because the interpretation of BMI depends on weight, height, age, and sex.

HOW CAN YOU TELL IF YOUR CHILD IS OVERWEIGHT OR HAS OBESITY?

The CDC and the American Academy of Pediatrics (AAP) recommend the use of BMI to screen for overweight and obesity in children and teens age 2 through 19 years. Although BMI is used to screen for overweight and obesity in children and teens, BMI is not a diagnostic tool. To determine whether the child has excess fat, further assessment by a trained health professional would be needed.

CAN YOU DETERMINE IF YOUR CHILD OR TEEN HAS OBESITY BY USING AN ADULT BMI CALCULATOR?

In general, this is not possible. The adult calculator provides only the BMI value and not the BMI percentile. Consequently, it is not appropriate to use the BMI categories for adults to interpret the BMI of children and teens.

However, if a child or teen has a BMI of 30 kg/m^2 or higher, the child almost certainly has obesity. A BMI of 30 kg/m^2 is approximately the 95th percentile among 17-year-old girls and 18-year-old boys.

WHAT ARE THE HEALTH CONSEQUENCES OF OBESITY DURING CHILDHOOD?

Obesity during childhood can harm the body in a variety of ways, now and in the future.

Section 4.7 | Screening Test for Child's Vision

This section includes text excerpted from "Get Your Child's Vision Checked," Office of Disease Prevention and Health Promotion (ODPHP), U.S. Department of Health and Human Services (HHS), March 19, 2021.

It is important for all children to have their vision checked at least once between ages 3 and 5. Even if children do not show signs of eye problems, they still need their vision checked. Finding and treating eye problems early on can save a child's sight.

Healthy eyes and vision are very important to a child's development. Growing children constantly use their eyes, both at play and in the classroom.

WHAT ARE COMMON EYE PROBLEMS IN CHILDREN?

These common eye problems can be treated if they are found early enough:

- Lazy eye (amblyopia)
- Crossed eyes (strabismus)

Other conditions – like being nearsighted or farsighted – can be corrected with glasses or contact lenses. Conditions like these are called "refractive errors."

IS YOUR CHILD AT RISK FOR VISION PROBLEMS?

If your family has a history of childhood vision problems, your child may be more likely to have eye problems. Talk to the doctor about eye problems in your family.

EYE EXAMS

Eye exams are part of regular checkups. The doctor will check your child's eyes during each checkup, beginning with your child's first well-baby visit.

Around age 3 or 4, the doctor will do a more complete eye exam to make sure your child's vision is developing normally. If there are any problems, the doctor may send your child to an eye doctor.

SEE A DOCTOR

Follow these steps to protect your child's vision.

Talk to your child's doctor.

Ask the doctor or nurse if there are any problems with your child's vision.

If the doctor recommends a visit to an eye-care professional:

- Ask the doctor for the name of an eye doctor who is good with kids. You can also use these tips to find an eye doctor.
- Write down any information about your child's vision problem.
- Plan your child's visit to the eye doctor.

COST AND INSURANCE

What about Cost

Under the Affordable Care Act (ACA), the health-care reform law passed in 2010, health insurance plans must cover vision screening for kids.

- If you have private insurance, your child may be able to get screened at no cost to you. Check with your insurance provider.
- Medicaid and Children's Health Insurance Program (CHIP) also cover vision care for kids.

EYE PROBLEMS

Look out for problems. Schedule an eye exam for your child if you see signs of an eye problem, like if your child's eyes:

- Look crossed
- Turn outwards
- Do not focus together
- Are red, crusted, or swollen around the eyelids

PREVENT EYE INJURIES

- Do not let your child play with toys that have sharp edges or points.
- Keep sharp or pointed objects, like knives and scissors, away from your child.
- Protect your child's eyes from the sun with kids' sunglasses that block 100 percent of ultraviolet A (UVA) and ultraviolet B (UVB) rays.
- Keep chemicals and sprays (such as cleaners and bug spray) in places that kids cannot reach.
- Make sure your child wears the right eye protection for sports.

VISION DEVELOPMENT

Help develop your child's vision. It takes skill to match up what we see with what we want to do – such as when we want to bounce a ball or read a book.

Here are some activities that can help your child develop vision skills:

- Read to your child and let your child see what you are reading.

- Play with your child using a chalkboard, finger paints, or blocks.
- Take your child to the playground to climb the jungle gym and walk on the balance beam.
- Play catch with your child.

Section 4.8 | Get Your Teen Screened for Depression

This section includes text excerpted from "Get Your Teen Screened for Depression," Office of Disease Prevention and Health Promotion (ODPHP), U.S. Department of Health and Human Services (HHS), October 15, 2020.

If your child is between ages 12 and 18, ask the doctor about screening (testing) for depression – even if you do not see signs of a problem.

WHY DO YOU NEED TO GET YOUR TEEN SCREENED FOR DEPRESSION?

Depression can be serious, and many teens with depression do not get the help they need.

The good news is that depression can be treated with counseling, medicine, or a combination of both. When you ask your child's doctor about screening for depression, find out what services are available in case your teen needs follow-up care.

WHAT IS DEPRESSION?

It can affect your thoughts, mood, and daily activities – and make you feel sad or down. But, depression is more than feeling sad for a few days.

Teen depression can be a serious mental illness. If your child is depressed, she may:

- Feel sad or irritable (easily upset) most of the time
- Lose interest in activities she used to enjoy
- Have aches and pains for no clear reason

- Have trouble concentrating, remembering things, or making decisions
- Sleep too much or be unable to sleep
- Eat too much or have trouble eating
- Use drugs or alcohol
- Think about death or suicide

It is normal for teens to have mood swings, and it can be hard to tell if your child is just feeling down or if she is depressed. That is why it is so important for all teens to be screened for depression.

CAUSES OF DEPRESSION

Depression can happen to anyone. It is not your fault or your teen's fault. Some experiences may make it more likely that a teen will develop depression, such as:

- Dealing with a big loss, such as a death or divorce in the family
- Living with someone who is depressed
- Having another mental-health problem, such as anxiety or an eating disorder (ED)
- Feeling stressed at school or at home
- Having a family history of depression

Teen girls are more likely to get depressed than teen boys.

WHAT TO EXPECT

What Happens during a Depression Screening

The doctor will ask your teen questions about her of his feelings and behaviors. This may include asking how often your teen:

- Feels hopeless or sad
- Has low energy or feels tired during the day
- Has trouble paying attention at school
- Eats too much or has trouble eating

Screening for depression usually takes about 5 minutes. It can be done as part of your teen's yearly checkup.

TREATMENT FOR DEPRESSION

What If the Doctor Finds Signs of Depression

If your child is showing signs of depression, the doctor will:

- Refer your teen to a therapist or doctor with special training in helping young people with emotional or behavioral problems
- Talk about medicines or other treatments – such as talk therapy – that could help your teen manage her or his depression
- Order tests to check for other health problems

Make sure to include your teen when you make any decisions about treatment.

SEE A DOCTOR

Take steps to protect your teen's mental health.

Talk to your teen's doctor about depression screening.

Ask the doctor to screen your child for depression. If you are worried about your teen, be sure to let the doctor know.

What about Cost

Screening for depression is covered under the Affordable Care Act (ACA). Depending on your insurance plan, your teen may be able to get screened at no cost to you. Check with your insurance company to find out what is included in your plan.

LOOK FOR CHANGES

Write down any concerns you have. Keep track of your teen's actions and words that make you think she or he might be depressed. If you see a change in your child's behavior, make a note about the change and when it happened. Include details such as:

- How long the behavior's been going on
- How often the behavior happens
- How serious you think it is

Share these notes with your teen's doctor. You can also use them to start a conversation with your teen.

SUICIDE WARNING SIGNS

Watch for signs that your teen may be thinking about suicide. Most people who are depressed do not attempt suicide, but depression can increase the risk of suicide and suicide attempts. Suicide is the second leading cause of death for young people ages 10 to 24.

These behaviors may be signs that your teen is thinking about suicide:

- Talking about wanting to kill or hurt himself
- Taking risks, like driving recklessly
- Spending less time with friends and family
- Talking about not being around in the future or "going away"
- Giving away prized possessions
- Increasing the use of alcohol or drugs
- Talking about feeling hopeless or very angry

If your child is showing some or all of these warning signs, get help right away. Visit the National Suicide Prevention Lifeline or call toll-free: 800-273-TALK (800-273-8255) to learn how to help.

If you think your child may be in immediate danger, call 911 or take him to the emergency room.

SUPPORT YOUR TEEN

Find resources for your teen. If your child is not ready to talk to you about her or his feelings, there are still things you can do. Help your teen find resources online and in the community.

Let her or him know that, in a crisis, she or he can get support anonymously (without giving her or his name) by:

- Texting the Crisis Text Line
- Chatting online with someone from the National Suicide Prevention Hotline
- Calling the National Suicide Prevention Hotline at toll-free: 800-273-TALK (800-273-8255)

Make a list with your teen of other people she can go to with problems or questions – like a teacher, guidance counselor, or another trusted adult.

Remind your teen that you are always there if she or he wants to talk.

Chapter 5 | Preventive Care and Screening Tests for Adults

Chapter Contents

Section 5.1 | Women's Health Screening Recommendations

This section includes text excerpted from "Get Recommended Screening Tests and Immunizations for Women," U.S. Department of Veterans Affairs (VA), July 20, 2021.

Screening tests are used to look for health conditions before there are symptoms. If you are having symptoms of a condition, please talk with your provider.

HEALTH CONDITIONS	18–29 years	30–39 years	40–49 years	50–59 years	60–69 years	70–79 years	80 years and older
Abdominal Aortic Aneurysm (AAA)	Not recommended (age 18–64)				Talk with your provider (age 65–75)	Not recommended (age 76 and older)	
Breast Cancer	Not recommended (age 18–39)		Recommended annually (45-54) Recommend biennial (55 and older or have opportunity to continue annually) Have opportunity to begin annual screening (40-44)			Recommended for some women – talk with your provider (age 75 and older)	
Cervical Cancer	Every 3 years (age 21–29)	Recommended. Every 3 or 5 years, depending on tests chosen (age 30–65)			Not recommended (age 66 and older)		
Colon Cancer	Not recommended (age 18–44)		Recommended. Frequency varies by test chosen (age 45–75)			Talk with your provider (age 76–85)	NR (age 86 and older)
Depression	Recommended every year						
Hepatitis B Infection	Recommended for some women – talk with your provider (age 18 and older)						
Hepatitis C Infection	Recommended in adults aged 18-79 years, and in all pregnant women, during each pregnancy						
High Blood Pressure	Recommended every year (age 18 and older)						
High Cholesterol	Talk with your provider (age 20 and older)						
HIV Infection	Recommended once (age 18 and older); in all pregnant Veterans; annually in Veterans with ongoing risk factors						
Lung Cancer	Not recommended (age 18–49)			Recommended for some women – talk with your provider (age 50–80)			Not recommended (age 81 and older)
Osteoporosis	Recommended for some women – talk with your provider (age 18–64)				Recommended once (age 65 and older)		
Overweight & Obesity	Recommended every year (age 18 and older)						
Sexually Transmitted Infections	Recommended. Test for gonorrhea and chlamydia every year (age 18–24). Talk with your provider about syphilis testing.	Talk with your provider about testing for gonorrhea, chlamydia, and syphilis (age 25 and older) Early screening for syphilis infection is recommended for all pregnant Veterans, regardless of age					

Figure 5.1. Screening Tests for Women

HEALTH CONDITIONS	18–29 years	30–39 years	40–49 years	50–59 years	60–69 years	70–79 years	80 years and older
Folic Acid for Pregnancy Planning	Recommended. Daily folic acid supplement for any woman who may become pregnant (age 18-55)			Not recommended after child-bearing age (age 55 and older)			
Aspirin to Prevent Stroke	Not recommended (age 18–49)			Talk with your provider (age 50–69)		Not recommended (age 70 and older)	

Figure 5.2. Medications for Women

HEALTH CONDITIONS	18–29 years	30–39 years	40–49 years	50–59 years	60–69 years	70–79 years	80 years and older
Tobacco Use	Recommended every visit (if using tobacco) (age 18 and older)						
Alcohol Use	Talk with your provider about healthy alcohol use (age 18 and older)						
Healthy Diet and Physical Activity	Talk with your provider about a healthy diet and physical activity (age 18 and older)						

Figure 5.3. Health Counseling for Women

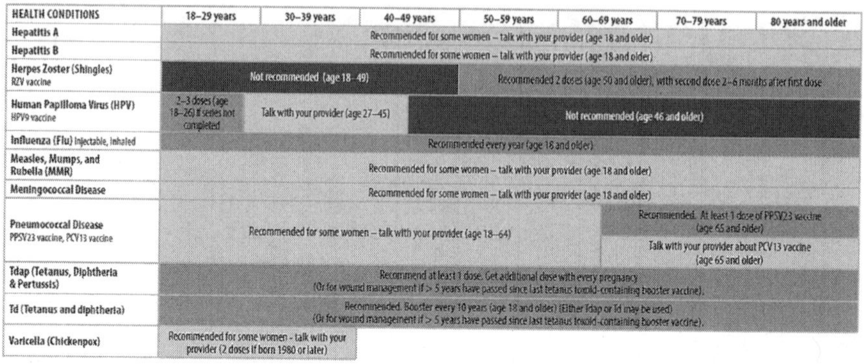

Figure 5.4. Vaccines for Women

Medium gray:	Recommended
Light gray:	Recommended for some women – talk with your provider
Dark gray:	Not recommended (NR)

Section 5.2 | **Men's Health Screening Recommendations**

This section includes text excerpted from "Get Recommended Screening Tests and Immunizations for Men," U.S. Department of Veterans Affairs (VA), August 31, 2021.

Screening tests are used to look for health conditions before there are symptoms. If you are having symptoms of a condition, please talk with your provider.

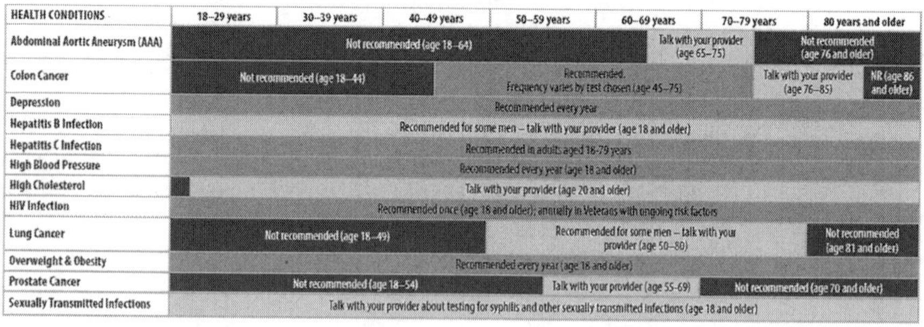

Figure 5.5. Screening Tests for Men

HEALTH CONDITIONS	18–29 years	30–39 years	40–49 years	50–59 years	60–69 years	70–79 years	80 years and older
Aspirin to Prevent Heart Attack	Not recommended (age 18–49)			Talk with your provider (age 50–69)		Not recommended (age 70 and older)	

Figure 5.6. Medications for Men

HEALTH CONDITIONS	18–29 years	30–39 years	40–49 years	50–59 years	60–69 years	70–79 years	80 years and older
Tobacco Use	Recommended every visit (if using tobacco) (age 18 and older)						
Alcohol Use	Talk with your provider about healthy alcohol use (age 18 and older)						
Healthy Diet and Physical Activity	Talk with your provider about a healthy diet and physical activity (age 18 and older)						

Figure 5.7. Health Counseling for Men

HEALTH CONDITIONS	18–29 years	30–39 years	40–49 years	50–59 years	60–69 years	70–79 years	80 years and older
Hepatitis A	Recommended for some men – talk with your provider (age 18 and older)						
Hepatitis B	Recommended for some men – talk with your provider (age 18 and older)						
Herpes Zoster (Shingles) RZV vaccine	Not recommended (age 18–49)			Recommended 2 doses (age 50 and older), with second dose 2–6 months after first dose			
Human Papilloma Virus (HPV) HPV9 vaccine	2–3 doses (age 18–26) if series not completed	Talk with your provider (age 27–45)	Not recommended (age 46 and older)				
Influenza (Flu) injectable, inhaled	Recommended every year (age 18 and older)						
Measles, Mumps, and Rubella (MMR)	Recommended for some men – talk with your provider (age 18 and older)						
Meningococcal Disease	Recommended for some men – talk with your provider (age 18 and older)						
Pneumococcal Disease PPSV23 vaccine, PCV13 vaccine	Recommended for some men – talk with your provider (age 18–64)				Recommended. At least 1 dose of PPSV23 vaccine (age 65 and older) Talk with your provider about PCV13 vaccine (age 65 and older)		
Tdap (Tetanus, Diphtheria & Pertussis)	Recommend at least 1 dose (age 18 and older) (Or for wound management if > 5 years have passed since last tetanus toxoid-containing booster vaccine).						
Td (Tetanus and diphtheria)	Recommended. Booster every 10 years (age 18 and older) (Either Tdap or Td may be used) (Or for wound management if > 5 years have passed since last tetanus toxoid-containing booster vaccine)						
Varicella (Chickenpox)	Recommended for some men – talk with your provider (2 doses if born 1980 or later)						

Figure 5.8. Vaccines for Men

Medium gray:	Recommended
Light gray:	Recommended for some men – talk with your provider
Dark gray:	Not recommended (NR)

Section 5.3 | Get Your Blood Pressure Checked

This section includes text excerpted from "High Blood Pressure," National Heart, Lung, and Blood Institute (NHLBI), May 8, 2020.

High blood pressure (HBP), also known as "hypertension," is a common disease that develops when blood flows through your arteries at higher-than-normal pressures. Your blood pressure is made up of two numbers: systolic and diastolic. Systolic pressure is the pressure when the ventricles pump blood out of the heart. Diastolic pressure is the pressure between heartbeats when the heart is filling with blood.

Your blood pressure changes throughout the day based on your activities. For most adults, a normal blood pressure is less than 120 over 80 millimeters of mercury, which is written as your systolic pressure reading over your diastolic pressure reading – 120/80 mm Hg. Your blood pressure is considered high when you have consistent systolic readings of 130 mm Hg or higher or diastolic readings of 80 mm Hg or higher.

To control or lower HBP, your doctor may recommend that you adopt a heart-healthy lifestyle. This includes choosing heart-healthy foods such as those in the DASH eating plan (www.nhlbi.nih.gov/health-topics/dash-eating-plan). You may also need to

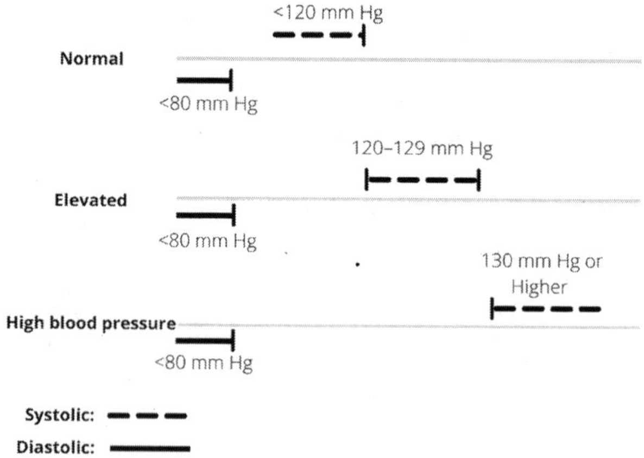

Figure 5.9. Blood Pressure Levels

take medicines. Controlling or lowering blood pressure can help prevent or delay serious health problems such as chronic kidney disease (CKD), heart attack, heart failure, stroke, and possibly vascular dementia. You usually do not have symptoms from HBP until it has caused serious health problems. About 1 in 3 U.S. adults with HBP are not even aware they have it and are not being treated to control their blood pressure. In fact, that is why it is important to have your blood pressure checked at least once a year.

RISK FACTORS OF HIGH BLOOD PRESSURE

Many factors raise your risk of HBP. Some risk factors, such as unhealthy lifestyle habits, can be changed. Other risk factors, such as age, family history and genetics, race and ethnicity, and sex, cannot be changed. A healthy lifestyle can lower your risk for developing HBP.

Age

Blood pressure tends to increase with age. The blood vessels naturally thicken and stiffen over time. These changes increase the risk for HBP.

However, the risk of HBP is increasing for children and teens, possibly because of rise in the number of children and teens who are living with overweight or obesity.

Family History and Genetics

High blood pressure often runs in families. Much of the understanding of the body systems involved in HBP has come from genetic studies. Many different genes are linked to a small increase in the risk of developing HBP. Research suggests that certain deoxyribonucleic acid (DNA) changes as an unborn baby grows in the womb may also lead to HBP later in life.

Some people have a high sensitivity to salt in their diet. This can also run in families.

Lifestyle Habits

Lifestyle habits can increase the risk of HBP. These habits include:

- Eating unhealthy foods often, especially those with too much sodium and not enough potassium. Some people, including African Americans, older adults, and people who have CKD, diabetes, or metabolic syndrome, are more sensitive to salt in their diet.
- Drinking too much alcohol or caffeine.
- Not getting enough physical activity.
- Smoking or using illegal drugs such as cocaine, "bath salts," and methamphetamine.
- Not getting enough good-quality sleep.

Medicines

Some prescription and over-the-counter (OTC) medicines can make it more difficult for your body to control your blood pressure. Medicines that can raise your blood pressure include antidepressants, decongestants (medicines to relieve a stuffy nose), hormonal birth control pills, and nonsteroidal anti-inflammatory drugs (NSAIDs) such as aspirin or ibuprofen.

Other Medical Conditions

Other medical conditions change the way your body controls fluids, sodium, and hormones in your blood. Other medical causes of HBP include:

- Certain tumors
- Chronic kidney disease
- Metabolic syndrome
- Overweight and obesity
- Sleep apnea
- Thyroid problems

Race or Ethnicity

High blood pressure is more common in African American and Hispanic adults than in white or Asian adults. Compared with other racial or ethnic groups, African Americans tend to have higher average blood pressure numbers and get HBP earlier in life. Experiencing discrimination has been tied to HBP. In addition, some HBP medicines may not work as well in African Americans.

During pregnancy, African-American women are more likely than white women to develop preeclampsia. Preeclampsia is a pregnancy disorder that causes sudden HBP and problems with the kidneys and liver.

Sex

Men are more likely than women to develop HBP throughout middle age. But, in older adults, women are more likely than men to develop HBP.

Women who have HBP during pregnancy are more likely to have HBP later in life.

Social and Economic Factors

Research has shown that factors such as income, your education, where you live, and the type of job you have may contribute to your risk of developing HBP. For example, working early or late shifts can raise your risk.

Experiencing danger or harm as a child has also been tied to a higher risk of developing HBP.

SCREENING AND PREVENTION OF HIGH BLOOD PRESSURE

Everyone age 3 or older should have their blood pressure checked by a health-care provider at least once a year. Your doctor will use a blood pressure test to see whether you have consistently HBP readings. Your doctor will talk to you about heart-healthy lifestyle changes to help prevent or manage your blood pressure.

How to Prepare for a Blood Pressure Test

Your doctor will use a blood pressure test to see if you have higher-than-normal blood pressure readings. The reading is made up of two numbers, with the systolic number above the diastolic number. These numbers are measures of pressure in mm Hg.

A blood pressure test is easy and painless and can be done in a doctor's office or clinic. A health-care provider will use a gauge, stethoscope, or electronic sensor and a blood pressure cuff to measure your blood pressure. To prepare, take the following steps:

- Do not exercise, drink coffee, or smoke cigarettes for 30 minutes before the test.
- Go to the bathroom before the test.
- For at least 5 minutes before the test, sit in a chair and relax.
- Make sure your feet are flat on the floor.
- Do not talk while you are relaxing or during the test.
- Uncover your arm for the cuff.
- Rest your arm on a table so it is supported and at the level of your heart.

If it is the first time your provider has measured your blood pressure, you may have readings taken on both arms.

You can also take your blood pressure at home or at a pharmacy.

What the Numbers Mean

For most adults, a normal blood pressure is less than 120/80 mm Hg. Your blood pressure is considered high when you have consistent systolic readings of 130 mm Hg or higher or diastolic readings of 80 mm Hg or higher.

For children younger than 13, blood pressure readings are compared with readings common for children of the same, age, sex, and height.

Talk to your doctor if your blood pressure readings are consistently higher than 120/80 mm Hg. The National Heart, Lung, and Blood Institute (NHLBI)-supported research indicates that systolic blood pressure greater than 120 mm Hg can be increasingly harmful to health. Note that readings above 180/120 mm Hg are dangerously high and require immediate medical attention.

How to Prevent High Blood Pressure

A heart-healthy lifestyle can help prevent HBP from developing. To live a healthy lifestyle:

- Choose heart-healthy foods that are lower in sodium (salt) and are rich in potassium. Fruits and vegetables are high in potassium.
- Avoid or limit alcohol
- Get regular physical activity. Even modest amounts can make a difference.
- Aim for a healthy weight
- Quit smoking
- Manage stress
- Get enough good-quality sleep

SIGNS, SYMPTOMS, AND COMPLICATIONS OF HIGH BLOOD PRESSURE

It is important to have regular blood pressure readings taken and to know your numbers, because HBP usually does not cause symptoms until it has caused serious problems.

Undiagnosed or uncontrolled HBP can lead to serious health problems:

- Aneurysm
- Stroke
- Chronic kidney disease
- Eye damage
- Heart attack
- Heart failure
- Peripheral artery disease or carotid artery disease
- Vascular dementia

High blood pressure in pregnancy can raise the risk of later heart and blood vessel problems for both the mother and her child.

DIAGNOSIS OF HIGH BLOOD PRESSURE

Your doctor may diagnose you with HBP based on your medical history and if your blood pressure readings are consistently at high levels. Your doctor may do more tests to look for medical conditions that could cause HBP, or to see if HBP has affected your kidneys.

Medical History

Your doctor will want to understand your risk factors and get general information about your health – such as your eating patterns, your physical activity level, and your family's health history to develop a treatment plan for you. Your doctor also will ask questions to see if HBP has caused you any health problems. This will help your doctor determine if you need to undergo any tests.

Confirming High Blood Pressure

To diagnose HBP, your doctor will take two or more readings at separate medical appointments.

For most adults, a normal blood pressure is less than 120/80 mm Hg. Your doctor may diagnose you with HBP when you have consistent systolic readings of 130 mm Hg or higher or diastolic readings of 80 mm Hg or higher.

For children younger than 13, blood pressure readings are compared with readings common for children of the same, age, sex, and height.

Talk to your doctor if your blood pressure readings are consistently at or above 130/80 mm Hg. Note that readings above 180/120 mm Hg are dangerously high and require immediate medical attention.

Even after taking these steps, your blood pressure reading may not be accurate for other reasons.

- **You are excited or nervous.** "White coat hypertension" refers to blood pressure readings that are higher in a doctor's office than readings at home or in a pharmacy, for example. Doctors can detect this type of HBP by reviewing readings from the office and from other places.

- **Your blood pressure tends to be lower when measured at the doctor's office.** This is called "masked high blood pressure." Doctors can diagnose this type of HBP by looking at readings taken at the office and at home, especially at night. When this happens, your doctor will have difficulty detecting HBP.
- **The wrong blood pressure cuff was used.** Your readings can appear different if the cuff is too small or too large. It is important for your health-care team to track your readings over time and ensure the correct pressure cuff is used for your sex and age.
- Get tips on how to prepare for a blood pressure test.

Diagnostic Tests

- **Blood tests.** Your doctor may recommend blood tests to check for kidney damage, high cholesterol or diabetes that may raise your risk of coronary heart disease (CHD), or other problems like thyroid disease that may be causing HBP.
- **Blood pressure monitor.** To gather more information about your blood pressure, your doctor may recommend wearing a blood pressure monitor to record readings over 24 hours. Your doctor may also teach you how to take blood pressure readings at home.

TREATMENT FOR HIGH BLOOD PRESSURE

For most people with HBP, a doctor will develop a treatment plan that may include heart-healthy lifestyle changes alone or with medicines. A risk calculator can help your doctor estimate your risk of complications and choose the right treatment. A health-care team can help you best manage your blood pressure and prevent complications. This team may include your doctor, a nutritionist, a pharmacist, and specialists for any conditions you may have, including those related to your heart.

If your HBP is caused by another medical condition or medicine, it may improve once the cause is treated or removed.

Risk Calculators

Your doctor may use a risk calculator to estimate your risk of having a stroke or heart attack or dying from a heart or blood vessel disease in the next 10 years or throughout your lifetime. This information can help your doctor choose the best treatment to prevent complications.

For example, the Atherosclerotic Cardiovascular Disease (ASCVD) Risk Estimator (tools.acc.org/ASCVD-Risk-Estimator-Plus) considers your cholesterol levels, age, sex, race, and blood pressure. It also factors in whether you smoke or take medicines to manage HBP or cholesterol.

Healthy Lifestyle Changes

If you have HBP, your doctor may recommend that you adopt a heart-healthy lifestyle to help lower and control HBP.

- **Choose heart-healthy foods such as those in the DASH eating plan.** NHLBI-funded research has shown that DASH combined with a low-salt eating plan can be as effective as medicines in lowering HBP.
- **Avoid or limit alcohol.** Talk to your doctor about how much alcohol you drink. Your doctor may recommend that you limit or stop drinking alcohol. You can find resources and support at the Alcohol Treatment Navigator (alcoholtreatment.niaaa.nih.gov) from the National Institute on Alcohol Abuse and Alcoholism (NIAAA).
- **Get regular physical activity.** Many health benefits result from being physically active and getting the recommended amount of physical activity each week. Studies have shown that physical activity can help lower and control HBP levels. Even modest amounts of physical activity may help. Before starting any exercise program, ask your doctor what level of physical activity is right for you.

- **Aim for a healthy weight.** If you are an adult who is living with overweight or obesity, losing 5 to 10 percent of your initial weight over about 6 months can improve your health. Even losing just 3 to 5 percent of your weight can improve blood pressure readings.
- **Quit smoking.** Visit Smoking and Your Heart (www.nhlbi.nih.gov/health-topics/smoking-and-your-heart) and Your Guide to a Healthy Heart (www.nhlbi.nih.gov/health-topics/all-publications-and-resources/your-guide-healthy-heart). Although these resources focus on heart health, they include basic information about how to quit smoking. For free help and support to quit smoking, you can call the National Cancer Institute's Smoking Quitline at toll-free: (877-44U-QUIT (877-448-7848)).
- **Manage stress.** Learning how to manage stress and cope with problems can improve your mental and physical health. Learning relaxation techniques, talking to a counselor, and finding a support group can all help.
- **Get enough good-quality sleep.** The recommended amount for adults is 7 to 9 hours of sleep a day. Develop healthy sleep habits by going to sleep and getting up at regular times, following a calming bedtime routine, and keeping your bedroom cool and dark.

Changing habits can be hard. To help make lifelong heart-healthy changes, try making one change at a time. Add another change when you feel comfortable with the previous one. You are more likely to manage your blood pressure when you practice several of these healthy lifestyle habits together and can keep them up.

Medicines

When healthy lifestyle changes alone do not control or lower HBP, your doctor may prescribe blood pressure medicines. These medicines act in different ways to lower blood pressure. When prescribing medicines, your doctor will also consider their effect on other conditions you might have, such as heart disease or kidney disease.

Keep up your healthy lifestyle changes while taking these medicines. The combination of the medicines and the heart-healthy lifestyle changes can help control and lower your HBP and prevent heart disease.

Talk to your doctor if you have any concerns about side effects from the medicines. She or he may change the dose or prescribe a new medicine. To manage HBP, many people need to take two or more medicines. This is more likely in African-American adults.

Possible HBP medicines include the following:

- Angiotensin-converting enzyme (ACE) inhibitors to keep your blood vessels from narrowing as much.
- Angiotensin II receptor blockers (ARBs) to keep blood vessels from narrowing.
- Calcium channel blockers to prevent calcium from entering the muscle cells of your heart and blood vessels. This allows blood vessels to relax.
- Diuretics to remove extra water and sodium (salt) from your body, reducing the amount of fluid in your blood. The main diuretic for HBP treatment is thiazide. Diuretics are often used with other HBP medicines, sometimes in one combined pill.
- Beta blockers to help your heart beat slower and with less force. As a result, your heart pumps less blood through your blood vessels. Beta blockers are typically used only as a backup option or if you have other conditions.

LIVING WITH HIGH BLOOD PRESSURE

If you have been diagnosed with HBP, it is important that you continue your treatment plan. You will need regular follow-up care and may want to learn how to monitor your condition at home. Your doctor may need to change or add medicines to your treatment plan over time.

Let your health-care team know if you are planning to become pregnant.

Manage Your Condition

Keep up your treatment plan, including healthy lifestyle changes, to help control your blood pressure and prevent heart disease. Making lifestyle changes and remembering your medicine every day can be hard, but there are ways to help.

- Ask your doctor, nurse, or pharmacist about apps for monitoring and tracking your blood pressure. They also may know a way to get texts to remind you to take your medicine every day and notify you when it is time to fill your prescription.
- Get support from loved ones and others in your community. You can share the Supporting Your Loved One with High Blood Pressure (millionhearts.hhs.gov/files/TipSheet_LovedOne_General.pdf) tip sheet with them.
- Have regular medical checkups and tests, as your doctor advises. Ask questions and discuss your progress. Let your doctor know if you have any new conditions or have been taking new medicines since your last appointment.
- Your doctor may want you to check your blood pressure at home or other locations that have blood pressure equipment. Return to screening for reminders on how to prepare for blood pressure testing and how to take your blood pressure yourself.
- Visit My Blood Pressure Wallet Card (www.nhlbi.nih.gov/health-topics/all-publications-and-resources/my-blood-pressure-wallet-card-0) to print out and keep a written log of all your results. Take the log to your doctor's appointments. You may be able to send the readings to your doctor's office electronically.

Know When to Call for Help for Complications

Readings above 180/120 mm Hg are dangerously high and require immediate medical attention. Blood pressure this high can damage your organs. Call 911 if you experience:

- A sudden, severe headache
- Difficulty breathing
- Sudden, severe pain in your abdomen, chest, or back

High blood pressure can also lead to heart attack or stroke. Call 911 if you suspect this is happening to you or someone else.

HEART ATTACK

The signs and symptoms of a heart attack include:

- **Nausea, vomiting, light-headedness or fainting, or breaking out in a cold sweat.** These symptoms of a heart attack are more common in women.
- **Prolonged or severe chest pain or discomfort not relieved by rest or nitroglycerin.** This involves uncomfortable pressure, squeezing, fullness, or pain in the center or left side of the chest that can be mild or strong. This pain or discomfort often lasts more than a few minutes or goes away and comes back.
- **Shortness of breath.** This may accompany chest discomfort or happen before it.
- **Upper body discomfort.** This can be felt in one or both arms, the back, neck, jaw, or upper part of the stomach.

STROKE

If you think someone may be having a stroke, act F.A.S.T. and perform the following simple test.

- F – Face: Ask the person to smile. Does one side of the face droop?
- A – Arms: Ask the person to raise both arms. Does one arm drift downward?
- S – Speech: Ask the person to repeat a simple phrase. Is their speech slurred or strange?
- T – Time: If you observe any of these signs, call for help immediately. Early treatment is essential.

Section 5.4 | Diabetes

This section contains text excerpted from the following sources: Text beginning with the heading "What Is Diabetes?" is excerpted from "What Is Diabetes?" Centers for Disease Control and Prevention (CDC), June 11, 2020; Text under the heading "Diabetes Tests" is excerpted from "Diabetes Tests," Centers for Disease Control and Prevention (CDC), August 10, 2021.

WHAT IS DIABETES?

Diabetes is a chronic (long-lasting) health condition that affects how your body turns food into energy.

Most of the food you eat is broken down into sugar (also called "glucose") and released into your bloodstream. When your blood sugar goes up, it signals your pancreas to release insulin. Insulin acts like a key to let the blood sugar into your body's cells for use as energy.

If you have diabetes, your body either does not make enough insulin or cannot use the insulin it makes as well as it should. When there is not enough insulin or cells stop responding to insulin, too much blood sugar stays in your bloodstream. Over time, that can cause serious health problems, such as heart disease, vision loss, and kidney disease.

There is not a cure yet for diabetes, but losing weight, eating healthy food, and being active can really help. Taking medicine as needed, getting diabetes self-management education and support, and keeping health-care appointments can also reduce the impact of diabetes on your life.

TYPES OF DIABETES

There are three main types of diabetes: type 1, type 2, and gestational diabetes (diabetes while pregnant).

Type 1 Diabetes

Type 1 diabetes is thought to be caused by an autoimmune reaction (the body attacks itself by mistake) that stops your body from making insulin. Approximately 5–10 percent of the people who have diabetes have type 1. Symptoms of type 1 diabetes often develop quickly. It is usually diagnosed in children, teens, and young adults.

If you have type 1 diabetes, you will need to take insulin every day to survive. Currently, no one knows how to prevent type 1 diabetes.

Type 2 Diabetes

With type 2 diabetes, your body does not use insulin well and cannot keep blood sugar at normal levels. About 90–95 percent of people with diabetes have type 2. It develops over many years and is usually diagnosed in adults (but more and more in children, teens, and young adults). You may not notice any symptoms, so it is important to get your blood sugar tested if you are at risk. Type 2 diabetes can be prevented or delayed with healthy lifestyle changes, such as losing weight, eating healthy food, and being active.

Gestational Diabetes

Gestational diabetes develops in pregnant women who have never had diabetes. If you have gestational diabetes, your baby could be at higher risk for health problems. Gestational diabetes usually goes away after your baby is born but increases your risk for type 2 diabetes later in life. Your baby is more likely to have obesity as a child or teen, and more likely to develop type 2 diabetes later in life too.

Prediabetes

In the United States, 88 million adults – more than 1 in 3 – have prediabetes. What is more, more than 84 percent of them do not know they have it. With prediabetes, blood sugar levels are higher than normal, but not high enough yet to be diagnosed as type 2 diabetes. Prediabetes raises your risk for type 2 diabetes, heart disease, and stroke. The good news is if you have prediabetes, a CDC-recognized lifestyle change program can help you take healthy steps to reverse it.

DIABETES TESTS

You will need to get your blood sugar tested to find out for sure if you have prediabetes or type 1, type 2, or gestational diabetes. Testing is simple, and results are usually available quickly.

Tests for Type 1 Diabetes, Type 2 Diabetes, and Prediabetes

Your doctor will have you take one or more of the following blood tests to confirm the diagnosis:

A1c TEST

The A1c test measures your average blood sugar level over the past 2 or 3 months. An A1c below 5.7 percent is normal, between 5.7 and 6.4 percent indicates you have prediabetes, and 6.5 percent or higher indicates you have diabetes.

FASTING BLOOD SUGAR TEST

This measures your blood sugar after an overnight fast (not eating). A fasting blood sugar level of 99 mg/dL or lower is normal, 100 to 125 mg/dL indicates you have prediabetes, and 126 mg/dL or higher indicates you have diabetes.

GLUCOSE TOLERANCE TEST

This measures your blood sugar before and after you drink a liquid that contains glucose. You will fast (not eat) overnight before the test and have your blood drawn to determine your fasting blood sugar level. Then you will drink the liquid and have your blood sugar level checked 1 hour, 2 hours, and possibly 3 hours afterward. At 2 hours, a blood sugar level of 140 mg/dL or lower is considered normal, 140 to 199 mg/dL indicates you have prediabetes, and 200 mg/dL or higher indicates you have diabetes.

RANDOM BLOOD SUGAR TEST

This measures your blood sugar at the time you are tested. You can take this test at any time and do not need to fast (not eat) first. A blood sugar level of 200 mg/dL or higher indicates you have diabetes.

If your doctor thinks you have type 1 diabetes, your blood may also tested for autoantibodies (substances that indicate your body is attacking itself) that are often present in type 1 diabetes but not in type 2 diabetes. You may have your urine tested for ketones

Table 5.1. Blood Sugar Test

Result*	A1c Test	Fasting Blood Sugar Test	Glucose Tolerance Test	Random Blood Sugar Test
Diabetes	6.5% or above	126 mg/dL or above	200 mg/dL or above	200 mg/dL or above
Prediabetes	5.7–6.4%	100–125 mg/dL	140–199 mg/dL	N/A
Normal	Below 5.7%	99 mg/dL or below	140 mg/dL or below	N/A

**Results for gestational diabetes can differ. Ask your health-care provider what your results mean if you are being tested for gestational diabetes.*
(Source: American Diabetes Association (ADA).)

(produced when your body burns fat for energy), which also indicate type 1 diabetes instead of type 2 diabetes.

Tests for Gestational Diabetes

Gestational diabetes is diagnosed using blood tests. You will probably be tested between 24 and 28 weeks of pregnancy. If your risk is higher for getting gestational diabetes (due to having more risk factors), your doctor may test you earlier. Blood sugar that is higher than normal early in your pregnancy may indicate you have type 1 or type 2 diabetes rather than gestational diabetes.

GLUCOSE SCREENING TEST

This measures your blood sugar at the time you are tested. You will drink a liquid that contains glucose, and then 1 hour later your blood will be drawn to check your blood sugar level. A normal result is 140 mg/dL or lower. If your level is higher than 140 mg/dL, you will need to take a glucose tolerance test.

GLUCOSE TOLERANCE TEST

This measures your blood sugar before and after you drink a liquid that contains glucose. You will fast (not eat) overnight before the test and have your blood drawn to determine your fasting blood sugar level. Then you will drink the liquid and have your blood sugar level checked 1 hour, 2 hours, and possibly 3 hours afterward. Results can differ depending on the size of the glucose drink and how often your blood sugar is tested. Ask your doctor what your test results mean.

Section 5.5 | Get Tested for Cholesterol

This section includes text excerpted from "Get Your Cholesterol Checked," Office of Disease Prevention and Health Promotion (ODPHP), U.S. Department of Health and Human Services (HHS), October 7, 2021.

It is important to get your cholesterol checked regularly. Too much cholesterol in your blood can cause a heart attack or a stroke.

The good news is that it is easy to get your cholesterol checked. If your cholesterol is high, you can take steps to lower it – such as eating healthy, getting more physical activity, and taking medicine if your doctor recommends it.

HOW OFTEN DO YOU NEED TO GET YOUR CHOLESTEROL CHECKED?

The general recommendation is to get your cholesterol checked every 4 to 6 years. Some people may need to get their cholesterol checked more or less often depending on their risk of heart disease.

For example, high cholesterol can run in families. If someone in your family has high cholesterol or takes medicine to control cholesterol, you might need to get tested more often. Talk to your doctor about what is best for you.

WHAT IS CHOLESTEROL?

Cholesterol is a waxy material that is found naturally in your blood. Your body makes cholesterol and uses it to do important things, such as making hormones and digesting fatty foods.

If you have too much cholesterol in your body, it can build up inside your blood vessels and make it hard for blood to flow through them. Over time, this can lead to heart disease.

CHOLESTEROL TEST

How Can You Tell If You Have High Cholesterol?

Most people who have high cholesterol do not have any signs or symptoms. That is why it is so important to get your cholesterol checked.

How Can You Get Your Cholesterol Checked?

Your doctor will check your cholesterol levels with a blood test called a "lipid profile." For this test, a nurse will take a small sample of blood from your finger or arm.

There are other blood tests that can check cholesterol, but a lipid profile gives the most information.

TYPES OF CHOLESTEROL

What Do the Test Results Mean?

If you get a lipid profile test, the results will show 4 numbers. A lipid profile measures:

- Total cholesterol
- Low-density lipoprotein (LDL) (bad) cholesterol
- High-density lipoprotein HDL (good) cholesterol
- Triglycerides

Total cholesterol is a measure of all the cholesterol in your blood. It is based on the LDL, HDL, and triglycerides numbers.

LDL cholesterol is the "bad" type of cholesterol that can block your arteries – so a lower level is better for you.

HDL cholesterol is the "good" type of cholesterol that helps clear LDL cholesterol out of your arteries – so a higher level is better for you. Having a low HDL cholesterol level can increase your risk for heart disease.

Triglycerides are a type of fat in your blood that can increase your risk for heart attack and stroke.

ARE YOU AT RISK?

What Can Cause Unhealthy Cholesterol Levels?

LDL cholesterol levels tend to increase as people get older. Other causes of high LDL (bad) cholesterol levels include:

- Family history of high LDL cholesterol
- High blood pressure (HBP) or type 2 diabetes
- Smoking
- Being overweight
- Not getting enough physical activity
- Eating too much saturated fat and *trans* fat – and not enough fruits and vegetables
- Taking certain medicines, like medicines to lower blood pressure

Causes of low HDL (good) cholesterol levels include:

- Smoking
- Being overweight
- Not getting enough physical activity
- Not eating enough fruits, vegetables, and unsaturated fat (like olive oil)

What If Your Cholesterol Levels Are Not Healthy?

As your LDL cholesterol gets higher, so does your risk of heart disease. Take these steps to lower your cholesterol and reduce your risk of heart disease:

- Eat heart-healthy foods.
- Get active.
- Stay at a healthy weight.
- If you smoke, quit.
- If you have type 2 diabetes or HBP, take steps to manage it.
- Ask your doctor about taking medicine to lower your risk of heart attack and stroke.

GET TESTED

Find out what your cholesterol levels are. If your cholesterol is high or you are at risk for heart disease, take steps to control your cholesterol levels.

Make an Appointment to Get Your Cholesterol Checked

Call your doctor's office or health center to schedule the test. Be sure to ask for a complete lipid profile – and find out what instructions you will need to follow before the test. For example, you may need to fast (not eat or drink anything except water) for 8 to 12 hours before the test.

What about Cost

Cholesterol testing is covered under the Affordable Care Act (ACA), the healthcare reform law passed in 2010. Depending on your insurance plan, you may be able to get your cholesterol checked at no cost to you.

Even if you do not have insurance, you can still get your cholesterol checked.

Keep Track of Your Cholesterol Levels

Remember to ask the doctor or nurse for your cholesterol levels each time you get your cholesterol checked. Write the levels down to keep track of your progress.

EAT HEALTHY

Making healthy choices to your diet can help lower your cholesterol. Try to:

- Cut down on saturated fats, which comes from animal products (such as cheese, fatty meats, and dairy desserts) and tropical oils (such as palm, palm kernel, and coconut oil). Use healthier oils (such as olive, peanut, or canola oil) instead.
- Choose foods with healthy fats, such as olives, avocados, nuts, and fish. Stay away from *trans* fats, which may be in foods such as stick margarines, coffee creamers, and some desserts.
- Limit foods that are high in sodium (salt) or added sugars
- Choose low-fat or fat-free milk, cheese, and yogurt

- Eat more foods that are high in fiber, such as oatmeal, oat bran, beans, and lentils
- Eat more vegetables and fruits

HEALTHY HABITS

Get Active

Getting active can help you lose weight, lower your LDL (bad) cholesterol, and raise your HDL (good) cholesterol. Aim for 2 hours and 30 minutes a week of moderate-intensity aerobic activity, such as:

- Walking briskly
- Dancing
- Yardwork

Or aim for 1 hour and 15 minutes a week of vigorous activity, such as:

- Jogging or running
- Swimming laps
- Jumping rope

Quit Smoking

Quitting smoking can help lower your cholesterol. If you smoke, make a plan to quit today. Call toll-free: (800-QUIT-NOW (800-784-8669)) for free support and to set up your quit plan.

Section 5.6 | **Depression**

This section includes text excerpted from "Depression Screening," MedlinePlus, National Institutes of Health (NIH), August 4, 2021.

WHAT IS DEPRESSION SCREENING?

A depression screening, also called a "depression test," helps find out if you have depression. Depression is a common, though serious, illness. Everyone feels sad at times, but depression is different than normal sadness or grief. Depression can affect how you think, feel, and behave. Depression makes it hard to function at home and work. You may lose interest in activities you once enjoyed. Some people with depression feel worthless and are at risk for harming themselves.

There are different types of depression. The most common types are:

- Major depression, which causes persistent feelings of sadness, anger, and/or frustration. Major depression lasts for several weeks or longer.
- Persistent depressive disorder, which causes depressive symptoms that last two years or more.
- **Postpartum depression.** Many new mothers feel sad, but postpartum depression causes extreme sadness and anxiety after childbirth. It can make it hard for mothers to care for themselves and/or their babies.
- **Seasonal affective disorder (SAD).** This form of depression usually happens in winter when there is less sunlight. Most people with SAD feel better in the spring and summer.
- Psychotic depression occurs with psychosis, a more serious psychiatric disorder. Psychosis can cause people to lose touch with reality.
- Bipolar disorder formerly called "manic depression." People with bipolar disorder have alternating episodes of mania (extreme highs or euphoria) and depression.

Fortunately, most people with depression feel better after treatment with medicine and/or talk therapy.

WHAT IS IT USED FOR?

A depression screening is used to help diagnose depression. Your primary care provider may give you a depression test if you are showing signs of depression. If the screening shows you have depression, you may need treatment from a mental-health provider. A mental-health provider is a health-care professional who specializes in diagnosing and treating mental-health problems. If you are already seeing a mental-health provider, you may get a depression test to help guide your treatment.

WHY DO YOU NEED DEPRESSION SCREENING?

You may need depression screening if you are showing signs of depression. Signs of depression include:

- Loss of interest or pleasure in daily living and/or other activities, such as hobbies, sports, or sex
- Anger, frustration, or irritability
- Sleep problems: trouble falling asleep and/or staying asleep (insomnia) or sleeping too much
- Fatigue and lack of energy
- Restlessness
- Trouble concentrating or making decisions
- Feelings of guilt or worthlessness
- Losing or gaining a lot of weight

One of the most serious signs of depression is thinking about or attempting suicide. If you are thinking about hurting yourself, or about suicide, seek help right away. There are many ways to get help. You can:

- Call 911 or go to your local emergency room
- Call your mental-health provider or other health-care provider
- Reach out to a loved one or close friend
- Call a suicide hotline. In the United States, you can call the National Suicide Prevention Lifeline at 800-273-TALK (800-273-8255)

WHAT HAPPENS DURING DEPRESSION SCREENING

Your primary care provider may give you a physical exam and ask you about your feelings, mood, sleep habits, and other symptoms. Your provider may also order a blood test to find out if a disorder, such as anemia or thyroid disease, may be causing your depression.

During a blood test, a health-care professional will take a blood sample from a vein in your arm, using a small needle. After the needle is inserted, a small amount of blood will be collected into a test tube or vial. You may feel a little sting when the needle goes in or out. This usually takes less than five minutes.

If you are being tested by a mental-health provider, she or he may ask you more detailed questions about your feelings and behaviors. You may also be asked to fill out a questionnaire about these issues.

ARE THERE ANY RISKS TO SCREENING?

There is no risk to having a physical exam or taking a questionnaire.

There is very little risk to having a blood test. You may have slight pain or bruising at the spot where the needle was put in, but most symptoms go away quickly.

WHAT DO THE RESULTS MEAN?

If you are diagnosed with depression, it is important to get treatment as soon as possible. The sooner you get treatment, the better chance you have of recovery. Treatment for depression may take a long time, but most people who get treated eventually feel better.

If your primary care provider diagnosed you, she or he may refer you to a mental-health provider. If a mental-health provider diagnosed you, she or he will recommend a treatment plan based on the type of depression you have and how serious it is.

Section 5.7 | **Hearing Tests**

This section includes text excerpted from "Hearing Tests for Adults," MedlinePlus, National Institutes of Health (NIH), March 3, 2021.

WHAT ARE HEARING TESTS?

Hearing tests measure how well you are able to hear. Normal hearing happens when sound waves travel into your ear, causing your eardrum to vibrate. The vibration moves the waves farther into the ear, where it triggers nerve cells to send sound information to your brain. This information is translated into the sounds you hear.

Hearing loss happens when there is a problem with one or more parts of the ear, the nerves inside the ear, or the part of the brain that controls hearing. There are three main types of hearing loss:

- **Sensorineural** (also called "nerve deafness"). This type of hearing loss is caused by a problem with the structure of the ear and/or with the nerves that control hearing. It may be present at birth or show up late in life. Sensorineural hearing loss is usually permanent. This type of hearing loss ranges from mild (the inability to hear certain sounds) to profound (the inability to hear any sounds).
- **Conductive.** This type of hearing loss is caused by a blockage of sound transmission into the ear. It can occur at any age, but it is most common in infants and young children and is often caused by ear infections or fluid in the ears. Conductive hearing loss is usually mild, temporary, and treatable.
- Mixed, a combination of both sensorineural and conductive hearing loss.

Hearing loss is common in older adults. About one-third of adults over the age of 65 have some hearing loss, most often the sensorineural type. If you are diagnosed with hearing loss, there are steps you can take that may help treat or manage the condition.

WHAT ARE THEY USED FOR?

Hearing tests are used to find out whether or not you have a hearing problem and, if so, how serious it is.

WHY DO YOU NEED A HEARING TEST?

You may need a hearing test if you have symptoms of hearing loss. These include:

- Trouble understanding what other people are saying, especially in a noisy environment
- Needing to ask people to repeat themselves
- Trouble hearing high-pitched sounds
- Needing to turn up the volume on the TV or music player
- A ringing sound in your ears

WHAT HAPPENS DURING A HEARING TEST

Your hearing test may be done by a primary health-care provider or one of the following types of providers:

- An audiologist, a health-care provider who specializes in diagnosing, treating, and managing hearing loss
- An otolaryngologist (ENT), a doctor specializing in treating diseases and conditions of the ears, nose, and throat.

There are several types of hearing tests. Most tests check for your response to tones or words delivered at different pitches, volumes, and/or noise environments. These are called "sound tests." Common sound tests include:

Acoustic reflex measures, also called "middle ear muscle reflex" (MEMR), test how well the ear responds to loud sounds. In normal hearing, a tiny muscle inside the ear tightens when you hear loud noises. This is called the "acoustic reflex." It happens without you knowing it. During the test:

- The audiologist or other provider will place a soft rubber tip inside the ear.
- A series of loud sounds will be sent through the tips and recorded onto a machine.

- The machine will show when or if the sound has triggered a reflex.
- If hearing loss is bad, the sound may have to be very loud to trigger a reflex, or it may not trigger the reflex at all.

Pure-tone test, also known as "audiometry." During this test:

- You will put on headphones.
- A series of tones will be sent to your headphones.
- The audiologist or other provider will change the pitch and loudness of the tones at different points during the test. At some points, the tones may be barely audible.
- The provider will ask you to respond whenever you hear the tones. Your response may be to raise your hand or press a button.
- The test helps find the quietest sounds you can hear at different pitches.

Tuning fork tests. A tuning fork is a two-pronged metal device that makes a tone when it vibrates. During the test:

- The audiologist or other provider will place the tuning fork behind your ear or on top of your head.
- The provider will hit the fork so that it makes a tone.
- You will be asked to tell the provider whenever you hear the tone at different volumes, or if you heard the sound in your left ear, right ear, or both equally.
- Depending on where the fork is placed and how you respond, the test can show if there is hearing loss in one or both ears. It can also show which type of hearing loss you have (conductive or sensorineural).

Speech and word recognition tests can show how well you can hear spoken language. During the test:

- You will put on headphones.
- The audiologist will talk to you through your headphones, and ask you to repeat a series of simple words, spoken at different volumes.

- The provider will record the softest speech you are able to hear.
- Some of the testing may be done in a noisy environment, because many people with hearing loss have trouble understanding speech in loud places.

Another type test, called "tympanometry," checks for how well your eardrum moves.

During a tympanometry test:

- The audiologist or other provider will place a small device inside the ear canal.
- The device will push air into the ear, making the eardrum move back and forth.
- A machine records the movement on graphs called "tympanograms."
- The test helps find out if there is an ear infection or other problems such as fluid or wax buildup, or a hole or tear in the eardrum.

WILL YOU NEED TO DO ANYTHING TO PREPARE FOR A HEARING TEST?

You do not need any special preparations for a hearing test.

ARE THERE ANY RISKS TO HEARING TESTS?

There is no risk to having a hearing test.

WHAT DO THE RESULTS MEAN?

Your results may show if you have a hearing loss, and whether the hearing loss is sensorineural or conductive.

If you are diagnosed with sensorineural hearing loss, your results may show that the hearing loss is:

- **Mild.** You cannot hear certain sounds, such as tones that are too high or too low.
- **Moderate.** You cannot hear many sounds, such as speech in a noisy environment.

- **Severe.** You cannot hear most sounds.
- **Profound.** You cannot hear any sounds.

Treatment and management of sensorineural hearing loss will depend on serious it is.

If you are diagnosed with conductive hearing loss, your provider may recommend medicine or surgery, depending on the cause of the loss.

If you have questions about the results, talk to your health-care provider.

IS THERE ANYTHING ELSE YOU NEED TO KNOW ABOUT HEARING TESTS?

Even mild hearing loss can make it difficult to understand normal speech. Because of this, many older adults will avoid social situations, leading to isolation and depression. Treating hearing loss can help prevent these problems. While hearing loss in older adults is usually permanent, there are ways to manage the condition. Treatment options include:

- **Hearing aids.** A hearing aid is a device that is worn either behind or inside the ear. A hearing aid amplifies (makes louder) sound. Some hearing aids have more advanced functions. Your audiologist can recommend the best option for you.
- **Cochlear implants.** This is a device that is implanted surgically in the ear. It is usually used in people with more severe hearing loss and who do not get much benefit from using a hearing aid. Cochlear implants send sound directly to the hearing nerve.
- **Surgery.** Some types of hearing loss can be treated with surgery. These include problems with the eardrum or in the tiny bones inside the ear.

Section 5.8 | **Vision Test**

This section includes text excerpted from "Keep an Eye on Your Vision Health," Centers for Disease Control and Prevention (CDC), October 1, 2020.

Going to the doctor, going to the dentist – all part of taking care of your health. But, going to the eye doctor? Also important! Eye exams at every age and life stage can help keep your vision strong.

Many people think their eyesight is just fine, but then they get that first pair of glasses or contact lenses and the world comes into clearer view – everything from fine print to street signs.

Improving your eyesight is important – about 11 million Americans over age 12 need vision correction – but it is just one of the reasons to get your eyes examined. Regular eye exams are also an important part of finding eye diseases early and preserving your vision.

ONLY YOUR EYE DOCTOR KNOWS FOR SURE

Eye diseases are common and can go unnoticed for a long time – some have no symptoms at first. A comprehensive dilated eye exam by an optometrist or ophthalmologist (eye doctor) is necessary to find eye diseases in the early stages when treatment to prevent vision loss is most effective.

During the exam, visual acuity (sharpness), depth perception, eye alignment, and eye movement are tested. Eye drops are used to make your pupils larger so your eye doctor can see inside your eyes and check for signs of health problems. Your eye doctor may even spot other conditions such as HBP or diabetes, sometimes before your primary care doctor does.

VISION CARE CAN CHANGE LIVES

Early treatment is critically important to prevent some common eye diseases from causing permanent vision loss or blindness:

- Cataracts (clouding of the lens), the leading cause of vision loss in the United States

- Diabetic retinopathy (causes damage to blood vessels in the back of the eye), the leading cause of blindness in American adults
- Glaucoma (a group of diseases that damages the optic nerve)
- Age-related macular degeneration (gradual breakdown of light-sensitive tissue in the eye)

Of the estimated 93 million U.S. adults at high risk for vision loss, only half visited an eye doctor in the past 12 months. Regular eye care can have a life-changing impact on preserving the vision of millions of people.

START EARLY

Though people tend to have more vision problems as they get older, children need eye exams to ensure healthy vision, too. But, only 39 percent of preschool children have had their vision tested, which is needed to diagnose eye diseases.

Amblyopia (reduced vision because the eye and brain are not working together properly) is the most common cause of vision loss in children – 2 to 3 out of 100 children. Amblyopia needs to be treated promptly to help avoid vision loss.

EYE EXAMS: HOW OFTEN?

- Children's eyes should be checked regularly by an eye doctor or pediatrician. The U.S. Preventive Services Task Force (USPSTF) recommends vision screening for all children at least once between age 3 and 5 years to detect amblyopia or risk factors for the disease.
- People with diabetes should have a dilated eye exam every year.
- Some people are at higher risk for glaucoma and should have a dilated eye exam every 2 years:
- African Americans 40 years and older
- All adults older than 60, especially Mexican Americans
- People with a family history of glaucoma

OTHER REASONS TO SEE YOUR EYE DOCTOR

If you have any of the following eye problems, do not wait for your next appointment – visit your eye doctor as soon as possible:

- Decreased vision
- Draining or redness of the eye
- Eye pain
- Double vision
- Floaters (tiny specks that appear to float before your eyes)
- Circles (halos) around lights
- Flashes of light

DIABETES AND YOUR EYES

Diabetic retinopathy is a common complication of diabetes. High blood sugar damages the blood vessels in the retina (a light-sensitive part of the eye), where scarring can cause permanent vision loss.

Diabetic retinopathy is also one of the most preventable causes of vision loss and blindness. Early detection and treatment can prevent or delay blindness due to diabetic retinopathy in 90 percent of people with diabetes, but 50 percent or more of them do not get their eyes examined or are diagnosed too late for effective treatment.

People with diabetes are also at higher risk for other eye diseases, including glaucoma and cataracts. If you have diabetes, an eye exam every year is necessary to protect and preserve your eyesight and eye health.

LOOKING AHEAD

Due to the aging population, the number of blind and visually impaired people in the United States is estimated to double by 2030 and triple by 2050. Encouraging people to take care of their vision health as part of their overall health and wellness could significantly reduce that number and improve quality of life for millions of Americans.

Section 5.9 | Testing for COVID-19

This section includes text excerpted from "COVID-19 Testing Overview," Centers for Disease Control and Prevention (CDC), October 21, 2021.

TYPES OF TESTS

Coronavirus disease (COVID-19) tests are available that can test for current infection or past infection.

- A viral test tells you if you have a current infection. Two types of viral tests can be used: nucleic acid amplification tests (NAATs) and antigen tests.
- An antibody test (also known as a "serology test") might tell you if you had a past infection. Antibody tests should not be used to diagnose a current infection.

WHO SHOULD GET TESTED FOR CURRENT INFECTION?

- People who have symptoms of COVID-19.
- Most people who have had close contact (within 6 feet for a total of 15 minutes or more over a 24-hour period) with someone with confirmed COVID-19.
    - Fully vaccinated people should be tested 3 to 5 days following a known exposure to someone with suspected or confirmed COVID-19 and wear a mask in public indoor settings for 14 days or until they receive a negative test result.
    - People who have tested positive for COVID-19 within the past 3 months and recovered do not need to get tested following an exposure as long as they do not develop new symptoms.
- Unvaccinated people who have taken part in activities that put them at higher risk for COVID-19 because they cannot physically distance as needed to avoid exposure, such as travel, attending large social or mass gatherings, or being in crowded or poorly-ventilated indoor settings.
- People who have been asked or referred to get tested by their health-care provider, or state, tribal, local, or territorial health department.

The Centers for Disease Control and Prevention (CDC) recommends that anyone with any signs or symptoms of COVID-19 get tested, regardless of vaccination status or prior infection. If you get tested because you have symptoms or were potentially exposed to the virus, you should stay away from others pending test results and follow the advice of your health-care provider or a public-health professional.

WHEN YOU ARE FULLY VACCINATED AND TRAVELING INTERNATIONALLY

International travelers need to pay close attention to the situation at their international destinations before traveling due to the spread of new variants and because the burden of COVID-19 varies globally.

- Fully vaccinated travelers do not need to get tested before leaving the United States unless required by their destination.
- Fully vaccinated air travelers coming to the United States from abroad, including U.S. citizens, are still required to have a negative SARS-CoV-2 viral test result or documentation of recovery from COVID-19 before they board a flight to the United States.
- International travelers arriving in the United States are still recommended to get a SARS-CoV-2 viral test 3 to 5 days after travel regardless of vaccination status.
- Fully vaccinated travelers do not need to self-quarantine in the United States following international travel.

HOW TO GET TESTED FOR CURRENT COVID-19 INFECTION

- Contact your health-care provider or visit your state, tribal, local, and territorial health department's website (www.cdc.gov/publichealthgateway/healthdirectories/index.html) to find the latest local information on testing. The type of viral COVID-19 tests offered may differ by location.

You and your health-care provider might also consider either an at-home collection kit or an at-home test if you have signs and symptoms of COVID-19 and if you cannot get tested by a health-care provider or public-health official.

HOW TO USE RESULTS OF VIRAL TESTS

- If you test positive, know what protective steps to take to prevent others from getting sick.
- If you test negative, you probably were not infected at the time your sample was collected. The test result only means that you did not have COVID-19 at the time of testing. Continue to take steps to protect yourself.

Section 5.10 | Get Tested for Sexually Transmitted Disease

This section contains text excerpted from the following sources: Text under the heading "What Are Sexually Transmitted Diseases?" is excerpted from "Sexually Transmitted Diseases (STDs) – Diseases and Related Conditions," Centers for Disease Control and Prevention (CDC), November 4, 2016. Reviewed October 2021; Text under the heading "Which STD Tests Should I Get?" is excerpted from "Which STD Tests Should You Get?" Centers for Disease Control and Prevention (CDC), July 22, 2021.

WHAT ARE SEXUALLY TRANSMITTED DISEASES?

Sexually transmitted diseases (STDs), also known as "sexually transmitted infections" (STIs), are very common. Millions of new infections occur every year in the United States.

STDs are passed from one person to another through sexual activity including vaginal, oral, and anal sex. They can also be passed from one person to another through intimate physical contact, such as heavy petting, though this is not very common.

STDs do not always cause symptoms or may only cause mild symptoms, so it is possible to have an infection and not know it. That is why it is important to get tested if you are having sex. If you are diagnosed with an STD, know that all can be treated with medicine and some can be cured entirely.

STDs are preventable. If you have sex, know how to protect yourself and your sexual partner from STDs.

Some common diseases, conditions, and infections are listed below.

- Bacterial vaginosis
- Chlamydia
- Gonorrhea
- Hepatitis
- Herpes
- Human immunodeficiency virus/acquired immunodeficiency syndrome (HIV/AIDS)
- Human papillomavirus (HPV) infection
- Pelvic inflammatory disease (PID)
- Syphilis
- Trichomoniasis

WHICH STD TESTS SHOULD YOU GET?

If you are sexually active, getting tested for STDs is one of the most important things you can do to protect your health. Make sure you have an open and honest conversation about your sexual history and STD testing with your doctor and ask whether you should be tested for STDs. If you are not comfortable talking with your regular health-care provider about STDs, there are many clinics that provide confidential and free or low-cost testing.

Below is a brief overview of STD testing recommendations.

- All adults and adolescents from ages 13 to 64 should be tested at least once for HIV.
- All sexually active women younger than 25 years should be tested for gonorrhea and chlamydia every year. Women 25 years and older with risk factors such as new or multiple sex partners or a sex partner who has an STD should also be tested for gonorrhea and chlamydia every year.
- All pregnant women should be tested for syphilis, HIV, hepatitis B, and hepatitis C starting early in pregnancy. At-risk pregnant women should also be tested for chlamydia and gonorrhea starting early in pregnancy.

Testing should be repeated as needed to protect the health of mothers and their infants.

- All sexually active gay, bisexual, and other men who have sex with men should be:
- Tested at least once a year for syphilis, chlamydia, and gonorrhea. Those who have multiple or anonymous partners should be tested more frequently (e.g., every 3 to 6 months).
- Tested at least once a year for HIV and may benefit from more frequent HIV testing (e.g., every 3 to 6 months).
- Tested at least once a year for hepatitis C, if living with HIV.
- Anyone who has unsafe sex or shares injection drug equipment should get tested for HIV at least once a year.
- People who have had oral or anal sex should talk with their health-care provider about throat and rectal testing options.

Section 5.11 | **Recommended Immunizations for Seniors**

This section includes text excerpted from "Get Shots to Protect Your Health (Adults Age 50 or Older)," Office of Disease Prevention and Health Promotion (ODPHP), U.S. Department of Health and Human Services (HHS), October 15, 2020.

Older adults need to get shots (vaccines) to prevent serious diseases. Protect your health by getting all your shots on schedule.

If you are age 50 or older:

- Get shots to prevent shingles. Shingles causes a painful rash that can last for months. Learn about shingles vaccines.

If you are age 65 or older:

- Get shots to prevent pneumococcal disease. Pneumococcal disease can include pneumonia, meningitis, and blood infections.

It is also important for all adults to:

- Get a flu vaccine every year. The seasonal flu vaccine is the best way to protect yourself and others from the flu.
- Get the Tdap shot to protect against tetanus, diphtheria, and whooping cough (pertussis). Everyone needs to get the Tdap shot once.
- After you get a Tdap shot, get a Td shot every 10 years to keep you protected against tetanus and diphtheria.

Ask your doctor, nurse, or pharmacist about other shots you may need to stay healthy.

HEALTH BENEFITS

Why Do You Need to Get These Shots?

Shots help protect you from diseases that can be serious – and sometimes deadly. Many of these diseases are common, but vaccines can prevent them.

Even if you have always gotten your shots on schedule, you still need to get some shots as an older adult. This is because:

- Older adults are more likely to get certain diseases.
- Older adults are at higher risk for serious complications from diseases.
- The protection from some shots can wear off over time.

Getting Your Shots Also Protects Other People

When you get shots, you do not just protect yourself – you also protect others. This is especially important if you spend time around anyone with a long-term health problem or a weakened immune system (the system in the body that fights infections).

Protect yourself and people around you by staying up-to-date on your shots.

OTHER SHOTS

Do You Need Any Other Shots to Help You Stay Healthy?

You may need other shots if you:

- Did not get all of your shots when you were a child

- Have a health condition like human immunodeficiency virus (HIV) that makes it harder for your body to fight off infections.
- Have a long-term health condition such as diabetes or heart, lung, or liver disease
- Are a man who has sex with men
- Smoke
- Spend time with infants or young children
- Travel outside the United States

And you may need other shots if you work in a:

- School
- Daycare
- Hospital
- Health clinic
- Nursing home
- Prison

Ask your doctor or nurse if you need any other shots.

MAKE A PLAN

Talk with a doctor, nurse, or pharmacist about getting up-to-date on your shots.

Make a Plan to Get Your Shots

Schedule an appointment with your doctor or nurse to get the shots you need. You may also be able to get shots at your local pharmacy.

Use the vaccine clinic locator (www.vaccines.gov) to find out where you can get shots.

Get a Seasonal Flu Shot Every Year

Remember, everyone age 6 months and older needs to get the seasonal flu vaccine every year.

What about Cost

Under the Affordable Care Act (ACA), most private insurance plans must cover recommended shots for adults. Depending on your insurance plan, you may be able to get your shots at no cost to you.

Medicare also covers most recommended shots for older adults, depending on your plan.

If you do not have insurance, you still may be able to get free shots.

- Find a free or low-cost vaccination program in your state.
- Find a health center near you and ask about affordable vaccine services.

KEEP A RECORD

Keep a copy of your vaccination record.

Ask your doctor to print out a record of all the shots you have had. Keep this record in a safe place. You may need it for certain jobs or if you travel outside the United States.

If you are not sure which shots you have had, try these tips for finding old vaccination records. If you still cannot find a record of your shots, talk with your doctor about getting some shots again.

Section 5.12 | **Fall Risk Assessment**

This section includes text excerpted from "Fall Risk Assessment," MedlinePlus, National Institutes of Health (NIH), September 13, 2021.

WHAT IS A FALL RISK ASSESSMENT?

Falls are common in adults 65 years of age and older. In the United States, about a third of older adults who live at home and about half of people living in nursing homes fall at least once a year. There are many factors that increase the risk of falling in older adults. These include mobility problems, balance disorders, chronic illnesses, and impaired vision. Many falls cause at least some injury. These range from mild bruising to broken bones, head injuries, and even death. In fact, falls are a leading cause of death in older adults.

A fall risk assessment checks to see how likely it is that you will fall. It is mostly done for older adults. The assessment usually includes:

- **An initial screening.** This includes a series of questions about your overall health and if you have had previous falls or problems with balance, standing, and/or walking.
- **A set of tasks, known as "fall assessment tools."** These tools test your strength, balance, and gait (the way you walk).

Other names include fall risk evaluation, fall risk screening, assessment, and intervention.

WHAT IS IT USED FOR?

A fall risk assessment is used to find out if you have a low, moderate, or high risk of falling. If the assessment shows you are at an increased risk, your health-care provider and/or caregiver may recommend strategies to prevent falls and reduce the chance of injury.

WHY DO I NEED A FALL RISK ASSESSMENT?

The Centers for Disease Control and Prevention (CDC) and the American Geriatric Society (AGS) recommend yearly fall assessment screening for all adults 65 years of age and older. If the screening shows you are at risk, you may need an assessment. The assessment includes performing a series of tasks called "fall assessment tools."

You also may need an assessment if you have certain symptoms. Falls often come without warning, but if you have any of the following symptoms, you may be at higher risk:

- Dizziness
- Light-headedness
- Irregular or rapid heartbeats

WHAT HAPPENS DURING A FALL RISK ASSESSMENT

Many providers use an approach developed by the CDC called "STEADI" (Stopping Elderly Accidents, Deaths, and Injuries).

STEADI includes screening, assessing, and intervention. Interventions are recommendations that may reduce your risk of falling.

During the screening, you may be asked several questions including:

- Have you fallen in the past year?
- Do you feel unsteady when standing or walking?
- Are you worried about falling?

During an assessment, your provider will test your strength, balance, and gait, using the following fall assessment tools:

- **Timed up-and-go (tug).** This test checks your gait. You will start in a chair, stand up, and then walk for about 10 feet at your regular pace. Then you will sit down again. Your health-care provider will check how long it takes you to do this. If it takes you 12 seconds or more, it may mean you are at higher risk for a fall.
- **30-second chair stand test.** This test checks strength and balance. You will sit in a chair with your arms crossed over your chest. When your provider says "go," you will stand up and sit down again. You will repeat this for 30 seconds. Your provider will count how many times you can do this. A lower number may mean you are at higher risk for a fall. The specific number that indicates a risk depends on your age.
- **4-stage balance test.** This test checks how well you can keep your balance. You will stand in four different positions, holding each one for 10 seconds. The positions will get harder as you go.
  - **Position 1.** Stand with your feet side-by-side.
  - **Position 2.** Move one foot halfway forward, so the instep is touching the big toe of your other foot.
  - **Position 3.** Move one foot fully in front of the other, so the toes are touching the heel of your other foot.
  - **Position 4.** Stand on one foot.

If you cannot hold position 2 or position 3 for 10 seconds or you cannot stand on one leg for 5 seconds, it may mean you are at higher risk for a fall.

There are many other fall assessment tools. If your provider recommends other assessments, she or he will let you know what to expect.

WILL YOU NEED TO DO ANYTHING TO PREPARE FOR A FALL RISK ASSESSMENT?

You do not need any special preparations for a fall risk assessment.

ARE THERE ANY RISKS TO A FALL RISK ASSESSMENT?

There is a small risk that you may fall as you do the assessment.

WHAT DO THE RESULTS MEAN?

The results may show you have a low, moderate, or high risk of falling. They also may show which areas need addressing (gait, strength, and/or balance). Based on your results, your health-care provider may make recommendations to reduce your risk of falling. These may include:

- Exercising to improve your strength and balance. You may be given instructions on specific exercises or be referred to a physical therapist.
- Changing or reducing the dose of medicines that may be affecting your gait or balance. Some medicines have side effects that cause dizziness, drowsiness, or confusion.
- Taking vitamin D to strengthen your bones
- Getting your vision checked by an eye doctor
- Looking at your footwear to see if any of your shoes might increase your risk of falling. You may be referred to a podiatrist (foot doctor).
- Reviewing your home for potential hazards. These may include poor lighting, loose rugs, and/or cords on the floor. This review may be done by yourself, a

partner, an occupational therapist, or other health-care provider.

If you have questions about your results and/or recommendations, talk to your health-care provider.

Chapter 6 | Genetic Testing

Chapter Contents

Section 6.1 | Frequently Asked Questions about Genetic Testing

This section includes text excerpted from "Genetic Testing," MedlinePlus, National Institutes of Health (NIH), July 28, 2021.

WHAT IS GENETIC TESTING?

Genetic testing is a type of medical test that identifies changes in genes, chromosomes, or proteins. The results of a genetic test can confirm or rule out a suspected genetic condition or help determine a person's chance of developing or passing on a genetic disorder. More than 77,000 genetic tests are currently in use, and others are being developed.

Genetic testing involves looking for changes in:

- **Genes.** Gene tests study deoxyribonucleic acid (DNA) sequences to identify variations (mutations) in genes that can cause or increase the risk of a genetic disorder. Gene tests can be narrow or large in scope, analyzing an individual DNA building block (nucleotide), one or more genes, or all of a person's DNA (which is known as their "genome").
- **Chromosomes.** Chromosomal genetic tests analyze whole chromosomes or long lengths of DNA to see if there are large genetic changes, such as an extra copy of a chromosome, that cause a genetic condition.
- **Proteins.** Biochemical genetic tests study the amount or activity level of proteins or enzymes; abnormalities in either can indicate changes to the DNA that result in a genetic disorder.

Genetic testing is voluntary. Because testing has benefits as well as limitations and risks, the decision about whether to be tested is a personal and complex one. A geneticist or genetic counselor can help by providing information about the pros and cons of the test and discussing the social and emotional aspects of testing.

WHAT ARE THE DIFFERENT TYPES OF GENETIC TESTS?

Many types of genetic tests are available to analyze changes in genes, chromosomes, or proteins. A health-care provider will consider several factors when selecting the appropriate test, including what condition or conditions are suspected and the genetic variations typically associated with those conditions. If a diagnosis is unclear, a test that looks at many genes or chromosomes may be used. However, if a specific condition is suspected, a more focused test may be done.

There are several types of genetic tests:

- Molecular tests look for changes in one or more genes. These types of tests determine the order of DNA building blocks (nucleotides) in an individual's genetic code, a process called "DNA sequencing." These tests can vary in scope:
    - **Targeted single variant.** Single variant tests look for a specific variant in one gene. The selected variant is known to cause a disorder (e.g., the specific variant in the *HBB* gene that causes sickle cell disease (SCD)). This type of test is often used to test family members of someone who is known to have a particular variant, to determine whether they have a familial condition. Also, direct-to-consumer genetic testing companies typically analyze a number of specific variants in particular genes (rather than finding all the variants in those genes) when providing health or disease risk information.
    - **Single gene.** These tests look for any genetic changes in one gene. These tests are typically used to confirm (or rule out) a specific diagnosis, particularly when there are many variants in the gene that can cause the suspected condition.
    - **Gene panel.** Panel tests look for variants in more than one gene. This type of test is often used to pinpoint a diagnosis when a person has symptoms that may fit a wide array of conditions, or when the suspected condition can be caused by variants in many genes. (E.g., there are hundreds of genetic causes of epilepsy.)

    - **Whole exome sequencing/whole genome sequencing.** These tests analyze the bulk of an individual's DNA to find genetic variations. Whole exome or whole genome sequencing is typically used when single gene or panel testing has not provided a diagnosis, or when the suspected condition or genetic cause is unclear. Whole exome or whole genome sequencing is often more cost- and time-effective than performing multiple single gene or panel tests.
- Chromosomal tests analyze whole chromosomes or long lengths of DNA to identify large-scale changes. Changes that can be found include an extra or missing copy of a chromosome (trisomy or monosomy, respectively), a large piece of a chromosome that is added (duplicated) or missing (deleted), or rearrangements (translocations) of segments of chromosomes. Certain genetic conditions are associated with specific chromosomal changes, and a chromosomal test can be used when one of these conditions is suspected. (E.g., Williams syndrome is caused by a deletion of a section of chromosome 7.)
- Gene expression tests look at which genes are turned on or off (expressed) in different types of cells. When a gene is turned on (active), the cell produces a molecule called "mRNA" from the instructions in the genes, and the mRNA molecule is used as a blueprint to make proteins. Gene expression tests study the mRNA in cells to determine which genes are active. Too much activity (overexpression) or too little activity (underexpression) of certain genes can be suggestive of particular genetic disorders, such as many types of cancer.
- Biochemical tests do not directly analyze DNA, but they study the amount or activity level of proteins or enzymes that are produced from genes. Abnormalities in these substances can indicate that there are changes in the DNA that underlie a genetic disorder. (E.g., low levels of

biotinidase enzyme activity is suggestive of biotinidase deficiency, which is caused by *BTD* gene variants.)

WHAT ARE THE USES OF GENETIC TESTING?

Genetic testing can provide information about a person's genetic background. The uses of genetic testing include:

Newborn Screening

Newborn screening is used just after birth to identify genetic disorders that can be treated early in life. Millions of babies are tested each year in the United States. The U.S. Health Resources and Services Administration (HRSA) recommends that states screen for a set of 35 conditions, which many states exceed.

Diagnostic Testing

Diagnostic testing is used to identify or rule out a specific genetic or chromosomal condition. In many cases, genetic testing is used to confirm a diagnosis when a particular condition is suspected based on physical signs and symptoms. Diagnostic testing can be performed before birth or at any time during a person's life, but is not available for all genes or all genetic conditions. The results of a diagnostic test can influence a person's choices about healthcare and the management of the disorder.

Carrier Testing

Carrier testing is used to identify people who carry one copy of a gene mutation that, when present in two copies, causes a genetic disorder. This type of testing is offered to individuals who have a family history of a genetic disorder and to people in certain ethnic groups with an increased risk of specific genetic conditions. If both parents are tested, the test can provide information about a couple's risk of having a child with a genetic condition.

Prenatal Testing

Prenatal testing is used to detect changes in a fetus's genes or chromosomes before birth. This type of testing is offered during pregnancy if there is an increased risk that the baby will have a genetic or chromosomal disorder. In some cases, prenatal testing can lessen a couple's uncertainty or help them make decisions about a pregnancy. It cannot identify all possible inherited disorders and birth defects, however.

Preimplantation Testing

Preimplantation testing, also called "preimplantation genetic diagnosis" (PGD), is a specialized technique that can reduce the risk of having a child with a particular genetic or chromosomal disorder. It is used to detect genetic changes in embryos that were created using assisted reproductive techniques (ARTs) such as invitro fertilization (IVF). IVF involves removing egg cells from a woman's ovaries and fertilizing them with sperm cells outside the body. To perform preimplantation testing, a small number of cells are taken from these embryos and tested for certain genetic changes. Only embryos without these changes are implanted in the uterus to initiate a pregnancy.

Predictive and Presymptomatic Testing

Predictive and presymptomatic types of testing are used to detect gene mutations associated with disorders that appear after birth, often later in life. These tests can be helpful to people who have a family member with a genetic disorder, but who have no features of the disorder themselves at the time of testing. Predictive testing can identify mutations that increase a person's risk of developing disorders with a genetic basis, such as certain types of cancer. Presymptomatic testing can determine whether a person will develop a genetic disorder, such as hereditary hemochromatosis (an iron overload disorder), before any signs or symptoms appear. The results of predictive and presymptomatic testing can provide information about a person's risk of developing a specific disorder and help with making decisions about medical care.

Forensic Testing

Forensic testing uses DNA sequences to identify an individual for legal purposes. Unlike the tests described above, forensic testing is not used to detect gene mutations associated with disease. This type of testing can identify crime or catastrophe victims, rule out or implicate a crime suspect, or establish biological relationships between people (e.g., paternity).

HOW IS GENETIC TESTING DONE?

Once a person decides to proceed with genetic testing, a health-care provider can arrange testing. Genetic testing is often done as part of a genetic consultation.

Genetic tests are performed on a sample of blood, hair, skin, amniotic fluid (the fluid that surrounds a fetus during pregnancy), or other tissue. For example, a procedure called a "buccal smear" uses a small brush or cotton swab to collect a sample of cells from the inside surface of the cheek. The sample is sent to a laboratory where technicians look for specific changes in chromosomes, DNA, or proteins, depending on the suspected disorder. The laboratory reports the test results in writing to a person's doctor or genetic counselor, or directly to the patient if requested.

Newborn screening tests are done on a small blood sample, which is taken by pricking the baby's heel. Unlike other types of genetic testing, a parent will usually only receive the result if it is positive. If the test result is positive, additional testing is needed to determine whether the baby has a genetic disorder.

Individuals interested in direct-to-consumer genetic testing do not need to go through a health-care provider to obtain a test, but they can get it directly from the testing company. After undergoing direct-to-consumer genetic testing, people who test positive for a condition or are found to be at higher risk of developing a disorder are encouraged to follow-up with a genetic counselor or other health-care provider.

WHAT IS INFORMED CONSENT?

Before a person has a genetic test, it is important to fully understand the testing procedure, the benefits and limitations of the test, and the possible consequences of the test results. The process of educating a person about the test and obtaining permission to carry out testing is called "informed consent." "Informed" means that the person has enough information to make an educated decision about testing; "consent" refers to a person's voluntary agreement to have the test done.

In general, informed consent can only be given by adults who are competent to make medical decisions for themselves. For children and others who are unable to make their own medical decisions (such as people with impaired mental status), informed consent can be given by a parent, guardian, or other person legally responsible for making decisions on that person's behalf.

Informed consent for genetic testing is generally obtained by a doctor or genetic counselor during an office visit. The health-care provider will discuss the test and answer any questions. If the person wishes to have the test, she or he will then usually read and sign a consent form.

Several factors are commonly included on an informed consent form:

- A general description of the test, including the purpose of the test and the condition for which the testing is being performed.
- How the test will be carried out (e.g., a blood sample).
- What the test results mean, including positive and negative results, and the potential for uninformative results or incorrect results such as false positives or false negatives.
- Any physical or emotional risks associated with the test.
- Whether the results can be used for research purposes.
- Whether the results might provide information about other family members' health, including the risk of developing a particular condition or the possibility of having affected children.
- How and to whom test results will be reported and under what circumstances results can be disclosed (e.g., to health insurance providers).
- What will happen to the test specimen after the test is complete.

- Acknowledgement that the person undergoing testing has had the opportunity to discuss the test with a health-care provider.
- The individual's signature, and possibly that of a witness.

The elements of informed consent may vary, because some states have laws that specify factors that must be included. (E.g., some states require disclosure that the test specimen will be destroyed within a certain period of time after the test is complete.)

Informed consent is not a contract, so a person can change their mind at any time after giving initial consent. A person may choose not to go through with genetic testing even after the test sample has been collected. A person simply needs to notify the health-care provider if the decision has been made to not continue with the testing process.

HOW CAN YOU BE SURE A GENETIC TEST IS VALID AND USEFUL?

Before undergoing genetic testing, it is important to be sure that the test is valid and useful. A genetic test is valid if it provides an accurate result. Two main measures of accuracy apply to genetic tests: analytical validity and clinical validity. Another measure of the quality of a genetic test is its usefulness, or clinical utility.

- Analytical validity refers to how well the test predicts the presence or absence of a particular gene or genetic change. In other words, can the test accurately detect whether a specific genetic variant is present or absent?
- Clinical validity refers to how well the genetic variant being analyzed is related to the presence, absence, or risk of a specific disease.
- Clinical utility refers to whether the test can provide helpful information about diagnosis, treatment, management, or prevention of a disease.

All laboratories that perform health-related testing, including genetic testing, are subject to federal regulatory standards called the "Clinical Laboratory Improvement Amendments" (CLIA) or even stricter state requirements. CLIA standards cover how tests are performed, the qualifications of laboratory personnel, and quality control and testing procedures for each laboratory. By controlling the quality of laboratory practices, CLIA standards are designed to ensure the analytical validity of genetic tests.

CLIA standards do not address the clinical validity or clinical utility of genetic tests. The U.S. Food and Drug Administration (FDA) requires information about clinical validity for some genetic tests, particularly those tests that have been produced by a lab (known as "laboratory-developed tests"). Additionally, states may require additional information on clinical validity for laboratory tests performed for people living in that state. Test takers, health-care providers, and health insurance companies are often the ones who determine the clinical utility of a genetic test.

It can be difficult to determine the quality of a genetic test sold directly to the public. Some providers of direct-to-consumer genetic tests are not CLIA-certified, so it can be difficult to tell whether their tests are valid. If providers of direct-to-consumer genetic tests offer easy-to-understand information about the scientific basis of their tests, it can help people make more informed decisions. It may also be helpful to discuss any concerns with health-care providers before ordering a direct-to-consumer genetic test and after receiving test results.

WHAT DO THE RESULTS OF GENETIC TESTS MEAN?

The results of genetic tests are not always straightforward, which often makes them challenging to interpret and explain. Therefore, it is important for patients and their families to ask questions about the potential meaning of genetic test results both before and after the test is performed. When interpreting test results, health-care providers consider a person's medical history, family history, and the type of genetic test that was done.

A positive test result means that the laboratory found a change in a particular gene, chromosome, or protein of interest. Depending on the purpose of the test, this result may confirm a diagnosis, indicate that a person is a carrier of a particular genetic variant, identify an increased risk of developing a disease (such as cancer), or suggest a need for further testing. Because family members have some genetic material in common, a positive test result may also have implications for certain blood relatives of the person undergoing testing. It is important to note that a positive result of a predictive or presymptomatic genetic test usually cannot establish the exact risk of developing a disorder. Also, health-care providers typically cannot use a positive test result to predict the course or severity of a condition. Rarely, tests results can be false positive, which occur when results indicate an increased risk for a genetic condition when the person is unaffected.

A negative test result means that the laboratory did not find a change that is known to affect health or development in the gene, chromosome, or protein under consideration. This result can indicate that a person is not affected by a particular disorder, is not a carrier of a specific genetic variant, or does not have an increased risk of developing a certain disease. It is possible, however, that the test missed a disease-causing genetic alteration because many tests cannot detect all genetic changes that can cause a particular disorder. Further testing, or retesting at a later date, may be required to confirm a negative result. Rarely, tests results can be false negative, which occur when the results indicate a decreased risk or a genetic condition when the person is actually affected.

In some cases, a test result might not give any useful information. This type of result is called "uninformative, indeterminate, inconclusive, or ambiguous." Uninformative test results sometimes occur because everyone has common, natural variations in their DNA, called "polymorphisms" that do not affect health. If a genetic test finds a change in DNA that has not been confirmed to play a role in the development of disease, known as a "variant of uncertain significance" (VUS or VOUS), it can be difficult to tell whether it is a natural polymorphism or a disease-causing variant. For these variants, there may not be enough scientific research to confirm or refute a disease association or the research may be conflicting. An uninformative result cannot confirm or rule out a specific diagnosis, and it cannot indicate whether a person has an increased risk of developing a disorder. In some cases, testing other affected and unaffected family members can help clarify this type of result.

WHAT IS THE COST OF GENETIC TESTING, AND HOW LONG DOES IT TAKE TO GET THE RESULTS?

The cost of genetic testing can range from under $100 to more than $2,000, depending on the nature and complexity of the test. The cost increases if more than one test is necessary or if multiple family members must be tested to obtain a meaningful result. For newborn screening, costs vary by state. Some states cover part of the total cost, but most charge a fee of $30 to $150 per infant.

From the date that a sample is taken, it may take a few days to weeks to receive the test results. Results for prenatal testing are usually available more quickly because time is an important consideration in making decisions about a pregnancy. The doctor or genetic counselor who orders a particular test can provide specific information about the cost and time frame associated with that test.

WILL HEALTH INSURANCE COVER THE COSTS OF GENETIC TESTING?

In many cases, health insurance plans will cover the costs of genetic testing when it is recommended by a person's doctor. Health insurance providers have different policies about which tests are covered, however. A person may wish to contact their insurance company before testing to ask about coverage.

Some people may choose not to use their insurance to pay for testing. Instead, they may opt to pay out of pocket for the test or pursue direct-to-consumer genetic testing, if available. People considering genetic testing may want to find out more about their state's privacy protection laws before they ask their insurance company to cover the costs.

WHAT ARE THE BENEFITS OF GENETIC TESTING?

Genetic testing has potential benefits whether the results are positive or negative for a gene mutation. Test results can provide a sense of relief from uncertainty and help people make informed decisions about managing their healthcare. For example, a negative result can eliminate the need for unnecessary checkups and screening tests in some cases. A positive result can direct a person toward available prevention, monitoring, and treatment options. Some test results can also help people make decisions about having children. Newborn screening can identify genetic disorders early in life so treatment can be started as early as possible.

WHAT ARE THE RISKS AND LIMITATIONS OF GENETIC TESTING?

The physical risks associated with most genetic tests are very small, particularly for those tests that require only a blood sample or buccal smear (a method that samples cells from the inside surface of the cheek). The procedures used for prenatal diagnostic testing (called "amniocentesis" and "chorionic villus sampling") carry a small, but real risk of losing the pregnancy (miscarriage) because they require a sample of amniotic fluid or tissue from around the fetus.

Many of the risks associated with genetic testing involve the emotional, social, or financial consequences of the test results. People may feel angry, depressed, anxious, or guilty about their results. In some cases, genetic testing creates tension within a family because the results can reveal information about other family members in addition to the person who is tested. The possibility of genetic discrimination in employment or insurance is also a concern.

Genetic testing can provide only limited information about an inherited condition. The test often cannot determine if a person will show symptoms of a disorder, how severe the symptoms will be, or whether the disorder will progress over time. Another major limitation is the lack of treatment strategies for many genetic disorders once they are diagnosed.

A genetics professional can explain in detail the benefits, risks, and limitations of a particular test. It is important that any person who is considering genetic testing understand and weigh these factors before making a decision.

Section 6.2 | Genetic Consultation

This section includes text excerpted from "Genetic Consultation," MedlinePlus, National Institutes of Health (NIH), September 10, 2020.

WHAT IS A GENETIC CONSULTATION?

A genetic consultation is a health service that provides information and support to people who have, or may be at risk for, genetic conditions. During a consultation, a genetics professional meets with an individual or family to discuss genetic risks or to diagnose, confirm, or rule out a genetic condition.

Genetics professionals include medical geneticists (doctors who specialize in genetics) and genetic counselors (certified health-care workers with experience in medical genetics and counseling). Other health-care professionals such as nurses, psychologists, and social workers trained in genetics can also provide genetic consultations.

Consultations usually take place in a doctor's office, hospital, genetics center, or other type of medical center. These meetings are most often in-person visits with individuals or families, but they are occasionally conducted in a group. Additionally, genetic consultations may be carried out using telemedicine (also known as "telehealth"), in which the meeting is done from a distance using computers, cameras, videoconferencing tools, or the telephone.

WHY MIGHT SOMEONE HAVE A GENETIC CONSULTATION?

Individuals or families who are concerned about an inherited condition may benefit from a genetic consultation. The reasons that a person might be referred to a genetic counselor, medical geneticist, or other genetics professional include:

- A personal or family history of a genetic condition, birth defect, chromosomal disorder, or hereditary cancer.
- Two or more pregnancy losses (miscarriages), a stillbirth, or a baby who died.
- A child with a known inherited disorder, a birth defect, intellectual disability, or developmental delay.

- A woman who is pregnant or plans to become pregnant at or after age 35. (Some chromosomal disorders occur more frequently in children born to older women.)
- Abnormal test results that suggest a genetic or chromosomal condition.
- An increased risk of developing or passing on a particular genetic disorder on the basis of a person's ethnic background.
- People related by blood (e.g., cousins) who plan to have children together. (A child whose parents are related may be at an increased risk of inheriting certain genetic disorders.)
- A person received results from direct-to-consumer genetic testing and they want to discuss the implications of the results.

A genetic consultation is also an important part of the decision-making process for genetic testing. A visit with a genetics professional may be helpful even if testing is not available for a specific condition, however.

WHAT HAPPENS DURING A GENETIC CONSULTATION

A genetic consultation provides information, offers support, and addresses a patient's specific questions and concerns. To help determine whether a condition has a genetic component, a genetics professional asks about a person's medical history and takes a detailed family health history (a record of health information about a person's immediate and extended family). The genetics professional may also perform a physical examination and recommend appropriate medical tests.

If a person is diagnosed with a genetic condition, the genetics professional provides information about the diagnosis, how the condition is inherited, the chance of passing the condition to future generations, and the options for testing and treatment.

During a consultation, a genetics professional will:

- Interpret and communicate complex medical information.

- Help each person make informed, independent decisions about their healthcare and reproductive options.
- Respect each person's individual beliefs, traditions, and feelings.

A genetics professional will not:

- Tell a person which decision to make.
- Coerce a couple about whether or not to have children.
- Recommend that a woman continue or end a pregnancy.
- Tell someone whether to undergo testing for a genetic disorder.

HOW CAN YOU FIND A GENETICS PROFESSIONAL IN YOUR AREA?

To find a genetics professional in your community, you may wish to ask your doctor for a referral. If you have health insurance, you can also contact your insurance company to find a medical geneticist or genetic counselor in your area who participates in your plan.

Several organizations have tips for finding a health-care professional:

- The Genetic and Rare Diseases Information Center (GARD), a service of the National Institutes of Health (NIH), provides a guide to finding specialists in particular genetic and rare conditions.
- The Tuberous Sclerosis Alliance provides advice on finding and choosing a doctor. Although this advice is written for adults with tuberous sclerosis, much of it applies to people with any chronic health condition.

Additional resources for locating a genetics professional in your community are available online:

- The National Society of Genetic Counselors (NSGC) offers a searchable directory of genetic counselors in the United States and Canada. You can search by location, name, area of practice/specialization, and/or ZIP Code.

- The American Board of Genetic Counseling (ABGC) provides a searchable directory of certified genetic counselors worldwide. You can search by practice area, name, organization, or location.
- The Canadian Association of Genetic Counsellors (CAGC) has a searchable directory of genetic counselors in Canada. You can search by name, distance from an address, province, or services.
- The American College of Medical Genetics and Genomics (ACMG) has a searchable database of medical genetics clinic services in the United States.
- The National Cancer Institute provides a Cancer Genetics Services Directory, which lists professionals who provide services related to cancer genetics. You can search by type of cancer or syndrome, location, and/or provider name.

If you have a health condition that has not been diagnosed, you may be interested in the Undiagnosed Diseases Network (UDN). They have information about how to apply for this multicenter research study.

WHAT IS THE PROGNOSIS OF A GENETIC CONDITION?

The prognosis of a genetic condition includes its likely course, duration, and outcome. When health professionals refer to the prognosis of a disease, they may also mean the chance of recovery; however, most genetic conditions are lifelong and are managed rather than cured.

Disease prognosis has multiple aspects, including:

- How long a person with the disorder is likely to live (life expectancy)
- When signs and symptoms develop and whether they worsen (and how quickly) or are stable over time
- Quality of life (QOL), such as independence in daily activities
- Potential for complications and associated health issues

The prognosis of a genetic condition depends on many factors, including the specific diagnosis and an individual's particular signs and symptoms. Sometimes the associated genetic variant, if known, can also give clues to the prognosis. Additionally, the course and outcome of a condition depends on the availability and effectiveness of treatment and management approaches. The prognosis of very rare diseases can be difficult to predict because so few affected individuals have been identified. Prognosis may also be difficult or impossible to establish if a person's diagnosis is unknown.

The prognoses of genetic disorders vary widely, often even among people with the same condition. This variability is likely caused by a combination of genetic, environmental, and lifestyle factors, many of which can be difficult to identify. Some genetic disorders cause physical and developmental problems that are so severe they are incompatible with life. These conditions may cause a miscarriage of an affected embryo or fetus, or an affected infant may be stillborn or die shortly after birth. People with less severe genetic conditions may live into childhood or adulthood, but have a shortened lifespan due to health problems related to their disorder. Genetic conditions with a milder course may be associated with a normal lifespan and few related health issues.

The prognosis of a disease is based on probability, which means that it is likely, but not certain that the disorder will follow a particular course. Your health-care provider is the best resource for information about the prognosis of your specific genetic condition. She or he can assess your medical history and signs and symptoms to give you the most accurate estimate of your prognosis.

HOW ARE GENETIC CONDITIONS DIAGNOSED?

A doctor may suspect a diagnosis of a genetic condition on the basis of a person's physical characteristics and family history, or on the results of a screening test.

Genetic testing is one of several tools that doctors use to diagnose genetic conditions. The approaches to making a genetic diagnosis include:

- **A physical examination.** Certain physical characteristics, such as distinctive facial features, can suggest the diagnosis of a genetic disorder. A geneticist will do a thorough physical examination that may include measurements such as the distance around the head (head circumference), the distance between the eyes, and the length of the arms and legs. Depending on the situation, specialized examinations such as nervous system (neurological) or eye (ophthalmologic) exams may be performed. The doctor may also use imaging studies including x-rays, computerized tomography (CT) scans, or magnetic resonance imaging (MRI) to see structures inside the body.

- **Personal medical history.** Information about an individual's health, often going back to birth, can provide clues to a genetic diagnosis. A personal medical history includes past health issues, hospitalizations and surgeries, allergies, medications, and the results of any medical or genetic testing that has already been done.
- **Family health history.** Because genetic conditions often run in families, information about the health of family members can be a critical tool for diagnosing these disorders. A doctor or genetic counselor will ask about health conditions in an individual's parents, siblings, children, and possibly more distant relatives. This information can give clues about the diagnosis and inheritance pattern of a genetic condition in a family.
- **Laboratory tests, including genetic testing.** Molecular, chromosomal, and biochemical genetic or genomic testing are used to diagnose genetic disorders. Other laboratory tests that measure the levels of certain substances in blood and urine can also help suggest a diagnosis.

Genetic testing is currently available for many genetic conditions. However, some conditions do not have a genetic test; either the genetic cause of the condition is unknown or a test has not yet been developed. In these cases, sequencing the entire genome may result in locating the responsible genetic variant. Additionally, a combination of the approaches listed above may be used to make a diagnosis. Even when genetic testing is available, the tools listed above are used to narrow down the possibilities (known as "a differential diagnosis") and choose the most appropriate genetic tests to pursue.

A diagnosis of a genetic disorder can be made anytime during life, from before birth to old age, depending on when the features of the condition appear and the availability of testing. Sometimes, having a diagnosis can guide treatment and management decisions. A genetic diagnosis can also suggest whether other family members may be affected by or at risk of a specific disorder. Even when no treatment is available for a particular condition, having a diagnosis can help people know what to expect and may help them identify useful support and advocacy resources.

HOW ARE GENETIC CONDITIONS TREATED OR MANAGED?

Many genetic disorders result from gene changes that are present in essentially every cell in the body. As a result, these disorders often affect many body systems, and most cannot be cured. However, approaches may be available to treat or manage some of the associated signs and symptoms.

For a group of genetic conditions called "inborn errors of metabolism," which result from genetic changes that disrupt the production of specific enzymes, treatments sometimes include dietary changes or replacement of the particular enzyme that is missing. Limiting certain substances in the diet can help prevent the buildup of potentially toxic substances that are normally broken down by the enzyme. In some cases, enzyme replacement therapy can help make up for the enzyme shortage. These treatments are used to manage existing signs and symptoms and may help prevent future complications. An example of an inborn error of metabolism is phenylketonuria (PKU).

For other genetic conditions, treatment and management strategies are designed to improve particular signs and symptoms associated with the disorder. These approaches vary by disorder and are specific to an individual's health needs. For example, a genetic disorder associated with a heart defect might be treated with surgery to repair the defect or with a heart transplant. Conditions that are characterized by defective blood cell formation, such as sickle cell disease (SCD), can sometimes be treated with a bone marrow transplant. Bone marrow transplantation can allow the formation of normal blood cells and, if done early in life, may help prevent episodes of pain and other future complications.

Some genetic changes are associated with an increased risk of future health problems, such as certain forms of cancer. One well-known example is familial breast cancer related to mutations in the *BRCA1* and *BRCA2* genes. Management may include more frequent cancer screening or preventive (prophylactic) surgery to remove the tissues at highest risk of becoming cancerous.

Genetic disorders may cause such severe health problems that they are incompatible with life. In the most severe cases, these conditions may cause a miscarriage of an affected embryo or fetus. In other cases, affected infants may be stillborn or die shortly after birth. Although few treatments are available for these severe genetic conditions, health professionals can often provide supportive care, such as pain relief or mechanical breathing assistance, to the affected individual.

Most treatment strategies for genetic disorders do not alter the underlying genetic mutation; however, a few disorders have been treated with gene therapy. This experimental technique involves changing a person's genes to prevent or treat a disease. Gene therapy, along with many other treatment and management approaches for genetic conditions, are under study in clinical trials.

Section 6.3 | **Genetic Testing for Breast Cancer Risk**

This section includes text excerpted from "BRCA Gene Mutations: Cancer Risk and Genetic Testing," National Cancer Institute (NCI), November 19, 2020.

WHAT ARE *BRCA1* AND *BRCA2*?

BRCA1 (BReast CAncer gene 1) and *BRCA2* (BReast CAncer gene 2) are genes that produce proteins that help repair damaged DNA. Everyone has two copies of each of these genes – one copy inherited from each parent. *BRCA1* and *BRCA2* are sometimes called "tumor suppressor genes" because when they have certain changes, called "harmful (or pathogenic) variants (or mutations)," cancer can develop.

People who inherit harmful variants in one of these genes have increased risks of several cancers – most notably breast and ovarian cancer, but also several additional types of cancer. People who have inherited a harmful variant in *BRCA1* and *BRCA2* also tend to develop cancer at younger ages than people who do not have such a variant.

A harmful variant in *BRCA1* or *BRCA2* can be inherited from either parent. Each child of a parent who carries any mutation in one of these genes has a 50 percent chance (or 1 in 2 chance) of inheriting the mutation. Inherited mutations – also called "germline mutations or variants" – are present from birth in all cells in the body.

Even if someone has inherited a harmful variant in *BRCA1* or *BRCA2* from one parent, they would have inherited a normal copy of that gene from the other parent (i.e., because in most cases, embryos with a harmful variant from each parent cannot develop). But, the normal copy can be lost or change in some cells in the body during that person's lifetime. Such a change is called a "somatic alteration." Cells that do not have any functioning BRCA1 or BRCA2 proteins can grow out of control and become cancer.

HOW MUCH DOES AN INHERITED HARMFUL VARIANT IN *BRCA1* OR *BRCA2* INCREASE A WOMAN'S RISK OF BREAST AND OVARIAN CANCER?

A woman's lifetime risk of developing breast and/or ovarian cancer is markedly increased if she inherits a harmful variant in *BRCA1* or *BRCA2*, but the degree of increase varies depending on the mutation.

Breast cancer. About 13 percent of women in the general population will develop breast cancer sometime during their lives. By contrast, 55 percent to 72 percent of women who inherit a harmful *BRCA1* variant and 45 percent to 69 percent of women who inherit a harmful *BRCA2* variant will develop breast cancer by 70 to 80 years of age. The risk for any one woman depends on a number of factors, some of which have not been fully characterized.

Like women with breast cancer in general, those with harmful *BRCA1* or *BRCA2* variants also have an increased risk of developing cancer in the opposite (contralateral) breast in the years following a breast cancer diagnosis. The risk of contralateral breast cancer increases with the time since a first breast cancer, reaching 20 percent to 30 percent at 10 years of follow-up and 40 percent to 50 percent at 20 years, depending on the gene involved.

Ovarian cancer. About 1.2 percent of women in the general population will develop ovarian cancer sometime during their lives. By contrast, 39 percent to 44 percent of women who inherit a harmful *BRCA1* variant and 11 percent to 17 percent of women who inherit a harmful *BRCA2* variant will develop ovarian cancer by 70 to 80 years of age.

WHAT OTHER CANCERS ARE LINKED TO HARMFUL VARIANTS IN *BRCA1* AND *BRCA2*?

Harmful variants in *BRCA1* and *BRCA2* increase the risk of several additional cancers. In women, these include fallopian tube cancer and primary peritoneal cancer, both of which start in the same cells as the most common type of ovarian cancer. Men with *BRCA2* variants, and to a lesser extent *BRCA1* variants, are also at increased risk of breast cancer and prostate cancer. Both men and women with harmful *BRCA1* or *BRCA2* variants are at increased risk of pancreatic cancer, although the risk increase is low.

In addition, certain variants in *BRCA1* and *BRCA2* can cause subtypes of Fanconi anemia, a rare syndrome that is associated with childhood solid tumors and development of acute myeloid leukemia. The mutations that cause these Fanconi anemia subtypes have a milder effect on protein function than the mutations that cause breast and ovarian cancer. Children who inherit one of these variants from each parent will develop Fanconi anemia.

ARE HARMFUL VARIANTS IN *BRCA1* AND *BRCA2* MORE COMMON IN CERTAIN RACIAL/ETHNIC POPULATIONS THAN OTHERS?

Yes. The likelihood of carrying an inherited mutation in *BRCA1* or *BRCA2* (the prevalence) varies across specific population groups. While the prevalence in the general population is about 0.2 percent to 0.3 percent (or about 1 in 400), about 2.0 percent of people of Ashkenazi Jewish descent carry a harmful variant in one of these two genes and the variants are usually one of three specific variants, called "founder mutations." Other populations, such as Norwegian, Dutch, and Icelandic peoples, also have founder mutations.

Different racial/ethnic and geographic populations also tend to carry different variants in these genes. For instance, African Americans have *BRCA1* variants that are not seen in other racial/ethnic groups in the United States. Most people of Ashkenazi Jewish descent in the United States who carry a BRCA variant have one of three specific variants (two in *BRCA1* and one in *BRCA2*). In the Icelandic population, a different variant in *BRCA1* is common among those who inherit a mutation in *BRCA1*.

WHO SHOULD CONSIDER GENETIC COUNSELING AND TESTING FOR *BRCA1* AND *BRCA2* VARIANTS?

Anyone who is concerned about the possibility that they may have a harmful variant in the *BRCA1* or *BRCA2* gene should discuss their concerns with their health-care provider or a genetic counselor.

Tests are available to see if someone has inherited a harmful variant in *BRCA1* and *BRCA2*. However, testing is not currently recommended for the general public. Instead, expert groups recommend that testing be focused on those who have a higher likelihood of carrying a harmful *BRCA1* or *BRCA2* variant, such as those who have a family history of certain cancers. Testing can be appropriate for both people without cancer as well as people who have been diagnosed with cancer. If someone knows they have a mutation in one of these genes, they can take steps to reduce their risk or detect cancer early. And if they have cancer, the information about their mutation may be important for selecting treatment.

Before testing is done, a person will usually have a risk assessment, in which they meet with a genetic counselor or other healthcare provider to review factors such as which of their relatives had cancer, what cancers they had, and at what ages they were diagnosed. If this assessment suggests that someone has an increased risk of carrying a harmful *BRCA1* or *BRCA2* gene variant, their genetic counselor can discuss the benefits and harms of testing with them and order the appropriate genetic test, if the individual decides to have genetic testing.

Some people may choose to have genetic testing via direct-to-consumer (DTC) testing. Genetic counseling is recommended for those people as well to help them understand the test results and to make sure the most appropriate test was done. People should be aware that DTC tests may not be comprehensive, in that some tests do not test for all of the harmful mutations in the two genes. So receiving a negative result with a DTC test may not mean that they do not have a harmful variant in *BRCA1* or *BRCA2*.

The United States Preventive Services Task Force recommends risk assessment for women who have a personal or family history of breast, ovarian, fallopian tube, or peritoneal cancer or whose ancestry is associated with having harmful *BRCA1* and *BRCA2* variants, as well as follow-up genetic counseling as appropriate.

The National Comprehensive Cancer Network (NCCN) has criteria for genetic testing of *BRCA1* and *BRCA2* as well as for several other genes (including *CDH1*, *PALB2*, *PTEN*, and *TP53*) that are associated with increased risk of breast and/or ovarian cancer. NCCN recommends risk assessment for people who have a blood relative with a known or likely harmful variant in any of these genes; who have certain personal and/or family histories of cancer (cancer diagnosed at a younger age, certain types of cancer, people with two or more cancer diagnoses, or families with multiple cases of cancer); or who have certain inherited cancer predisposition disorders, such as Cowden syndrome, Peutz-Jeghers syndrome, Li-Fraumeni syndrome, or Fanconi anemia.

The American Society of Clinical Oncology recommends that all women diagnosed with epithelial ovarian cancer be offered genetic testing for inherited variants in *BRCA1*, *BRCA2*, and other ovarian cancer susceptibility genes, regardless of the clinical features of their disease or their family history.

Professional societies do not recommend that children under age 18 undergo genetic testing for *BRCA1* and *BRCA2* variants. This is because there are no risk-reduction strategies that are specifically meant for children, and children are very unlikely to develop a cancer related to an inherited BRCA variant.

Testing for inherited *BRCA1* and *BRCA2* variants may be done using a blood sample or a saliva sample. That is because blood cells and cells that are present in saliva, like every cell in the body, contain the *BRCA1* and *BRCA2* genes. Sometimes people with cancer find out that they have a *BRCA1* or *BRCA2* mutation when their tumor is tested to see if they are a candidate for treatment with a particular targeted therapy. Because harmful BRCA variants reported in the tumor may be of somatic or germline origin, someone with such a variant in their tumor should consider having a germline genetic (blood) test to determine if the variant was inherited.

When a family history suggests the possibility that someone without cancer may have inherited a harmful variant in *BRCA1* or *BRCA2*, it is best for a family member who has already been diagnosed with cancer to be tested, if such a person is alive and willing to get tested. If such testing reveals a known harmful variant, then testing the individual for that variant will provide a clear indication of whether they also carry it. If all family members with cancer are deceased or are unwilling or unable to have genetic testing, testing family members who have not been diagnosed with cancer may still be of value and provide good information.

DOES HEALTH INSURANCE COVER THE COST OF GENETIC TESTING FOR *BRCA1* AND *BRCA2* VARIANTS?

People considering *BRCA1* and *BRCA2* variant testing may want to confirm their insurance coverage for genetic counseling and testing. Genetic counselors can often help answer questions about insurance coverage for genetic testing.

Some genetic testing companies may offer testing for inherited *BRCA1* and *BRCA2* variants at no charge to patients who lack insurance and meet specific financial and medical criteria.

WHAT DO *BRCA1* AND *BRCA2* GENETIC TEST RESULTS MEAN?

BRCA1 and *BRCA2* mutation testing can give several possible results: A positive result, a negative result, or a variant of uncertain significance (VUS) result.

Positive result. A positive test result indicates that a person has inherited a known harmful variant in *BRCA1* or *BRCA2* (these are typically called "pathogenic" or "likely pathogenic" variants on laboratory test reports) and has an increased risk of developing certain cancers. However, a positive test result cannot tell whether or when the tested individual will develop cancer. Some people who inherit a harmful *BRCA1* or *BRCA2* variant never develop cancer.

A positive test result may also have important implications for family members, including future generations.

- Both men and women who inherit a harmful *BRCA1* or *BRCA2* variant, whether or not they develop cancer themselves, may pass the variant to their children. Each child has a 50 percent chance of inheriting a parent's variant.
- All blood relatives of a person who has inherited a harmful *BRCA1* or *BRCA2* variant are at some increased risk of having the variant themselves. For example, each of that person's full siblings has a 50 percent chance of having inherited the variant as well.
- Very rarely, an individual may test positive for a harmful variant not inherited from either parent. This is called a "*de novo*" (or "new") variant. Such a variant is one that arose in a germ cell (sperm or egg) of one of the parents and is present in all the cells of the person who grew from that cell. The children of someone with a *de novo* variant (but not her or his siblings) are at risk of inheriting the variant.

Negative result. A negative test result can have several meanings, depending on the personal and family medical history of the person who is tested and whether or not a harmful mutation has already been identified in the family. If a close blood relative of the tested person is known to carry a harmful *BRCA1* or *BRCA2* variant, a negative test result is clear: it means the tested person did not inherit the harmful variant that is present in the family and cannot pass it to their children. A person with such a test result, called "a true negative," has a risk of cancer that is similar to that of someone in the general population. However, there are other factors besides genetic factors that may increase the risk of cancer, such as radiation exposures at an early age, and those factors should be considered in assessing their risk of cancer.

If the tested person has no personal history of cancer and their family is not known to carry a harmful variant, then in this case, a negative test result is considered to be "uninformative." There are several possible reasons why someone could have an uninformative negative test result:

- Without testing family members who have had cancer, it is uncertain whether the negative test means that the person did not inherit a *BRCA1* or *BRCA2* mutation that is present in the family or whether the family history might be due to a mutation in another gene that was not tested or to other, nongenetic risk factors.
- The individual may have a harmful variant that is not detectable by current testing technologies.
- Rarely, there could be an error in the testing, either because inappropriate tests were recommended or ordered, genetic variants were interpreted incorrectly, or the wrong results were relayed to patients.

Variant of uncertain significance (VUS) result. Sometimes, a genetic test finds a change in *BRCA1* or *BRCA2* that has not been previously associated with cancer and is uncommon in the general population. This type of test result is called "a variant of uncertain significance," or VUS, because it is not known whether this specific genetic change is harmful.

As more research is conducted and more people are tested for *BRCA1* and *BRCA2* variants, scientists will learn more about uncertain changes and cancer risk. Clinicians and scientists are actively working to share information on these mutations so that they can be reclassified as either clearly harmful or clearly not harmful.

Genetic counseling can help a person understand what a VUS in *BRCA1* or *BRCA2* may mean in terms of their cancer risk. Until the interpretation of the variant is clarified, management of risk should be based on family history and other risk factors. However, it is important that a person who has a VUS test result regularly obtains updated information from the testing provider in case that VUS is reclassified as a harmful or likely harmful variant. Testing providers have different policies about notifying a tested person of a change in the interpretation of a VUS test result. Some will contact the tested person directly, whereas others place the responsibility on the tested person to check back in on a regular basis to learn of updates to the interpretation of their VUS test result.

HOW CAN A PERSON WHO HAS INHERITED A HARMFUL *BRCA1* OR *BRCA2* GENE VARIANT REDUCE THEIR RISK OF CANCER?

Several options are available for reducing cancer risk in individuals who have inherited a harmful *BRCA1* or *BRCA2* variant. These include enhanced screening, risk-reducing surgery (sometimes referred to as prophylactic surgery), and chemoprevention.

Enhanced screening. Some women who test positive for harmful *BRCA1* and *BRCA2* variants may choose to start breast cancer screening at younger ages, have more frequent screening than is recommended for women with an average risk of breast cancer, or have screening with magnetic resonance imaging (MRI) in addition to mammography.

No effective ovarian cancer screening methods are known. Some groups recommend transvaginal ultrasound, blood tests for the CA-125 antigen (which can be present at higher-than-normal levels in women with ovarian cancer), and clinical examinations for ovarian cancer screening in women with harmful *BRCA1* or *BRCA2* variants. However, none of these methods appear to detect ovarian tumors at an early enough stage to improve long-term survival.

The benefits of screening men who carry harmful variants in *BRCA1* or *BRCA2* for breast and other cancers are not known. Some expert groups recommend that such men undergo regular annual clinical breast exams starting at age 35. The National Comprehensive Cancer Network (NCCN) guidelines recommend that men with harmful germline variants in *BRCA1* or *BRCA2* consider having a discussion with their doctor about prostate-specific antigen (PSA) testing for prostate cancer screening starting at age 40.

Some experts recommend the use of ultrasound or magnetic resonance imaging (MRI)/magnetic retrograde cholangiopancreatography (MRCP) to screen for pancreatic cancer in people who are known to carry a harmful *BRCA1* or *BRCA2* variant and who have a close blood relative with pancreatic cancer. However, it is not yet clear whether pancreatic cancer screening and early pancreatic cancer detection reduces the overall risk of dying from a pancreatic cancer.

All of these screening approaches have potential harms as well as possible benefits. For example, MRI is more likely than mammography to result in false-positive findings. And there is some concern that women who have a harmful BRCA variant might be particularly sensitive to the DNA-damaging effects of tests that involve radiation (such as mammography) because they already have a defect in DNA repair.

Risk-reducing surgery. Risk-reducing, or prophylactic, surgery involves removing as much of the "at-risk" tissue as possible. Women may choose to have both breasts removed (bilateral risk-reducing mastectomy) to reduce their risk of breast cancer. Surgery to remove a woman's ovaries and fallopian tubes (bilateral risk-reducing salpingo-oophorectomy) can help reduce her risk of ovarian cancer. (Ovarian cancers often originate in the fallopian tubes, so it is essential that they be removed along with the ovaries.) Removing the ovaries may also reduce the risk of breast cancer in premenopausal women by eliminating a source of hormones that can fuel the growth of some types of breast cancer.

These surgeries are irreversible, and each has potential complications or harms. These include bleeding or infection, anxiety and concerns about body image (bilateral risk-reducing mastectomy), and early menopause in premenopausal women (bilateral risk-reducing salpingo-oophorectomy).

Risk-reducing surgery does not guarantee that cancer will not develop because not all at-risk tissue can be removed by these procedures. That is why these surgical procedures are described as "risk-reducing" rather than "preventive." Some women have developed breast cancer, ovarian cancer, or primary peritoneal carcinomatosis (a type of cancer similar to ovarian cancer) even after risk-reducing surgery. Nevertheless, these surgical procedures greatly reduce risk. For example, in several studies women who underwent bilateral salpingo-oophorectomy had a nearly 80 percent reduction in risk of dying from ovarian cancer, a 56 percent reduction in risk of dying from breast cancer, and a 77 percent reduction in risk of dying from any cause during the studies' follow-up periods.

The reduction in breast and ovarian cancer risk from removal of the ovaries and fallopian tubes appears to be similar for carriers of *BRCA1* and *BRCA2* variants.

Chemoprevention. It is the use of medicines to reduce the risk of cancer. Two chemopreventive drugs (tamoxifen (Nolvadex) and raloxifene (Evista)) have been approved by the U.S. Food and Drug Administration (FDA) to reduce the risk of breast cancer in women at increased risk, but the role of these drugs in women with harmful *BRCA1* or *BRCA2* variants is not yet clear. Data from three studies suggest that tamoxifen may be able to help lower the risk of breast cancer in women who carry harmful variants in *BRCA2* and of cancer in the opposite breast among *BRCA1* and *BRCA2* variant carriers previously diagnosed with breast cancer. Studies have not examined the effectiveness of raloxifene in *BRCA1* and *BRCA2* variant carriers specifically.

However, these medications may be an option for women who choose not to, or who cannot, undergo surgery. The potential harms of these drugs include menopausal symptoms, blood clots, stroke, increased risk of endometrial cancer (tamoxifen), and allergic reactions (raloxifene).

Both women in the general population, as well as those with harmful *BRCA1* or *BRCA2* variants, who have ever used oral contraceptives (birth control pills) have about a 50 percent lower risk of ovarian cancer than women who have never used oral contraceptives. Potential harms of oral contraceptives include increased risk of breast cancer, increased risk that a human papillomavirus (HPV) infection will become cervical cancer, and possible cardiovascular effects among older reproductive-age women.

WHAT ARE THE BENEFITS OF GENETIC TESTING FOR *BRCA1* AND *BRCA2* VARIANTS?

There can be benefits to genetic testing, regardless of whether a person receives a positive or a negative result.

The potential benefits of a true negative result include a sense of relief regarding the future risk of cancer, learning that one's children are not at risk of inheriting the family's cancer susceptibility, and the possibility that special checkups, tests, or risk-reducing surgeries may not be needed.

A positive test result may allow people to make informed decisions about their future healthcare, including taking steps to reduce their cancer risk.

WHAT ARE THE POSSIBLE HARMS OF GENETIC TESTING FOR *BRCA1* AND *BRCA2* VARIANTS?

The direct medical harms of genetic testing are minimal, but knowledge of test results, whether positive or negative, may have harmful effects on a person's emotions, social relationships, finances, and medical choices.

Dealing with uncertainty of an uninformative negative or a VUS test result is another potential harm. For this reason, it is important to have genetic counseling before undergoing genetic testing.

Results of genetic tests are normally included in a person's medical records, particularly if a doctor or other health-care provider has ordered the test or has been consulted about the test results. Therefore, people considering genetic testing must understand that their results may become known to other people or organizations that have legitimate, legal access to their medical records, such as their insurance company or employer, if their employer provides the patient's health insurance as a benefit.

WHAT ARE THE TREATMENT IMPLICATIONS OF HAVING A HARMFUL *BRCA1* OR *BRCA2* VARIANT FOR PATIENTS WHO HAVE ALREADY DEVELOPED CANCER?

Because the *BRCA1* and *BRCA2* genes are involved in DNA repair, tumors with alterations in either gene are particularly sensitive to anticancer agents that act by damaging DNA, such as cisplatin.

A class of drugs called "PARP inhibitors," which block the repair of DNA damage, have been found to arrest the growth of cancer cells that have harmful *BRCA1* or *BRCA2* variants. Four PARP inhibitors – olaparib (Lynparza), rucaparib (Rubraca), niraparib (Zejula), and talazoparib (Talzenna) – are approved by the FDA to treat certain cancers bearing harmful variants in *BRCA1* or *BRCA2*. (In some cases, these are used whether or not a *BRCA1* or *BRCA2* mutation is present.)

Breast cancers with harmful *BRCA1* variants are more likely to be "triple-negative cancers" (i.e., the breast cancer cells do not have estrogen receptors, progesterone receptors, or large amounts of HER2/neu protein) than sporadic breast cancers or breast cancers with harmful *BRCA2* variants. Triple-negative cancers are harder to treat and have a poorer prognosis than other types of breast cancers.

If someone has tumor genetic testing that reveals the presence of a harmful *BRCA1* or *BRCA2* variant in the tumor, they should consider having a germline genetic (blood) test to determine if the variant was inherited. Knowing if the variant was inherited is important for that individual to understand their risks to potentially develop other cancers in the future. It can also determine if other family members may be at risk of inheriting the harmful variant.

Chapter 7 | **Required Medical Screening of Immigrants to the United States**

WHAT IS THE ROLE IN MEDICAL EXAMINATIONS?

The Centers for Disease Control and Prevention (CDC) is responsible for providing the technical instructions to Civil Surgeons and Panel Physicians who conduct medical examinations for immigration. These instructions are developed in order to implement the Immigration and Nationality Act (INA) regulations regarding the health-related grounds for inadmissibility of persons applying for admission into the United States.

WHAT IS THE PURPOSE OF THE MEDICAL EXAMINATION?

The purpose of the medical examination is to identify applicants with inadmissible health-related conditions for the Department of State (DOS) and U.S. Citizenship and Immigration Services (USCIS). The health-related grounds for inadmissibility include persons who have a communicable disease of public-health significance, who fail to present documentation of having received vaccination against vaccine-preventable diseases, who have or have had a physical or mental disorder with associated harmful behavior, or who are a drug abuser or an addict.

This chapter includes text excerpted from "Immigrant, Refugee, and Migrant Health – Medical Examination: Frequently Asked Questions (FAQs)," Centers for Disease Control and Prevention (CDC), March 12, 2021.

Table 7.1. Who Is Required to Have a Medical Examination for Migration to the United States?

Category	Medical Examination	Examination Site	Examination Location
Immigrants	Yes	Panel Physicians	Overseas
Refugees	Yes	Panel Physicians	Overseas
Status adjusters	Yes	Civil Surgeons	U.S.
Nonimmigrants	No	—	—
Short-term Transit	No	—	—
Others*	No	—	—

(Source: U.S. Department of Homeland Security (DHS).)

Note: *Others include migrants who entered the United States without inspection, including those who entered with and without proper documentation.

All immigrants, refugees and certain nonimmigrants, including fiancés, coming to the United States must have a physical and mental examination abroad by a Panel Physician. Persons in the United States applying for adjustment of status to a permanent resident of the United States must have a physical and mental examination in the United States by a Civil Surgeon.

WHAT DOES A MEDICAL EXAMINATION ENTAIL?

The medical examination procedure consists of a physical examination, an evaluation (skin test/chest x-ray examination) for tuberculosis (TB), and blood test for syphilis. The vaccination requirements include vaccines recommended by the Advisory Committee on Immunization Practices (ACIP).

The technical instructions indicating the required testing, the diseases currently listed as being communicable diseases of public-health significance, and the vaccination requirements are available on the CDC website (www.cdc.gov/immigrantrefugeehealth/index.html).

WHAT ARE THE COMMUNICABLE DISEASES OF PUBLIC-HEALTH SIGNIFICANCE THAT WOULD CAUSE AN APPLICANT TO FAIL A MEDICAL EXAMINATION OR BE INADMISSIBLE?

Communicable diseases of public-health significance include:

- Tuberculosis
- Syphilis
- Gonorrhea
- Hansen disease (leprosy)

And the following two disease categories:

- Quarantinable diseases designated by any Presidential Executive Order. Current diseases include: cholera, diphtheria, infectious tuberculosis, plague, smallpox, yellow fever, viral hemorrhagic fevers, severe acute respiratory syndromes, and influenza caused by novel or reemergent influenza (pandemic flu).
- Events that are reportable as a public-health emergency of international concern (PHEIC) to the World Health Organization (WHO) under the International Health Regulations (IHR) of 2005 (currently polio, smallpox, SARS, influenza, and other public-health emergencies of international concern).

Some health-related waivers may be available for these diseases.

WHAT VACCINES/BOOSTERS ARE REQUIRED FOR IMMIGRANTS AND THOSE APPLYING FOR ADJUSTMENT OF STATUS IN THE UNITED STATES?

As part of the medical examination for immigration, all immigrants are required to have an assessment for the following vaccine-preventable diseases: mumps, measles, rubella, polio, tetanus and diphtheria toxoids, pertussis, *Haemophilus influenzae type b*, rotavirus, hepatitis A, hepatitis B, meningococcal disease, varicella, influenza, and *pneumococcal pneumonia*. Persons already in the United States applying for adjustment of status for permanent residency, including refugees, are also required to be assessed for these vaccine-preventable diseases.

Each set of technical instructions for medical examination of aliens has an addendum regarding the vaccination requirements for immigrants.

Part 2 | **Laboratory Tests**

Chapter 8 | Understanding Laboratory Tests

WHAT ARE LAB TESTS?

Laboratory tests are medical devices that are intended for use on samples of blood, urine, or other tissues or substances taken from the body to help diagnose disease or other conditions.

WHY DOES YOUR DOCTOR USE LAB TESTS?

Your doctor uses laboratory tests to help:

- Identify changes in your health condition before any symptoms occur,
- Diagnose or aid in diagnosing a disease or condition,
- Plan your treatment for a disease or condition,
- Evaluate your response to a treatment, or
- Monitor the course of a disease over time.

HOW ARE LAB TESTS ANALYZED?

After your doctor collects a sample from your body, it is sent to a laboratory. Laboratories perform tests on the sample to see if it contains different substances, and how much. Depending on the test, the presence, absence, or amount of an analyte may mean you do have a particular condition or it may mean that you do not have

This chapter contains text excerpted from the following sources: Text beginning with the heading "What Are Lab Tests?" is excerpted from "Tests Used in Clinical Care," U.S. Food and Drug Administration (FDA), September 27, 2018. Reviewed October 2021; Text under the heading "How Do You Prepare for a Lab Test?" is excerpted from "How to Prepare for a Lab Test," MedlinePlus, National Institutes of Health (NIH), March 8, 2021; Text under the heading "How to Understand Your Lab Results" is excerpted from "How to Understand Your Lab Results," MedlinePlus, National Institutes of Health (NIH), December 3, 2020.

the particular condition. Sometimes laboratories compare your results to results obtained from previous tests, to see if there has been a change in your condition.

WHAT DO LAB TESTS SHOW?

Some types of lab tests show whether or not your results fall within normal ranges. Normal test values are usually given as a range, rather than as a specific number, because normal values vary from person to person. What is normal for one person may not be normal for another person.

Other types show whether there is a particular substance present or absent, such as a mutation in a gene, or an infectious organism, which indicates whether you have a disease, an infection, or may or may not respond to a therapy.

Some laboratory tests are precise, reliable indicators of specific health problems, while others provide more general information that gives doctors clues to your possible health problems. Information obtained from laboratory tests may help doctors decide whether other tests or procedures are needed to make a diagnosis or to develop or revise a previous treatment plan. All laboratory test results must be interpreted within the context of your overall health and should be used along with other exams or tests.

WHAT FACTORS AFFECT YOUR LAB TEST RESULTS?

Many factors can affect test results, including:

- Sex
- Age
- Race
- Medical history
- General health
- Specific foods
- Drugs you are taking
- How closely you follow preparatory instructions
- Variations in laboratory techniques
- Variation from one laboratory to another

HOW DO YOU PREPARE FOR A LAB TEST?

For any type of lab test, you should prepare for it by:

- Following all the instructions given to you by your health-care provider
- Telling your provider or lab professional if you did not follow these instructions exactly. It is important to be honest. Even a minor change from the instructions can have a big effect on your results. For example, some medicines raise or lower blood sugar levels. Taking them too close to a blood sugar test could affect your results.
- Telling your provider about any medicines, vitamins, or supplements that you are taking

Taking these steps can help ensure your results will be accurate and reliable.

Will You Need to Take Other Steps to Prepare for Your Lab Test?

For many lab tests, you do not need to do anything other than answer questions from your provider and/or lab professional. But, for others, you may need do some specific preparations before the test.

One of the most common lab test preparations is fasting. Fasting means you should not eat or drink anything except water for up to several hours or overnight before your test. This is done because nutrients and ingredients in food are absorbed in the bloodstream. This can affect certain blood test results. The length of fasting can vary. So if you do need to fast, make sure you ask your provider how long you should do it.

Other common test preparations include:

- Avoiding specific foods and drinks such as cooked meats, herbal tea, or alcohol
- Making sure not to overeat the day before a test
- Not smoking
- Avoiding specific behaviors such as strenuous exercise or sexual activity

- Avoiding certain medicines and/or supplements. Be sure to talk to your provider about what you are currently taking, including over-the-counter (OTC) medicines, vitamins, and supplements.

For some blood tests, you may be asked to drink extra water to help keep more fluid in your veins. You may also be asked to drink water 15 to 20 minutes before certain urine tests.

What Types of Lab Tests Require Special Preparation?

Some of the most common lab tests that require fasting include:

- Blood glucose test
- Cholesterol levels test
- Triglycerides test
- Calcitonin test

Some of the most common lab tests that require other special preparations include:

- **Creatinine test.** This test may require fasting or avoiding cooked meats.
- **Cortisol test.** For this test, you may need to rest for a bit before your sample is taken. You may also have to avoid eating, drinking, or brushing your teeth for a certain time period before your test.
- **Fecal occult blood test.** For this test, you may need to avoid certain foods or medicines.
- **5-HIAA test.** For this test, you may be asked to avoid a variety of specific foods. These include avocados, bananas, pineapples, walnuts, and eggplants.
- **Pap smear.** A woman may be instructed not to douche, use tampons, or have sex for 24 to 48 hours before this test.

Is There Anything Else You Should Know about Preparing for a Lab Test?

If you have questions or concerns about test preparations, talk to your health-care provider. Be sure you understand your preparation instructions before the day of your test.

HOW TO UNDERSTAND YOUR LAB RESULTS

Why Do You Need a Lab Test?

Lab tests are used in many different ways. Your health-care provider may order one or more lab tests to:

- Diagnose or rule out a specific disease or condition
  - An HPV test is an example of this type of test. It can show you whether or not you have an HPV infection.
- **Screen for a disease.** A screening test can show if you are at a higher risk for getting a specific disease. It can also find out if you have a disease, even if you have no symptoms.
  - A Pap test is a type of screening test for cervical cancer.
- **Monitor a disease and/or treatment.** If you have already been diagnosed with a disease, lab tests can show if your condition is getting better or worse. It can also show if your treatment is working.
  - A blood glucose test is a type of test that is used to monitor diabetes and diabetes treatment. It is also sometimes used to diagnose the disease.
- **Check your overall health.** Lab tests are often included in a routine checkup. Your provider may order tests of various organs and systems to see if there have been changes in your health over time. Testing can help find health problems before symptoms appear.
  - A complete blood count is a type of routine test that measures different substances in your blood. It can give your health-care provider important information about your overall health and risk for certain diseases.

What Do Your Results Mean?

Lab results are often shown as a set of numbers known as a "reference range." A reference range may also be called "normal values." You may see something like this on your results: "normal: 77-99mg/dL" (milligrams per deciliter). Reference ranges are based on the normal test results of a large group of healthy people. The range helps show what a typical normal result looks like.

But, not everyone is typical. Sometimes, healthy people get results outside the reference range, while people with health problems can have results in the normal range. If your results fall outside the reference range, or if you have symptoms despite a normal result, you will likely need more testing.

Your lab results may also include one of these terms:

- Negative or normal, which means the disease or substance being tested was not found
- Positive or abnormal, which means the disease or substance was found
- Inconclusive or uncertain, which means there was not enough information in the results to diagnose or rule out a disease. If you get an inconclusive result, you will probably get more tests.

Tests that measure various organs and systems often give results as reference ranges, while tests that diagnose or rule out diseases often use the terms listed above.

What Are False Positive and False Negative Results?

A false positive result means your test shows you have a disease or condition, but you do not actually have it.

A false negative result means your test shows you do not have a disease or condition, but you actually do.

These incorrect results do not happen often, but they are more likely to happen with certain of types tests, or if testing was not done right. Even though false negatives and positives are uncommon, your provider may need to do multiple tests to make sure your diagnosis is correct.

What Factors Can Affect Your Results?

There are many factors that can affect the accuracy of your test results. These include:

- Certain foods and drinks

- Medicines
- Stress
- Vigorous exercise
- Variations in lab procedures
- Having an illness

If you have any questions about your lab tests or what your results mean, talk to your health-care provider.

Chapter 9 | **Blood Tests**

Chapter Contents

Section 9.1 | **Common Blood Tests**

This section includes text excerpted from "Blood Tests," National Heart, Lung, and Blood Institute (NHLBI), September 27, 2021.

WHAT ARE BLOOD TESTS?

Blood tests help doctors check for certain diseases and conditions. They also help check the function of your organs and show how well treatments are working.

Specifically, blood tests can help doctors:

- Evaluate how well organs – such as the kidneys, liver, thyroid, and heart – are working
- Diagnose diseases and conditions such as cancer, human immunodeficiency virus/acquired immunodeficiency syndrome (HIV/AIDS), diabetes, anemia, and coronary heart disease
- Find out whether you have risk factors for heart disease
- Check whether medicines you are taking are working
- Assess how well your blood is clotting

Blood tests are very common. When you have routine checkups, your doctor may recommend blood tests to see how your body is working.

Many blood tests do not require any special preparations. For some, you may need to fast (not eat any food) for 8 to 12 hours before the test. Your doctor will let you know how to prepare for blood tests.

During a blood test, a small sample of blood is taken from your body. It is usually drawn from a vein in your arm using a needle. A finger prick also might be used.

The procedure usually is quick and easy, although it may cause some short-term discomfort. Most people do not have serious reactions to having blood drawn.

Laboratory (lab) workers draw the blood and analyze it. They use either whole blood to count blood cells, or they separate the blood cells from the fluid that contains them. This fluid is called "plasma" or "serum."

The fluid is used to measure different substances in the blood. The results can help detect health problems in early stages, when treatments or lifestyle changes may work best.

Doctors cannot diagnose many diseases and medical problems with blood tests alone. Your doctor may consider other factors to confirm a diagnosis. These factors can include your signs and symptoms, your medical history, your vital signs (blood pressure, breathing, pulse, and temperature), and results from other tests and procedures.

Blood tests have few risks. Most complications are minor and go away shortly after the tests are done.

WHAT TO EXPECT WITH BLOOD TESTS

Many blood tests do not require any special preparation and take only a few minutes.

Other blood tests require fasting (not eating any food) for 8 to 12 hours before the test. Your doctor will tell you how to prepare for your blood test(s).

During Blood Tests

Blood usually is drawn from a vein in your arm or other part of your body using a needle. It also can be drawn using a finger prick.

The person who draws your blood might tie a band around the upper part of your arm or ask you to make a fist. Doing this can make the veins in your arm stick out more, which makes it easier to insert the needle.

The needle that goes into your vein is attached to a small test tube. The person who draws your blood removes the tube when it is full, and the tube seals on its own. The needle is then removed from your vein. If you are getting a few blood tests, more than one test tube may be attached to the needle before it is withdrawn.

Some people get nervous about blood tests because they are afraid of needles. Others may not want to see blood leaving their bodies.

If you are nervous or scared, it can help to look away or talk to someone to distract yourself. You might feel a slight sting when the needle goes in or comes out.

Drawing blood usually takes less than 3 minutes.

After Blood Tests

Once the needle is withdrawn, you will be asked to apply gentle pressure with a piece of gauze or bandage to the place where the needle was inserted. This helps stop bleeding. It also helps prevent swelling and bruising.

Most of the time, you can remove the pressure after a minute or two. You may want to keep a bandage on for a few hours.

Usually, you do not need to do anything else after a blood test. Results can take anywhere from a few minutes to a few weeks to come back. Your doctor should get the results. It is important that you follow up with your doctor to discuss your test results.

WHAT ARE THE RISKS OF BLOOD TESTS?

The main risks of blood tests are discomfort and bruising at the site where the needle goes in. These complications usually are minor and go away shortly after the tests are done.

WHAT DO BLOOD TESTS SHOW?

Blood tests show whether the levels of different substances in your blood fall within a normal range.

For many blood substances, the normal range is the range of levels seen in 95 percent of healthy people in a certain group. For many tests, normal ranges vary depending on your age, gender, race, and other factors.

Your blood test results may fall outside the normal range for many reasons. Abnormal results might be a sign of a disorder or disease. Other factors – such as diet, menstrual cycle, physical activity level, alcohol intake, and medicines (both prescription and over the counter) – also can cause abnormal results.

Your doctor should discuss any unusual or abnormal blood test results with you. These results may or may not suggest a health problem.

Many diseases and medical problems cannot be diagnosed with blood tests alone. However, blood tests can help you and your doctor learn more about your health. Blood tests also can help find potential problems early, when treatments or lifestyle changes may work best.

Table 9.1. Normal Ranges for Different Parts of the Complete Blood Count Test

Test	Normal Range Results*
Red blood cell (varies with altitude)	Male: 5 to 6 million cells/mcL Female: 4 to 5 million cells/mcL
White blood cell	4,500 to 10,000 cells/mcL
Platelets	140,000 to 450,000 cells/mcL
Hemoglobin (varies with altitude)	Male: 14 to 17 gm/dL Female: 12 to 15 gm/dL
Hematocrit (varies with altitude)	Male: 41% to 50% Female: 36% to 44%
Mean corpuscular volume	80 to 95 femtoliter†

**Cells/mcL = cells per microliter; gm/dL = grams per deciliter.*
†A femtoliter is a measure of volume.

Result Ranges for Common Blood Tests

This section presents the result ranges for some of the most common blood tests.

NOTE: All values in this section are for adults only. They do not apply to children. Talk to your child's doctor about values on blood tests for children.

Complete Blood Count

The table 9.1 shows some normal ranges for different parts of the complete blood count (CBC) test. Some of the normal ranges differ between men and women. Other factors, such as age and race, also may affect normal ranges.

Your doctor should discuss your results with you. She or he will advise you further if your results are outside the normal range for your group.

Blood Glucose

Figure 9.1 shows the ranges for blood glucose levels after 8 to 12 hours of fasting (not eating). It shows the normal range and the abnormal ranges that are a sign of prediabetes or diabetes.

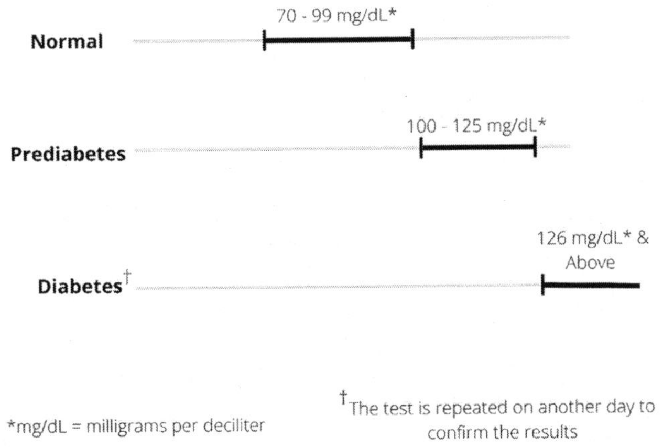

Figure 9.1. Blood Glucose Levels after 8- to 12-Hours of Fasting

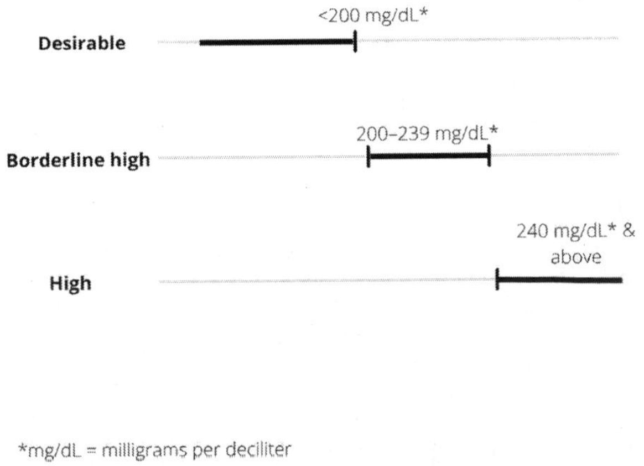

Figure 9.2. Range for Total Cholesterol

Lipoprotein Panel

Figures 9.3 and 9.4 shows ranges for total cholesterol, LDL ("bad") cholesterol, and HDL ("good") cholesterol levels after 9 to 12 hours of fasting. High blood cholesterol is a risk factor for coronary heart disease.

Your doctor should discuss your results with you. She or he will advise you further if your results are outside the desirable range.

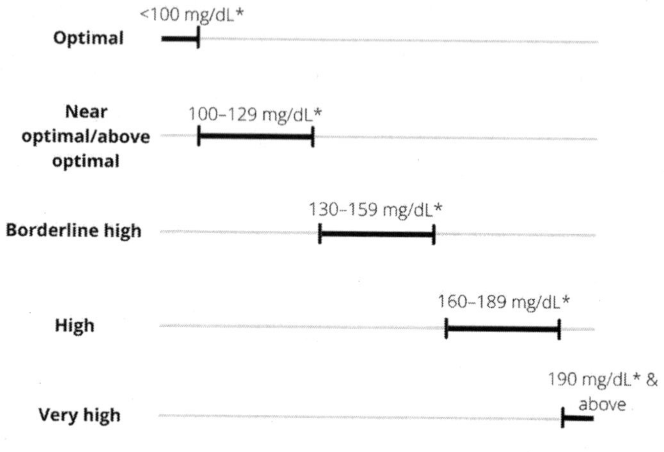

*mg/dL = milligrams per deciliter

Figure 9.3. LDL ("Bad") Cholesterol Level

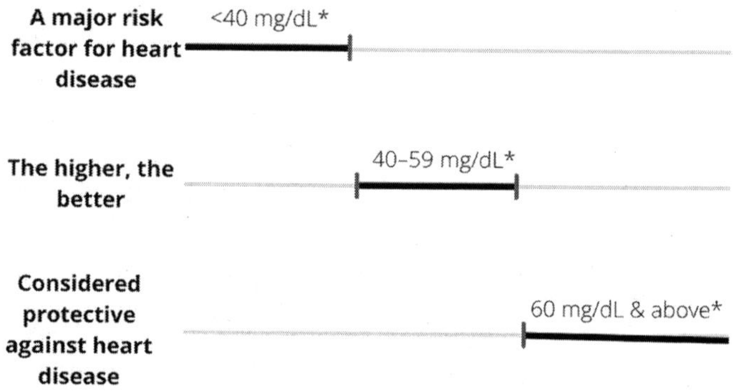

*mg/dL = milligrams per deciliter

Figure 9.4. HDL ("Good") Cholesterol Level

Section 9.2 | Biochemical Analysis

This section includes text excerpted from "Comprehensive Metabolic Panel (CMP)," MedlinePlus, National Institutes of Health (NIH), September 9, 2021.

WHAT IS A COMPREHENSIVE METABOLIC PANEL?

A comprehensive metabolic panel (CMP) is a test that measures 14 different substances in your blood. It provides important information about your body's chemical balance and metabolism. Metabolism is the process of how the body uses food and energy. A CMP includes tests for the following:

- Glucose, a type of sugar and your body's main source of energy
- Calcium, one of the body's most important minerals. Calcium is essential for proper functioning of your nerves, muscles, and heart.
- Sodium, potassium, carbon dioxide, and chloride. These are electrolytes, electrically charged minerals that help control the amount of fluids and the balance of acids and bases in your body.
- Albumin, a protein made in the liver
- Total protein, which measures the total amount of protein in the blood
- ALP (alkaline phosphatase), ALT (alanine transaminase), and AST (aspartate aminotransferase). These are different enzymes made by the liver.
- Bilirubin, a waste product made by the liver
- BUN (blood urea nitrogen) and creatinine, waste products removed from your blood by your kidneys

Abnormal levels of any of these substances or combination of them can be a sign of a serious health problem.

WHAT IS IT USED FOR?

A CMP is used to check several body functions and processes, including:

- Liver and kidney health

- Blood sugar levels
- Blood protein levels
- Acid and base balance
- Fluid and electrolyte balance
- Metabolism

A CMP may also be used to monitor the side effects of certain medicines.

WHY DO YOU NEED A CMP?

A CMP is often done as part of a regular checkup. You may also need this test if your health-care provider thinks you have liver or kidney disease.

WHAT HAPPENS DURING A CMP

A health-care professional will take a blood sample from a vein in your arm, using a small needle. After the needle is inserted, a small amount of blood will be collected into a test tube or vial. You may feel a little sting when the needle goes in or out. This usually takes less than five minutes.

WILL YOU NEED TO DO ANYTHING TO PREPARE FOR THE TEST?

You may need to fast (not eat or drink) for at least 8 hours before the test.

ARE THERE ANY RISKS TO THE TEST?

There is very little risk to having a blood test. You may have slight pain or bruising at the spot where the needle was put in, but most symptoms go away quickly.

WHAT DO THE RESULTS MEAN?

If any one result or combination of CMP results were not normal, it can indicate a number of different conditions. These include liver disease, kidney failure, or diabetes. You will likely need more tests to confirm or rule out a specific diagnosis.

If you have questions about your results, talk to your healthcare provider.

IS THERE ANYTHING ELSE YOU NEED TO KNOW ABOUT A CMP?

There is a similar test to a CMP called a "basic metabolic panel" (BMP). A BMP includes eight of the same tests as a CMP. It does not include the liver and protein tests. Your provider may choose a CMP or a BMP depending on your health history and needs.

Section 9.3 | **Hematological Analysis**

This section contains text excerpted from the following sources: Text in this section begins with excerpts from "Hematologic Exam: Introduction," Surveillance, Epidemiology, and End Results (SEER) Program, National Cancer Institute (NCI), September 7, 2016. Reviewed October 2021; Text under the heading "Complete Blood Count" is excerpted from "Blood Tests," National Heart, Lung, and Blood Institute (NHLBI), September 27, 2021.

A hematologic examination is the microscopic examination of the cells of the blood or blood-forming tissues (especially bone marrow), looking for changes in the structure of and/or numbers of various types of blood cells, including immature cells.

Peripheral blood is circulating blood obtained from the extremities or from the circulatory system remote from the heart. One of the most frequently used procedures for obtaining blood for a complete blood count is the fingerstick method.

There are three main types of blood cells-erythrocytes, leukocytes, and thrombocytes (platelets) – all suspended in a fluid portion called "plasma."

COMPLETE BLOOD COUNT

The complete blood count (CBC) is one of the most common blood tests. It is often done as part of a routine checkup.

The CBC can help detect blood diseases and disorders, such as anemia, infections, clotting problems, blood cancers, and immune system disorders. This test measures many different parts of your blood, as discussed in the following paragraphs.

Red Blood Cells

Red blood cells (RBCs) carry oxygen from your lungs to the rest of your body. Abnormal red blood cell levels may be a sign of anemia, dehydration (too little fluid in the body), bleeding, or another disorder.

White Blood Cells

White blood cells (WBCs) are part of your immune system, which fights infections and diseases. Abnormal white blood cell levels may be a sign of infection, blood cancer, or an immune system disorder.

A CBC measures the overall number of white blood cells in your blood. A CBC with differential looks at the amounts of different types of white blood cells in your blood.

Platelets

Platelets are blood cell fragments that help your blood clot. They stick together to seal cuts or breaks on blood vessel walls and stop bleeding.

Abnormal platelet levels may be a sign of a bleeding disorder (not enough clotting) or a thrombotic disorder (too much clotting).

Hemoglobin

Hemoglobin is an iron-rich protein in red blood cells that carries oxygen. Abnormal hemoglobin levels may be a sign of anemia, sickle cell anemia, thalassemia, or other blood disorders.

If you have diabetes, excess glucose in your blood can attach to hemoglobin and raise the level of hemoglobin A1c.

Hematocrit

Hematocrit is a measure of how much space red blood cells take up in your blood. A high hematocrit level might mean you are dehydrated. A low hematocrit level might mean you have anemia.

Abnormal hematocrit levels also may be a sign of a blood or bone marrow disorder.

Mean Corpuscular Volume

Mean corpuscular volume (MCV) is a measure of the average size of your red blood cells. Abnormal MCV levels may be a sign of anemia or thalassemia.

Section 9.4 | Microbial Diagnosis of Bloodstream Infection

Microbiology testing services are a critical need in many sectors because the presence and growth of microorganisms such as bacteria, yeast, and molds can have a detrimental impact on goods, processes, and human health. Although most microorganisms are nonhazardous, some can cause considerable pollution, damage, and risk to human health.

Some microorganisms can use our product as a food source, breaking it down into nutrients and permanently altering the product, while others can ruin food and severely impact industrial settings, goods, and infrastructure. They have the potential to cause serious sickness or pollute sterile surroundings. Food, consumer items, cosmetics and skincare products, medical equipment, fuels, drinking water, and oil exploration all benefit from microbiological testing services.

BLOOD CULTURE

A blood culture test can tell a health-care practitioner whether a person has an infection in their bloodstream or not. This is known as "bacteremia" and is referred to as a systemic infection by doctors. The test examines a blood sample for bacteria or yeast that may be causing the illness.

If an infection is severe or if the immune system is unable to withstand it, the microorganisms can travel to the blood and become systemic.

This sort of infection affects the blood that flows throughout the body. Blood infections are frequently caused by bacteria that begin on the skin or in the lungs, urinary tract, or gastrointestinal system.

WHY BLOOD CULTURES ARE NEEDED

When a doctor believes that a person has a blood infection, she or he will request a blood culture. Blood infections must be tested since they might cause significant consequences. Sepsis is one such consequence of a blood infection.

The bacteria cause infection in the body's natural defenses and hinder the immune system from functioning correctly. Toxins are also produced by infections, which can harm vital organs.

The findings of the test can assist the doctor in determining which organism or bacterium causes the blood infection and how to effectively treat it.

If you have any of the following symptoms, your doctor may prescribe the blood test.

- Chills or fever
- Fatigue
- Nausea
- Confusion
- Increased heartbeat or breathing rate
- Inflammation in parts of the body
- Small blood clots in the blood vessels
- A significant decline in your blood pressure
- Failure of an organ

HOW BLOOD CULTURES ARE DONE

A nurse or phlebotomist will clean the person's skin before inserting a tiny needle into a vein to draw blood. To obtain the most precise findings, the procedure will be repeated using a different vein.

The blood samples will be combined with a specific substance known as a "culture" in a lab. If bacteria or yeast are already present in your blood, it promotes their growth. You may be able to obtain early results from your blood testing within 24 hours. However, you may need to wait 48–72 hours to find out what type of yeast or bacteria is causing your infection.

Your doctor may discuss "positive" and "negative" outcomes. If your blood culture test yields a "positive" result, it typically implies you have bacteria or yeast in your blood. "Negative" indicates that there is no evidence of them.

If two or more of your blood cultures test positive for the same type of bacteria or fungus, it is probable that bacteria or fungus is the cause of your infection. A blood infection is quite dangerous and might require emergency medical attention.

POST BLOOD CULTURE

If your doctor obtains results that you have a blood infection, she or he may start treatment immediately with intravenous broad-spectrum antibiotics. While you wait for the results of the blood culture or susceptibility tests, the antibiotics can begin combating a wide spectrum of germs.

Blood infections can cause significant problems, so it is import ant to consult your health-care practitioner if you think you are at risk or if you are experiencing any symptoms. A doctor or other health-care practitioner should be seen if a fever lasts more than three days. If a child under the age of three months gets a fever, she or he should be taken to a doctor immediately.

References

1. "What Is a Blood Culture Test?" WebMD, December 16, 2020.
2. Krans, Brian. "Blood Culture," Healthline, September 17, 2018.
3. "Blood Culture," Oxford University Hospitals (OUH), NHS Foundation Trust, October 21, 2015.
4. "Microbiology Testing Services," Intertek, October 8, 2016.

Section 9.5 | Immunological Tests

This section includes text excerpted from "Immunoglobulins Blood Test," MedlinePlus, National Institutes of Health (NIH), December 10, 2020.

WHAT IS AN IMMUNOGLOBULINS BLOOD TEST?

This test measures the amount of immunoglobulins, also known as "antibodies," in your blood. Antibodies are proteins made by the immune system to fight disease-causing substances, such as viruses and bacteria. Your body makes different types of immunoglobulins to fight different types of these substances.

An immunoglobulins test usually measures three specific types of immunoglobulins. They are called "igG," "igM," and "IgA." If your levels of igG, igM, or IgA are too low or too high, it may be a sign of a serious health problem.

WHAT IS IT USED FOR?

An immunoglobulins blood test may be used to help diagnose a variety of conditions, including:

- Bacterial or viral infections
- Immunodeficiency, a condition that reduces the body's ability to fight infections and other diseases
- An autoimmune disorder, such as rheumatoid arthritis or lupus. An autoimmune disorder causes your immune system to attack healthy cells, tissues, and/or organs by mistake.
- Certain types of cancer, such as multiple myeloma
- Infections in newborns

WHY DO YOU NEED AN IMMUNOGLOBULINS BLOOD TEST?

You may need this test if your health-care provider thinks your immunoglobulin levels might be too low or too high.

Symptoms of levels that are too low include:

- Frequent and/or unusual bacterial or viral infections
- Chronic diarrhea
- Sinus infections

- Lung infections
- Family history of immunodeficiency

If your immunoglobulin levels are too high, it may be a sign of an autoimmune disease, a chronic illness, an infection, or a type of cancer. Symptoms of these conditions vary greatly. Your health-care provider may use information from your physical exam, medical history, and/or other tests to see if you are at risk for one of these diseases.

WHAT HAPPENS DURING AN IMMUNOGLOBULINS BLOOD TEST

A health-care professional will take a blood sample from a vein in your arm, using a small needle. After the needle is inserted, a small amount of blood will be collected into a test tube or vial. You may feel a little sting when the needle goes in or out. This usually takes less than five minutes.

WILL YOU NEED TO DO ANYTHING TO PREPARE FOR THE TEST?

You do not need any special preparations for an immunoglobulins blood test.

ARE THERE ANY RISKS TO THE TEST?

There is very little risk to having a blood test. You may have slight pain or bruising at the spot where the needle was put in, but most symptoms go away quickly.

WHAT DO THE RESULTS MEAN?

If your results show lower than normal levels of immunoglobulins, it may indicate:

- Kidney disease
- Severe burn injury
- Complications from diabetes
- Malnutrition
- Sepsis
- Leukemia

If your results show higher than normal levels of immunoglobulins, it may indicate:

- An autoimmune disease
- Hepatitis
- Cirrhosis
- Mononucleosis
- A chronic infection
- A viral infection such as HIV or cytomegalovirus
- Multiple myeloma
- Non-Hodgkin lymphoma

If your results are not normal, it does not necessarily mean you have a medical condition needing treatment. The use of certain medicines, alcohol, and recreational drugs can affect your results. If you have questions about your results, talk to your health-care provider.

IS THERE ANYTHING ELSE YOU NEED TO KNOW ABOUT AN IMMUNGLOBULINS BLOOD TEST?

Your health-care provider may order other tests to help make a diagnosis. These tests might include urinalysis, other blood tests, or a procedure called a "spinal tap." During a spinal tap, a health-care provider will use a special needle to remove a sample of a clear liquid, called "cerebrospinal fluid," from your back.

Chapter 10 | **Surgical Pathology**

Chapter Contents

Section 10.1 | Bone Marrow Tests

This section includes text excerpted from "Bone Marrow Tests," MedlinePlus, National Institutes of Health (NIH), November 30, 2020.

WHAT ARE BONE MARROW TESTS?

Bone marrow is a soft, spongy tissue found in the center of most bones. Bone marrow makes different types of blood cells. These include:

- Red blood cells (also called "erythrocytes"), which carry oxygen from your lungs to every cell in your body
- White blood cells (also called "leukocytes"), which help you fight infections
- Platelets, which help with blood clotting

Bone marrow tests check to see if your bone marrow is working correctly and making normal amounts of blood cells. The tests can help diagnose and monitor various bone marrow disorders, blood disorders, and certain types of cancer. There are two types of bone marrow tests:

- Bone marrow aspiration, which removes a small amount of bone marrow fluid
- Bone marrow biopsy, which removes a small amount of bone marrow tissue

Bone marrow aspiration and bone marrow biopsy tests are usually performed at the same time.

WHAT ARE THEY USED FOR?

Bone marrow tests are used to:

- Find out the cause of problems with red blood cells, white bloods, or platelets
- Diagnose and monitor blood disorders, such as anemia, polycythemia vera, and thrombocytopenia
- Diagnose bone marrow disorders

- Diagnose and monitor certain types of cancers, including leukemia, multiple myeloma, and lymphoma
- Diagnose infections that may have started or spread to the bone marrow

WHY DO YOU NEED A BONE MARROW TEST?

Your health-care provider may order a bone marrow aspiration and a bone marrow biopsy if other blood tests show your levels of red blood cells, white blood cells, or platelets are not normal. Too many or too few of these cells may mean you have a medical disorder, such as cancer that starts in your blood or bone marrow. If you are being treated for another type of cancer, these tests can find out if the cancer has spread to your bone marrow.

WHAT HAPPENS DURING A BONE MARROW TEST

Bone marrow aspiration and bone marrow biopsy tests are usually given at the same time. A doctor or other health-care provider will perform the tests. Before the tests, the provider may ask you to put on a hospital gown. The provider will check your blood pressure, heart rate, and temperature. You may be given a mild sedative, a medicine that will help you relax. During the test:

- You will lie down on your side or your stomach, depending on which bone will be used for testing. Most bone marrow tests are taken from the hip bone.
- Your body will be covered with cloth, so that only the area around the testing site is showing.
- The site will be cleaned with an antiseptic.
- You will get an injection of a numbing solution. It may sting.
- Once the area is numb, the health-care provider will take the sample. You will need to lie very still during the tests.
  - For a bone marrow aspiration, which is usually performed first, the health-care provider will insert a needle through the bone and pull out bone marrow fluid and cells. You may feel a sharp but brief pain when the needle is inserted.

- For a bone marrow biopsy, the health-care provider will use a special tool that twists into the bone to take out a sample of bone marrow tissue. You may feel some pressure on the site while the sample is being taken.

- It takes about ten minutes to perform both tests.
- After the test, the health-care provider will cover the site with a bandage.
- Plan to have someone drive you home, since you may be given a sedative before the tests, which may make you drowsy.

WILL YOU NEED TO DO ANYTHING TO PREPARE FOR THE TEST?

You will be asked to sign a form that gives permission to perform bone marrow tests. Be sure to ask your provider any questions you have about the procedure.

ARE THERE ANY RISKS TO THE TEST?

Many people feel a little uncomfortable after bone marrow aspiration and bone marrow biopsy testing. After the test, you may feel stiff or sore at the injection site. This usually goes away in a few days. Your health-care provider may recommend or prescribe a pain reliever to help. Serious symptoms are very rare, but may include:

- Long-lasting pain or discomfort around the injection site
- Redness, swelling, or excessive bleeding at the site
- Fever

If you have any of these symptoms, call your health-care provider.

WHAT DO THE RESULTS MEAN?

It may take several days or even several weeks to get your bone marrow test results. The results may show whether you have a bone marrow disease, a blood disorder, or cancer. If you are being treated for cancer, the results may show:

- Whether your treatment is working
- How advanced your disease is

If your results are not normal, your health-care provider will likely order more tests or discuss treatment options. If you have questions about your results, talk to your health-care provider.

Section 10.2 | Lumbar Puncture

A lumbar puncture or spinal tap is a procedure where a hollow needle is inserted in the lower back, the lumbar region, to either diagnose or treat a condition. With the help of a hollow needle, a health-care professional will withdraw some cerebrospinal fluid (CSF) or inject medicine. CSF is a clear fluid that surrounds the spine and brain and is made up of water, cells, protein, sugars, and other substances essential to the nervous system. A lab tests the fluid sample for:

- Blood sugar levels
- White blood cell (WBC) levels and type
- Protein types and levels
- Presence of fungi, bacteria, or abnormal cells

WHEN IS A LUMBAR PUNCTURE REQUIRED?

The most common reason for a lumbar puncture is to withdraw CSF for diagnosing:

- Leukemia or other cancers
- Meningitis
- Encephalitis
- Intracranial hemorrhage
- Myelitis
- Reye syndrome
- Guillain-Barré syndrome

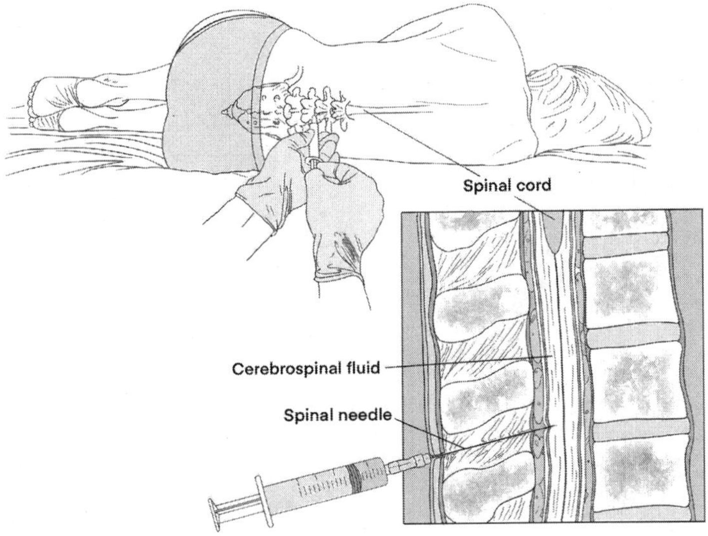

Figure 10.1. Lumbar Puncture Procedure

- Headaches of unknown cause
- Dementia
- Multiple sclerosis (MS)
- Idiopathic intracranial hypertension (IIH) or pseudotumor cerebri
- Normal-pressure hydrocephalus

Additionally, a lumbar puncture may also be done to administer:

- Regional anesthesia such as an epidural
- Chemotherapy drugs for cancer treatment
- Contrast dye for x-ray study
- Relieve intracranial pressure

WHAT ARE THE RISKS OF A LUMBAR PUNCTURE?

Although the procedure is generally safe, some risks may include:

- **Post-lumbar puncture headache.** A small amount of CSF may leak from the needle insertion site and into the nearby tissues, resulting in a headache. If the leak continues, the headaches can grow severe and can last

from a few hours to a week or more. The headache may be accompanied by vomiting and nausea.
- The patient may experience pain or discomfort in the lower back, and it may radiate down to the back of the legs.
- Infection at the incision area provides a way for bacteria to enter.
- Bleeding in the spinal canal
- **Brainstem herniation.** After removing the CSF, a brain tumor or other lesion that occupies space can lead to increased intracranial pressure.

HOW TO PREPARE FOR A LUMBAR PUNCTURE

The health-care provider will give the patient-specific instructions regarding food, drink, and medications. The neuroradiology physician needs to be informed of the following:
- If the patient is using blood thinners or other anticoagulant medicines
- A list of other medicines and supplements
- If the patient is allergic to povidone-iodine or procaine
- If a female patient thinks she might be pregnant

WHAT TO EXPECT DURING THE LUMBAR PUNCTURE PROCEDURE

A lumbar puncture may be performed as an outpatient procedure or in the hospital, depending upon the situation. The procedure takes 15–30 minutes, and if it is an outpatient procedure, someone needs to drive the patient home afterward. The patient will be asked to lie on their left side with their knees drawn up to the chest (fetal position), or they may be asked to sit and lean forward with their arms and head resting on a table. These positions help widen the space between vertebrae, making it easier for the needle to be inserted.

Before the procedure, the patient may be asked to empty their bladder. The site of the insertion will be cleaned with an antiseptic, and local anesthesia will be administered in the lower back. A slight burning sensation might be felt. Next, a hollow needle will be inserted between two spinal columns to draw CSF or inject medicine. Once the needle is withdrawn, the site will be cleaned with an antiseptic and bandaged.

WHAT TO EXPECT AFTER A LUMBAR PUNCTURE PROCEDURE

After the procedure, the patient will be required to remain in the fetal position or lie down if they were seated for at least an hour. Refrain from strenuous activities for 24 to 48 hours after the procedure. The patient may be allowed to go back to work if no strenuous physical activity is involved. Getting rest and rehydrating are important. Notify the health-care provider if any of the following occur:

- Headaches
- Bleeding from the injection site
- Inability to urinate
- Numbness or tingling in the legs
- Signs of infection, such as fever

The health-care provider may give other specific instructions based on the patient's case.

References

1. "Lumbar Puncture," Johns Hopkins Medicine, June 29, 2011.
2. "Lumbar Puncture (Spinal Tap)," Mayo Clinic, August 14, 2020.
3. "Spinal Tap (Lumbar Puncture)," Cleveland Clinic, October 23, 2020.

Section 10.3 | **Cytology**

This section includes text excerpted from "Cytology and Its Procedures," Surveillance, Epidemiology, and End Results (SEER) Program, National Cancer Institute (NCI), September 7, 2016. Reviewed October 2021.

The study of cells, their origin, structure, function, and pathology is called "cytology." Cells are continually shed (exfoliated) from tissues that line the cavities and hollow organs of the body. These exfoliated cells may float in the fluid and mucous material bathes or passes through these cavities. These cells can be examined microscopically to determine their tissue of origin and whether or not they are malignant. The term exfoliative cytology refers to "microscopic examination of cells contained within body fluids."

The three body cavities, the pleura (enclosing the lungs), the peritoneum (enclosing the intestinal tract), and the pericardium (enclosing the heart), may be checked for fluid. The normal fluids within the body cavities are limited to an insignificant lubricating layer that cannot be aspirated. Therefore, fluid in any body cavity which can be aspirated indicates a pathological process, commonly malignant and metastatic. It is believed that the formation of malignant ascites (fluid in the abdominal cavity), for example, is brought about by colonies of cancer cells which damage the capillaries and lymphatics resulting in leakage of cancer cells and plasma directly into the abdominal cavity.

The list below shows the sources of some of the specimens that are examined histologically and some that are examined cytologically.

- Sputum
- Breast secretion
- Gastric fluid
- Peritoneal fluid
- Pleural fluid
- Bone marrow aspiration (cells)
- Bronchial brushing
- Bronchial washing
- Prostate secretion
- Spinal fluid
- Urinary sediment

- Cervical and vaginal smears
- Tracheal washing

CYTOLOGY AND ITS PROCEDURES

There are a variety of procedures employed to obtain material for the cytologic examination, from fine-needle aspiration of superficial or internal lesions to exfoliated cells obtained by aspiration, washing, brushing, smears, or scraping of vaginal secretions, sputum, urine, abdominal fluid, prostate secretions, etc. The more common techniques include:

- **Brushings.** The procedure of brushing the lining of an organ for the purpose of obtaining cells.
- **Punctures.** Inserting a hollow needle into a cavity or organ for the purpose of removal of some portion of the contents (fluid, bone marrow, tissue).
  - **Paracentesis.** Surgical puncture of a cavity for aspiration of fluid, such as the abdominal cavity.
  - **Thoracentesis.** Surgical puncture for aspiration of fluid from the chest.
- **Scrapings.** The procedure of scraping the lining of a structure with an instrument for the purpose of obtaining cells.
- **Swabs.** Using a swab or similar device to obtain fluid and secretions which then can be used to make a smear.
- **Washings.** The removal of fluid from a hollow organ or structure for the purpose of collecting any cells in the fluid which may be exfoliated.

Section 10.4 | **Biopsy**

This section contains text excerpted from the following sources: Text in this section begins with excerpts from "Biopsy," MedlinePlus, National Institutes of Health (NIH), May 2, 2017. Reviewed October 2021; Text under the heading "Open Biopsy" is excerpted from "Open Biopsy," National Cancer Institute (NCI), May 8, 2006. Reviewed October 2021; Text under the heading "Bone Marrow Biopsy" is excerpted from "Bone Marrow Biopsy," National Cancer Institute (NCI), March 30, 2010. Reviewed October 2021; Text under the heading "Punch Biopsy" is excerpted from "Punch Biopsy," National Cancer Institute (NCI), January 5, 2014. Reviewed October 2021.

A biopsy is a procedure that removes cells or tissue from your body. A doctor called a "pathologist" looks at the cells or tissue under a microscope to check for damage or disease. The pathologist may also do other tests on it.

Biopsies can be done on all parts of the body. In most cases, a biopsy is the only test that can tell for sure if a suspicious area is cancer. But biopsies are performed for many other reasons too.

There are different types of biopsy procedures and a few common types are discussed below.

OPEN BIOPSY

A procedure in which a cut is made through the skin to remove abnormal tissue so it can be checked under a microscope for signs of disease. Also called surgical biopsy. The two types of open biopsy are

1. Excisional Biopsy*

A surgical procedure in which a cut is made through the skin to remove an entire lump or suspicious area so it can be checked under a microscope for signs of disease. A small amount of healthy tissue around the abnormal area may also be removed.

**Excerpted from "Excisional Biopsy," National Cancer Institute (NCI), February 3, 2017. Reviewed October 2021.*

2. Incisional Biopsy#

A surgical procedure in which a cut is made through the skin to remove a sample of abnormal tissue or part of a lump or suspicious area. The tissue is then checked under a microscope for signs of disease.

#*Excerpted from "Incisional Biopsy," National Cancer Institute (NCI), July 9, 2021.*

BONE MARROW BIOPSY

A procedure in which a small sample of bone with bone marrow inside it is removed, usually from the hip bone. A small area of skin and the surface of the bone underneath are numbed with an anesthetic. Then, a special, wide needle is pushed into the bone and rotated to remove a sample of bone with the bone marrow inside it. The sample is sent to a laboratory to be looked at under a microscope. This procedure may be done at the same time as a bone marrow aspiration.

PUNCH BIOPSY

A procedure in which a small round piece of tissue about the size of a pencil eraser is removed using a sharp, hollow, circular instrument. The tissue is then checked under a microscope for signs of disease. A punch biopsy may be used to check for certain types of cancer, including skin, vulvar, and cervical cancer. It may also be used to check for certain skin conditions and changes that may lead to cancer.

Chapter 11 | Types of Biopsies

Chapter Contents

Section 11.1 | **Breast Biopsy**

This section includes text excerpted from "Breast Biopsy," MedlinePlus, National Institutes of Health (NIH), December 3, 2020.

WHAT IS A BREAST BIOPSY?

A breast biopsy is a procedure that removes a small sample of breast tissue for testing. The tissue is looked at under a microscope to check for breast cancer. There are different ways to do a breast biopsy procedure. One method uses a special needle to remove tissue. Another method removes tissue in a minor, outpatient surgery. A breast biopsy can determine whether you have breast cancer. But, most women who have a breast biopsy do not have cancer.

WHAT IS IT USED FOR?

A breast biopsy is used to confirm or rule out breast cancer. It is done after other breast tests, such as a mammogram, or a physical breast exam, show there might be a chance of breast cancer.

WHY DO YOU NEED A BREAST BIOPSY?

You may need a breast biopsy if:

- You or your health-care provider felt a lump in your breast
- Your mammogram, magnetic resonance imaging (MRI), or ultrasound tests show a lump, shadow, or other area of concern
- You have changes in your nipple, such as bloody discharge

If your health-care provider has ordered a breast biopsy, it does not necessarily mean you have breast cancer. The majority of breast lumps that are tested are benign, which means noncancerous.

WHAT HAPPENS DURING A BREAST BIOPSY

There are three main types of breast biopsy procedures:

- Fine needle aspiration biopsy, which uses a very thin needle to remove a sample of breast cells or fluid
- Core needle biopsy, which uses a larger needle to remove a sample
- Surgical biopsy, which removes a sample in a minor, outpatient procedure

Fine needle aspiration and core needle biopsies usually include the following steps.

- You will lay on your side or sit on an exam table.
- A health-care provider will clean the biopsy site and inject it with an anesthetic, so you will not feel any pain during the procedure.
- Once the area is numb, the provider will insert either a fine aspiration needle or core biopsy needle into the biopsy site and remove a sample of tissue or fluid.
- You may feel a little pressure when the sample is withdrawn.
- Pressure will be applied to the biopsy site until the bleeding stops.
- Your provider will apply a sterile bandage at the biopsy site.

In a surgical biopsy, a surgeon will make a small cut in your skin to remove all or part of a breast lump. A surgical biopsy is sometimes done if the lump cannot be reached with a needle biopsy. Surgical biopsies usually include the following steps.

- You will lie on an operating table. An IV (intravenous line) may be placed in your arm or hand.
- You may be given medicine, called a "sedative," to help you relax.
- You will be given local or general anesthesia, so you will not feel pain during the procedure.
    - For local anesthesia, a health-care provider will inject the biopsy site with medicine to numb the area.
    - For general anesthesia, a specialist called an "anesthesiologist" will give you medicine, so you will be unconscious during the procedure.

- The biopsy area is numb or you are unconscious, the surgeon will make a small cut into the breast and remove part or all of a lump. Some tissue around the lump may also be removed.
- The cut in your skin will be closed with stitches or adhesive strips.
- The type of biopsy you have will depend on different factors, including the size of the lump and what the lump or area of concern looks like on a breast test.

WILL YOU NEED TO DO ANYTHING TO PREPARE FOR THE TEST?

You would not need any special preparations if you are getting local anesthesia (numbing of the biopsy site). If you are getting general anesthesia, you will probably need to fast (not eat or drink) for several hours before surgery. Your surgeon will give you more specific instructions. Also, if you are getting a sedative or general anesthesia, be sure to arrange for someone to drive you home. You may be groggy and confused after you wake up from the procedure.

ARE THERE ANY RISKS TO THE TEST?

You may have a little bruising or bleeding at the biopsy site. Sometimes the site gets infected. If that happens, you will be treated with antibiotics. A surgical biopsy may cause some additional pain and discomfort. Your health-care provider may recommend or prescribe medicine to help you feel better.

WHAT DO THE RESULTS MEAN?

It may take several days to a week to get your results. Typical results may show:

- **Normal.** No cancer or abnormal cells were found.
- **Abnormal, but benign.** These show breast changes that are not cancer. These include calcium deposits and cysts. Sometimes more testing and/or follow-up treatment may be needed.
- **Cancer cells found.** Your results will include information about the cancer to help you and your

health-care provider develop a treatment plan that best meets your needs. You will probably be referred to a provider who specializes in breast cancer treatment.

IS THERE ANYTHING ELSE YOU NEED TO KNOW ABOUT A BREAST BIOPSY?

In the United States, tens of thousands of women and hundreds of men die of breast cancer every year. A breast biopsy, when appropriate, can help find breast cancer at an early stage, when it is most treatable. If breast cancer is found early, when it is confined to the breast only, the five-year survival rate is 99 percent. This means, on average, that 99 out of 100 people with breast cancer that was detected early are still alive 5 years after being diagnosed. If you have questions about breast cancer screening, such as mammograms or a breast biopsy, talk to your health-care provider.

Section 11.2 | **Kidney Biopsy**

This section includes text excerpted from "Kidney Biopsy," National Institute of Diabetes and Digestive and Kidney Diseases (NIDDK), November 2015. Reviewed October 2021.

WHAT IS A KIDNEY BIOPSY?

A kidney biopsy is a procedure that involves taking a small piece of kidney tissue for examination with a microscope. A pathologist – a doctor who specializes in diagnosing diseases – examines the kidney tissue sample in a lab. The pathologist looks for signs of kidney disease or infection. If the kidney has been transplanted and is not working, a kidney biopsy may help identify the cause.

One of the following specialists will perform the kidney biopsy at a hospital or an outpatient center:

- **A nephrologist.** A doctor who specializes in treating kidney disease
- **A urologist.** A doctor who specializes in treating urologic and sexual problems

- **A transplant surgeon.** A doctor who specializes in performing organ transplants
- **An interventional radiologist.** A doctor who performs procedures using imaging equipment

WHY IS A KIDNEY BIOPSY PERFORMED?

A health-care provider will perform a kidney biopsy to evaluate any of the following conditions:

- **Hematuria.** Blood in the urine, which can be a sign of kidney disease or other urinary problems.
- **Albuminuria.** A condition in which the urine has more-than-normal amounts of a protein called "albumin." Albuminuria may be a sign of kidney disease.
- Changes in kidney function, which can cause the buildup of waste products in the blood.

The kidney tissue sample can show inflammation, scarring, infection, or unusual deposits of a protein called "immunoglobulin." If a person has chronic kidney disease – any condition that causes reduced kidney function over a period of time – the biopsy may show how quickly the disease is advancing. A biopsy can also help explain why a transplanted kidney is not working properly.

Health-care providers may use a kidney biopsy to diagnose cancer. If cancer is present, there is a small chance that the biopsy needle will spread the cancer. In addition, the biopsy specimen is very small and may miss the cancer and, therefore, may not provide the right diagnosis.

WHAT SHOULD A PERSON DO DAYS BEFORE A KIDNEY BIOPSY?

Days before the procedure, a person should prepare for a kidney biopsy by:

- Talking with a health-care provider
- Arranging for a ride home

Talking with a Health-Care Provider

People should talk with their health-care provider about medical conditions they have and all prescribed and over-the-counter (OTC) medications, vitamins, and supplements they take, including:

- Aspirin or medications that contain aspirin
- Nonsteroidal anti-inflammatory medications such as ibuprofen and naproxen
- Blood thinners
- Arthritis medications

People should also tell their health-care provider about any allergies they have to medications or foods.

The health-care provider should discuss the risks of the procedure, and the person should ask questions or bring up concerns. Two weeks before the biopsy, the health-care provider may instruct a person to stop taking certain medications that cause thinning of the blood because this may increase the risk of bleeding after the kidney biopsy. The health-care provider may also tell the person not to eat or drink anything for 8 hours before the biopsy.

Arranging for a Ride Home after the Procedure

For safety reasons, people cannot drive for 24 hours after the procedure because they are given a sedative to help them relax just before the procedure. A health-care provider will ask a person to make advance arrangements for getting home after the procedure.

WHAT CAN A PERSON EXPECT ON THE DAY OF THE KIDNEY BIOPSY?

A person should arrive 90 minutes to 2 hours before the kidney biopsy to have time for several preliminary procedures, including:

- Signing a consent form
- Having blood tests
- Receiving intravenous (IV) fluids and medications

Signing a Consent Form

A health-care provider will ask the person to sign a consent form that states that she or he understands the risks of the procedure and gives permission for the health-care provider to perform the kidney biopsy.

Having Blood Tests

Shortly before the procedure, a health-care provider will perform blood and urine tests to make sure the person does not have a condition that would make having a biopsy risky, such as a bleeding problem or high blood potassium.

Receiving Intravenous Fluids and Medications

A nurse or technician will insert an IV line into a vein in the person's arm to give fluids and medications, including sedatives.

HOW IS A KIDNEY BIOPSY PERFORMED?

The procedure typically takes about an hour and includes the following steps:

- Most people will lie on their abdomen on an examination table. The technician will place a firm pillow or sandbag under a person's body to support the abdomen and help push the kidneys up toward the person's back and the surface of the skin. People who have a transplanted kidneys lie on their backs because surgeons place transplanted kidneys in the front-lower part of the abdomen, to one side of the bladder.
- A nurse or technician will give the person sedatives through the IV.
- The health-care provider will mark the point where the needle will enter the skin, clean the area, and inject a local anesthetic to numb the area.
- Next, the health-care provider uses imaging techniques, such as ultrasound, to guide the biopsy needle into the kidney. Ultrasound uses a device called a "transducer"

that bounces safe, painless sound waves off organs to create an image of their structure. Sometimes the health-care provider uses a computerized tomography (CT) scan or magnetic resonance imaging (MRI) to guide the needle into the kidney.

- The health-care provider will ask the person to hold her or his breath and stay still as the health-care provider inserts the biopsy needle and removes the kidney tissue. When the health-care provider takes the biopsy, the instrument will make a clicking or popping noise. The health-care provider may need to insert the needle three or four times. People most often will need to hold their breath for about 30 seconds or a little longer for each insertion.

For people with bleeding problems, the health-care provider uses a laparoscope – a thin tube with a video camera. This procedure is surgery that requires general anesthesia. The surgeon makes a small incision into the back and inserts the laparoscope to see the kidney. The surgeon can insert tiny tools through the laparoscope to collect tissue samples and can watch after the procedure through the camera to make sure that if there is any bleeding, she or he can stop it.

WHAT CAN A PERSON EXPECT AFTER A KIDNEY BIOPSY?

After a kidney biopsy, a person can expect to:

- Lie on her or his back in the clinic or hospital for a few hours. During this time, the staff will monitor the person's blood pressure, pulse, urine, and blood test results.
- Go home the same day, in most cases; however, a person will need to rest at home for 12 to 24 hours after the biopsy. Sometimes a person may need to stay overnight at the hospital.
- Have some pain or soreness near the point where the needle went through the skin.
- Receive written instructions for ensuring a healthy recovery from the procedure. Most people need to wait

2 weeks before resuming strenuous activities, such as heavy lifting or participating in contact sports.

A health-care provider most often receives the complete biopsy results from the pathologist in about a week. In urgent cases, a person may receive a preliminary report within 24 hours. The health-care provider will review the results with the person during a follow-up visit.

WHAT ARE THE RISKS OF A KIDNEY BIOPSY?

The risks of a kidney biopsy include:

- **Bleeding.** The most common complication of a kidney biopsy. Bleeding may come from the kidney or the puncture site. Bleeding from the kidney rarely requires a blood transfusion.
- **Infection.** A rare complication of a kidney biopsy. Health-care providers prescribe bacteria-fighting medications called "antibiotics" to treat infections.

Section 11.3 | **Liver Biopsy**

This section includes text excerpted from "Liver Biopsy," National Institute of Diabetes and Digestive and Kidney Diseases (NIDDK), August 2019.

WHAT IS A LIVER BIOPSY?

A liver biopsy is a procedure in which a doctor takes a small piece of tissue from your liver. A pathologist will examine the tissue with a microscope to look for signs of damage or disease.

ARE THERE DIFFERENT TYPES OF LIVER BIOPSY?

Yes. In each type of liver biopsy, doctors take the sample of liver tissue in a different way. Common types of liver biopsy are described below.

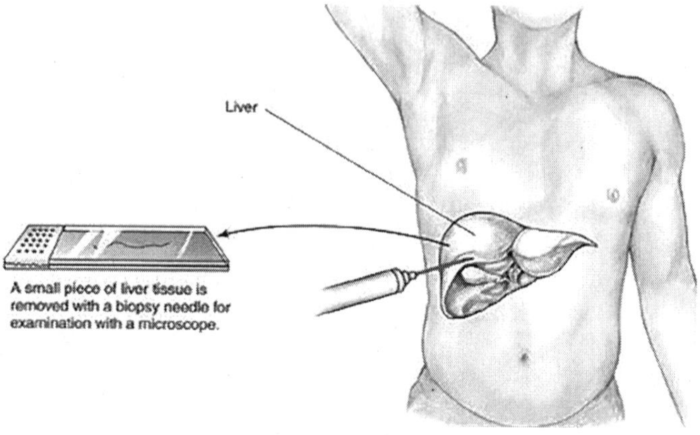

Figure 11.1. Percutaneous Liver Biopsy

Percutaneous Liver Biopsy

In a percutaneous liver biopsy, the doctor inserts a needle through your skin in the upper part of the abdomen to take a small piece of your liver tissue.

Percutaneous liver biopsy is the most common type of liver biopsy and has been performed routinely for many years. Your doctor may perform an ultrasound or computed tomography (CT) scan to be sure that the needle is positioned in the correct place.

Transjugular Liver Biopsy

In transjugular liver biopsy, a doctor inserts a needle into a vein in your neck called the "jugular vein." The doctor passes the needle through your veins to your liver to take a small piece of tissue.

Doctors usually perform transjugular biopsy in people who have a higher risk of problems with percutaneous liver biopsy. For example, bleeding after a percutaneous biopsy is more likely in people who have problems with blood clotting. In people who have ascites – a buildup of fluid in the abdomen that is a complication of cirrhosis – percutaneous biopsy is difficult because the liver is too far away from the skin and hard to target.

Transjugular biopsy also allows doctors to measure pressure in the veins of the liver at the same time that they perform the biopsy.

Surgical Liver Biopsy

If you need a liver biopsy and you are having surgery for other reasons, a doctor may perform a liver biopsy during the surgery.

WHY DO DOCTORS USE LIVER BIOPSY?

Doctors use liver biopsy to:

- Diagnose liver diseases when doctors cannot confirm a diagnosis with blood or imaging tests
- Find out how severe the liver damage or disease is
- Help determine the best treatment for liver damage or disease
- Find out how a treatment for liver disease is working

HOW DO YOU PREPARE FOR A LIVER BIOPSY?

To prepare for a liver biopsy talk with your doctor, have blood and imaging tests if needed, arrange for a ride home after the procedure, and follow your doctor's instructions about fasting before the procedure.

Talk with Your Doctor

Talk with your doctor about what you can expect before, during, and after the liver biopsy.

Also talk with your doctor about any allergies and medical conditions you have and all the prescribed and over-the-counter (OTC) medicines, vitamins, and supplements you take, including:

- Aspirin or medicines that contain aspirin
- Blood thinners
- Complementary or alternative medicines
- Diabetes medicines
- Dietary supplements
- Nonsteroidal anti-inflammatory drugs (NSAIDs), such as ibuprofen and naproxen, or medicines that contain NSAIDs

Your doctor may ask you to temporarily stop taking medicines that affect blood clotting or interact with sedatives. You may receive sedatives during a liver biopsy to help you relax and stay comfortable.

Have Blood and Imaging Tests

Before you have a liver biopsy, your doctor may order blood tests to find out how well your blood clots. For blood tests, a health-care professional will take blood samples and send the samples to a lab.

Severe liver disease, inherited bleeding disorders such as hemophilia, and other health conditions may cause problems with blood clotting. If you have problems with blood clotting, your doctor may give you a transfusion of platelets or clotting factors just before a liver biopsy. Your doctor may also recommend a transjugular liver biopsy instead of a percutaneous liver biopsy.

Your doctor may also order imaging tests to view your liver and surrounding organs and find the best place to insert the biopsy needle. Imaging tests may include:

- Ultrasound, which uses a device called a "transducer" that bounces safe, painless sound waves off organs to create images of their structure
- Computed tomography (CT) scan, which uses a combination of x-rays and computer technology to create images

Arrange for a Ride Home

For safety reasons, most people cannot drive home after a liver biopsy. You will need to make plans for getting a ride home after a liver biopsy.

Follow Your Doctor's Instructions about Fasting before the Procedure

Doctors may ask people to fast – not eat or drink anything – for several hours before a liver biopsy. In some cases, doctors ask patients to eat a small snack a few hours before a liver biopsy. Instructions about fasting vary, and doctors may give different instructions for different types of biopsy. Follow your doctor's instructions.

HOW DO DOCTORS PERFORM A LIVER BIOPSY?

Doctors perform a liver biopsy at a hospital or outpatient center.

Percutaneous Liver Biopsy

The doctor will find the best place to insert the biopsy needle by tapping on your abdomen or by using ultrasound or a CT scan. Doctors may also use ultrasound or CT scans to guide the biopsy needle during the procedure.

You will receive a local anesthetic to numb the area where the doctor will insert the biopsy needle. If needed, you may also receive sedatives and pain medicine.

You will be asked to lie on your back and rest your right hand above your head. The doctor will make a small cut in the right side of your abdomen and insert the biopsy needle. You may be asked to breathe out and hold your breath while the sample of liver tissue is taken.

After the biopsy, the doctor will place a bandage over the cut on your abdomen. You may be asked to lie on your right side after the biopsy, and you will need to remain lying down for a few hours. Health-care professionals will typically check your vital signs regularly for 2–4 hours after the procedure.

Transjugular Liver Biopsy

The doctor will use ultrasound to find the best place on your neck to access your jugular vein. During the procedure, the doctor will use ultrasound to view your jugular vein and will use fluoroscopy, a type of x-ray imaging, to view the veins between your neck and your liver.

You will receive a local anesthetic to numb the area on your neck where the doctor will insert the biopsy needle. You may also receive sedatives and pain medicine.

You will be asked to lie on your back and turn your head to the side. The doctor will make a small cut on your neck and use a needle to make a small hole in your jugular vein. The doctor will insert a thin, flexible tube, called a "catheter," through your veins to your liver. The doctor will thread a biopsy needle through the catheter and into your liver to take a tissue sample.

After the biopsy, the doctor will place a bandage over the cut on your neck. You will need to remain lying down and have your vital signs regularly checked for at least 4 hours after the procedure.

Surgical Liver Biopsy

You will receive anesthesia for surgery. Doctors can perform a liver biopsy during open surgery or laparoscopic surgery. In open surgery, doctors make a large cut to open the abdomen. In laparoscopic surgery, doctors make small cuts in the abdomen and insert special tools to view or repair organs and tissues.

WHAT SHOULD YOU EXPECT AFTER A LIVER BIOPSY?

Following a liver biopsy, you – or a friend or family member who is with you if you are still groggy – will receive instructions on how to care for yourself after the procedure. You should follow all instructions. Instructions may vary, depending on the type of liver biopsy you had.

Talk with your doctor about when you can resume your usual activities. After a liver biopsy, doctors often recommend avoiding intense activity and heavy lifting for up to 1 week.

After a liver biopsy, a pathologist will examine the biopsy tissue with a microscope to look for signs of damage or disease. Biopsy results typically take a few days or longer to come back.

WHAT ARE THE RISKS OF LIVER BIOPSY?

The risks of liver biopsy include complications such as the following.

Bleeding

Internal bleeding is a serious complication of liver biopsy. Bleeding may cause signs and symptoms such as pain that is severe or that lasts more than a few hours after the biopsy, low blood pressure, and a fast heartbeat. You may need treatment at a hospital, blood transfusions, and sometimes surgery or another procedure to stop the bleeding.

Bleeding occurs in about 1 out of every 500 liver biopsies. Severe bleeding occurs in 1 out of every 2,500 to 10,000 liver biopsies.

Pain

Pain is the most common complication after a liver biopsy. Pain often occurs in the upper right abdomen or right shoulder. In most cases, the pain is mild and goes away within a few hours after the biopsy. If pain is severe or lasts longer, it could be a sign of internal bleeding.

Talk with your doctor if you have any pain after a liver biopsy. Your doctor may recommend or prescribe medicines for pain. If the pain is not mild or does not go away within several hours after the biopsy, your doctor may order tests to find the cause of the pain.

Other Complications

Uncommon complications that may occur after a liver biopsy include:

- Infection, which may lead to sepsis
- A collapsed lung, called a "pneumothorax"
- A buildup of blood in the space between the lung and the chest wall, called "hemothorax"
- Injury to other organs

SEEK CARE RIGHT AWAY

If you have any of the following symptoms after a liver biopsy, seek medical help right away.

- Bleeding, pain, redness, or swelling at the biopsy site or where the doctor made a cut to insert the biopsy needle
- Dizziness, fainting, or weakness
- Fever
- Nausea or vomiting
- Pain in your abdomen, shoulder, or chest
- Problems breathing or shortness of breath
- Racing or pounding of your heart
- Stool that contains blood or is black and tarry
- Swelling or bloating of your abdomen

Section 11.4 | Sentinel Lymph Node Biopsy

This section includes text excerpted from "Sentinel Lymph Node Biopsy," National Cancer Institute (NCI), June 25, 2019.

WHAT ARE LYMPH NODES?

Lymph nodes are small round organs that are part of the body's lymphatic system. The lymphatic system is a part of the immune system. It consists of a network of vessels and organs that contains lymph, a clear fluid that carries infection-fighting white blood cells (WBCs) as well as fluid and waste products from the body's cells and tissues. In a person with cancer, lymph can also carry cancer cells that have broken off from the main tumor.

Lymph is filtered through lymph nodes, which are found widely throughout the body and are connected to one another by lymph vessels. Groups of lymph nodes are located in the neck, underarms, chest, abdomen, and groin. The lymph nodes contain white blood cells (B lymphocytes and T lymphocytes) and other types of immune system cells. Lymph nodes trap bacteria and viruses, as well as some damaged and abnormal cells, helping the immune system fight disease.

Many types of cancer spread through the lymphatic system, and one of the earliest sites of spread for these cancers is nearby lymph nodes.

WHAT IS A SENTINEL LYMPH NODE?

A sentinel lymph node is defined as the first lymph node to which cancer cells are most likely to spread from a primary tumor. Sometimes, there can be more than one sentinel lymph node.

WHAT IS A SENTINEL LYMPH NODE BIOPSY?

A sentinel lymph node biopsy (SLNB) is a procedure in which the sentinel lymph node is identified, removed, and examined to determine whether cancer cells are present. It is used in people who have already been diagnosed with cancer.

A negative SLNB result suggests that cancer has not yet spread to nearby lymph nodes or other organs.

A positive SLNB result indicates that cancer is present in the sentinel lymph node and that it may have spread to other nearby lymph nodes (called "regional lymph nodes") and, possibly, other organs. This information can help a doctor determine the stage of cancer (extent of the disease within the body) and develop an appropriate treatment plan.

WHAT HAPPENS DURING A SENTINEL LYMPH NODE BIOPSY

First, the sentinel lymph node (or nodes) must be located. To do so, a surgeon injects a radioactive substance, a blue dye, or both near the tumor. The surgeon then uses a device to detect lymph nodes that contain the radioactive substance or looks for lymph nodes that are stained with the blue dye. Once the sentinel lymph node is located, the surgeon makes a small incision (about 1/2 inch) in the overlying skin and removes the node.

The sentinel node is then checked for the presence of cancer cells by a pathologist. If cancer is found, the surgeon may remove additional lymph nodes, either during the same biopsy procedure or during a follow-up surgical procedure. SLNB may be done on an outpatient basis or may require a short stay in the hospital.

Sentinel lymph node biopsy is usually done at the same time the primary tumor is removed. In some cases the procedure can also be done before or even after (depending on how much the lymphatic vessels have been disrupted) removal of the tumor.

WHAT ARE THE BENEFITS OF SENTINEL LYMPH NODE BIOPSY?

Sentinel lymph node biopsy helps doctors stage cancers and estimate the risk that tumor cells have developed the ability to spread to other parts of the body. If the sentinel node is negative for cancer, a patient may be able to avoid more extensive lymph node surgery, reducing the potential complications associated with having many lymph nodes removed.

WHAT ARE THE POSSIBLE HARMS OF SENTINEL LYMPH NODE BIOPSY?

All surgery to remove lymph nodes, including SLNB, can have harmful side effects, although removal of fewer lymph nodes is usually associated with fewer side effects, particularly serious ones such as lymphedema. The potential side effects include:

- **Lymphedema or tissue swelling.** During lymph node surgery, lymph vessels leading to and from the sentinel node or group of nodes are cut. This disrupts the normal flow of lymph through the affected area, which may lead to an abnormal buildup of lymph fluid that can cause swelling. Lymphedema may cause pain or discomfort in the affected area, and the overlying skin may become thickened or hard.

The risk of lymphedema increases with the number of lymph nodes removed. There is less risk with the removal of only the sentinel lymph node. In the case of extensive lymph node removal in an armpit or groin, the swelling may affect an entire arm or leg. In addition, there is an increased risk of infection in the affected area or limb. Very rarely, chronic lymphedema due to extensive lymph node removal may cause a cancer of the lymphatic vessels called "lymphangiosarcoma."

- Seroma, or a mass or lump caused by the buildup of lymph fluid at the site of the surgery
- Numbness, tingling, swelling, bruising, or pain at the site of the surgery, and an increased risk of infection
- Difficulty moving the affected body part
- Skin or allergic reactions to the blue dye used in SNLB
- A false-negative biopsy result – that is, cancer cells are not seen in the sentinel lymph node even though they have already spread to regional lymph nodes or other parts of the body. A false-negative biopsy result gives the patient and the doctor a false sense of security about the extent of cancer in the patient's body.

IS SENTINEL LYMPH NODE BIOPSY USED TO HELP STAGE ALL TYPES OF CANCER?

No. SLNB is most commonly used to help stage breast cancer and melanoma. It is sometimes used to stage penile cancer and endometrial cancer. However, it is being studied with other cancer types, including vulvar and cervical cancers, and colorectal, gastric, esophageal, head and neck, thyroid, and non-small cell lung cancers.

WHAT HAS RESEARCH SHOWN ABOUT THE USE OF SENTINEL LYMPH NODE BIOPSY IN BREAST CANCER?

Breast cancer cells are most likely to spread first to lymph nodes located in the axilla, or armpit area, next to the affected breast. However, in breast cancers close to the center of the chest (near the breastbone), cancer cells may spread first to lymph nodes inside the chest (under the breastbone, called "internal mammary nodes") before they can be detected in the axilla.

The number of lymph nodes in the axilla varies from person to person; the usual range is between 20 and 40. Historically, all of these axillary lymph nodes were removed (in an operation called "axillary lymph node dissection," or "ALND") in women diagnosed with breast cancer. This was done for two reasons: To help stage the breast cancer and to help prevent a regional recurrence of the disease. (Regional recurrence of breast cancer occurs when breast cancer cells that have migrated to nearby lymph nodes give rise to a new tumor.)

However, because removing multiple lymph nodes at the same time increases the risk of harmful side effects, clinical trials were launched to investigate whether just the sentinel lymph nodes could be removed. The National Cancer Institute (NCI)-sponsored randomized phase 3 clinical trials have shown that SLNB without ALND is sufficient for staging breast cancer and for preventing regional recurrence in women who have no clinical signs of axillary lymph node metastasis, such as a lump or swelling in the armpit that may cause discomfort, and who are treated with surgery, adjuvant systemic therapy, and radiation therapy.

In one trial, involving 5,611 women, researchers randomly assigned participants to receive just SLNB, or SLNB plus ALND, after surgery. Those women in the two groups whose sentinel lymph node(s) were negative for cancer (a total of 3,989 women) were then followed for an average of 8 years. The researchers found no differences in overall survival or disease-free survival between the two groups of women.

The other trial included 891 women with tumors up to 5 cm in the breast and one or two positive sentinel lymph nodes. Patients were randomly assigned to receive SLNB only or to receive ALND after SLNB. All of the women were treated with lumpectomy, and most also received adjuvant systemic therapy and external-beam radiation therapy to the affected breast. After extended follow-up, the two groups of women had similar 10-year overall survival, disease-free survival, and regional recurrence rates.

WHAT HAS RESEARCH SHOWN ABOUT THE USE OF SENTINEL LYMPH NODE BIOPSY IN MELANOMA?

Research indicates that patients with melanoma who have undergone SLNB and whose sentinel lymph node is found to be negative for cancer and who have no clinical signs that cancer has spread to other lymph nodes can be spared more extensive lymph node surgery at the time of primary tumor removal. A meta-analysis of 71 studies with data from 25,240 patients found that the risk of regional lymph node recurrence in patients with a negative SLNB was 5 percent or less.

Findings from the Multicenter Selective Lymphadenectomy Trial II (MSLT-II) also confirmed the safety of SLNB in people with melanoma with positive sentinel lymph nodes and no clinical evidence of other lymph node involvement. This large, randomized phase 3 clinical trial, which included more than 1,900 patients, compared the potential therapeutic benefit of SLNB plus the immediate removal of the remaining regional lymph nodes (called "completion lymph node dissection," or "CLND") with SNLB plus active surveillance, which included regular ultrasound examination of the remaining regional lymph nodes and treatment with CLND if signs of additional lymph node metastasis were detected.

After a median follow-up of 43 months, patients who had undergone immediate CLND did not have better melanoma-specific survival than those who had undergone SLNB with CLND only if signs of additional lymph node metastasis appear (86 percent of participants in both groups had not died from melanoma at 3 years).

Section 11.5 | **Other Biopsies**

This section contains text excerpted from the following sources: Text beginning with the heading "Fine-Needle Aspiration Biopsy of the Thyroid" is excerpted from "Thyroid Cancer Treatment (Adult) (PDQ®) – Patient Version," National Cancer Institute (NCI), January 13, 2021; Text under the heading "Fine-Needle Aspiration Biopsy of the Lung" is excerpted from "Small Cell Lung Cancer Treatment (PDQ®) – Patient Version," National Cancer Institute (NCI), May 7, 2021; Text under the heading "Bone Marrow Aspiration and Biopsy" is excerpted from "Myelodysplastic Syndromes Treatment (PDQ®) – Patient Version," National Cancer Institute (NCI), September 20, 2021; Text under the heading "Skin Biopsy" is excerpted from "Skin Cancer Treatment (PDQ®) – Patient Version," National Cancer Institute (NCI), August 27, 2021.

FINE-NEEDLE ASPIRATION BIOPSY OF THE THYROID

The removal of thyroid tissue using a thin needle. The needle is inserted through the skin into the thyroid. Several tissue samples are removed from different parts of the thyroid. A pathologist views the tissue samples under a microscope to look for cancer cells. Because the type of thyroid cancer can be hard to diagnose, patients should ask to have biopsy samples checked by a pathologist who has experience diagnosing thyroid cancer.

SURGICAL BIOPSY

The removal of the thyroid nodule or one lobe of the thyroid during surgery so the cells and tissues can be viewed under a microscope by a pathologist to check for signs of cancer. Because the type of thyroid cancer can be hard to diagnose, patients should ask to have biopsy samples checked by a pathologist who has experience diagnosing thyroid cancer.

FINE-NEEDLE ASPIRATION BIOPSY OF THE LUNG

The removal of tissue or fluid from the lung, using a thin needle. A computed tomography (CT) scan, ultrasound, or other imaging procedure is used to find the abnormal tissue or fluid in the lung. A small incision may be made in the skin where the biopsy needle is inserted into the abnormal tissue or fluid. A sample is removed with the needle and sent to the laboratory. A pathologist then views the sample under a microscope to look for cancer cells. A chest x-ray is done after the procedure to make sure no air is leaking from the lung into the chest.

BONE MARROW ASPIRATION AND BIOPSY

The removal of bone marrow, blood, and a small piece of bone by inserting a hollow needle into the hipbone or breastbone. A pathologist views the bone marrow, blood, and bone under a microscope to look for abnormal cells.

SKIN BIOPSY

All or part of the abnormal-looking growth is cut from the skin and viewed under a microscope by a pathologist to check for signs of cancer. There are four main types of skin biopsies:

- **Shave biopsy.** A sterile razor blade is used to "shave-off" the abnormal-looking growth.
- **Punch biopsy.** A special instrument called a "punch" or a "trephine" is used to remove a circle of tissue from the abnormal-looking growth.
- **Incisional biopsy.** A scalpel is used to remove part of a growth.
- **Excisional biopsy.** A scalpel is used to remove the entire growth.

Chapter 12 | **Urine Tests**

Chapter Contents

Section 12.1 | **Urine Test: Basics**

This section contains text excerpted from the following sources: Text in this section begins with excerpts from "Urine and Urination," MedlinePlus, National Institutes of Health (NIH), May 10, 2021; Text under the heading "Urinalysis" is excerpted from "Urinalysis," MedlinePlus, National Institutes of Health (NIH), May 5, 2016. Reviewed October 2021.

Your kidneys make urine by filtering wastes and extra water from your blood. The waste is called "urea." Your blood carries it to the kidneys. From the kidneys, urine travels down two thin tubes called "ureters" to the bladder. The bladder stores urine until you are ready to urinate. It swells into a round shape when it is full and gets smaller when empty. If your urinary system is healthy, your bladder can hold up to 16 ounces (2 cups) of urine comfortably for 2 to 5 hours.

You may have problems with urination if you have:

- Kidney failure
- Urinary tract infections
- An enlarged prostate
- Bladder control problems such as incontinence, overactive bladder, or interstitial cystitis
- A blockage that prevents you from emptying your bladder

Some conditions may also cause you to have blood or protein in your urine. If you have a urinary problem, see your health-care provider. Urinalysis and other urine tests can help to diagnose the problem. Treatment depends on the cause.

URINALYSIS

A urinalysis is a test of your urine. It is often done to check for a urinary tract infections, kidney problems, or diabetes. You may also have one during a checkup, if you are admitted to the hospital, before you have surgery, or if you are pregnant. It can also monitor some medical conditions and treatments.

A urinalysis involves checking the urine for:

- Its color

- Its appearance (whether it is clear or cloudy)
- Any odor
- The pH level (acidity)
- Whether there are substances that are not normally in urine, such as blood, too much protein, glucose, ketones, and bilirubin
- Whether there are cells, crystals, and casts (tube-shaped proteins)
- Whether it contains bacteria or other germs

Section 12.2 | Mucus in Urine

This section includes text excerpted from "Mucus in Urine," MedlinePlus, National Institutes of Health (NIH), July 31, 2020.

HOW DO YOU TEST FOR MUCUS IN URINE?

Mucus is a thick, slimy substance that coats and moistens certain parts of the body, including the nose, mouth, throat, and urinary tract. A small amount of mucus in your urine is normal. An excess amount may indicate a urinary tract infection (UTI) or other medical condition. A test called "urinalysis" can detect whether there is too much mucus in your urine.

Other names include microscopic urine analysis, microscopic examination of urine, urine test, and urine analysis.

WHAT IS IT USED FOR?

A mucus in urine test may be part of a urinalysis. A urinalysis may include a visual check of your urine sample, tests for certain chemicals, and an examination of urine cells under a microscope. A mucus in urine test is part of a microscopic exam of urine.

WHY DO YOU NEED A MUCUS IN URINE TEST?

A urinalysis is often part of a routine checkup. Your health-care provider may include a mucus in urine test in your urinalysis if you have symptoms of a UTI. These include:

- Frequent urge to urinate, but little urine is passed
- Painful urination
- Dark, cloudy, or reddish-colored urine
- Bad smelling urine
- Weakness
- Fatigue

WHAT HAPPENS DURING A MUCUS IN URINE TEST

Your health-care provider will need to collect a sample of your urine. You will receive a container to collect the urine and special instructions to make sure that the sample is sterile. These instructions are often called the "clean catch method." The clean catch method includes the following steps:

- Wash your hands.
- Clean your genital area with a cleansing pad given to you by your provider. Men should wipe the tip of their penis. Women should open their labia and clean from front to back.
- Start to urinate into the toilet.
- Move the collection container under your urine stream.
- Collect at least an ounce or two of urine into the container. The container will have markings to indicate the amounts.
- Finish urinating into the toilet.
- Return the sample container as instructed by your health-care provider.

WILL YOU NEED TO DO ANYTHING TO PREPARE FOR THE TEST?

You do not need any special preparations for this test. If your health-care provider has ordered other urine or blood tests, you may need to fast (not eat or drink) for several hours before the test. Your health-care provider will let you know if there are any special instructions to follow.

ARE THERE ANY RISKS TO THE TEST?

There is no known risk to having a urinalysis or a test for mucus in urine.

WHAT DO THE RESULTS MEAN?

If your results show a small or moderate amount of mucus in your urine, it is mostly likely due to normal discharge. A large amount of mucus may indicate one of the following conditions:

- A UTI
- A sexually transmitted disease (STD)
- Kidney stones
- Irritable bowel syndrome (IBS)
- Bladder cancer

To learn what your results mean, talk to your health-care provider.

Section 12.3 | **Glucose in Urine**

This section includes text excerpted from "Glucose in Urine Test," MedlinePlus, National Institutes of Health (NIH), July 31, 2020.

WHAT IS A GLUCOSE IN URINE TEST?

A glucose in urine test measures the amount of glucose in your urine. Glucose is a type of sugar. It is your body's main source of energy. A hormone called "insulin" helps move glucose from your bloodstream into your cells. If too much glucose gets into the blood, the extra glucose will be eliminated through your urine. A urine glucose test can be used to help determine if blood glucose levels are too high, which may be a sign of diabetes.

Other names include urine sugar test, urine glucose test, and glucosuria test.

WHAT IS IT USED FOR?

A glucose in urine test may be part of a urinalysis, a test that measures different cells, chemicals, and other substances in your urine. Urinalysis is often included as part of a routine exam. A glucose in urine test may also be used to screen for diabetes. However, a urine glucose test is not as accurate as a blood glucose test. It may be ordered if blood glucose testing is difficult or not possible. Some people cannot get blood drawn because their veins are too small or too scarred from repeated punctures. Other people avoid blood tests due to extreme anxiety or fear of needles.

WHY DO YOU NEED A GLUCOSE IN URINE TEST?

You may get a glucose in urine test as part of your regular checkup or if you have symptoms of diabetes and cannot take a blood glucose test. Symptoms of diabetes include:

- Increased thirst
- More frequent urination
- Blurred vision
- Fatigue

You may also need a urinalysis, which includes a glucose in urine test, if you are pregnant. If high levels of glucose in urine are found, it may indicate gestational diabetes. Gestational diabetes is form of diabetes that happens only during pregnancy. Blood glucose testing can be used to confirm a diagnosis of gestational diabetes. Most pregnant women are tested for gestational diabetes with a blood glucose test, between their 24th and 28th weeks of pregnancy.

WHAT HAPPENS DURING A GLUCOSE IN URINE TEST

Your health-care provider will need to collect a sample of your urine. During your office visit, you will receive a container in which to collect the urine and special instructions to ensure the sample is sterile. These instructions are often referred to as the "clean catch method." The clean catch method includes the following steps:

- Wash your hands.
- Clean your genital area with a cleansing pad. Men should wipe the tip of their penis. Women should open their labia and clean from front to back.
- Start to urinate into the toilet.
- Move the collection container under your urine stream.

- Collect at least an ounce or two of urine into the container, which should have markings to indicate the amount.
- Finish urinating into the toilet.
- Return the sample container as instructed by your health-care provider.

Your health-care provider may ask you to monitor your urine glucose at home with a test kit. She or he will provide you with either a kit or a recommendation of which kit to buy. Your urine glucose test kit will include instructions on how to perform the test and a package of strips for testing. Be sure to follow the kit instructions carefully, and talk to your health-care provider if you have any questions.

WILL YOU NEED TO DO ANYTHING TO PREPARE FOR THE TEST?

You do not need any special preparations for this test.

ARE THERE ANY RISKS TO THE TEST?

There is no known risk to having a glucose in urine test.

WHAT DO THE RESULTS MEAN?

Glucose is not normally found in urine. If results show glucose, it may be a sign of:

- Diabetes
- Pregnancy. As many half of all pregnant women have some glucose in their urine during pregnancy. Too much glucose may indicate gestational diabetes.
- A kidney disorder

A urine glucose test is only a screening test. If glucose is found in your urine, your provider will order a blood glucose test to help make a diagnosis.

Section 12.4 | **Blood in Urine**

This section includes text excerpted from "Blood in Urine," MedlinePlus, National Institutes of Health (NIH), July 30, 2020.

WHY DO YOU NEED A BLOOD IN URINE TEST?

Your health-care provider may have ordered a urinalysis as part of a routine exam. You may also need this test if you have seen blood in your urine or have other symptoms of a urinary disorder. These symptoms include:

- Painful urination
- Frequent urination
- Back pain
- Abdominal pain

WHAT HAPPENS DURING A BLOOD IN URINE TEST

Your health-care provider will need to collect a sample of your urine. During your office visit, you will receive a container to collect the urine and special instructions to make sure that the sample is sterile. These instructions are often called the "clean catch method." It includes the following steps:

- Wash your hands.
- Clean your genital area with a cleansing pad given to you by your provider. Men should wipe the tip of their penis. Women should open their labia and clean from front to back.
- Start to urinate into the toilet.
- Move the collection container under your urine stream.
- Collect at least an ounce or two of urine into the container, which should have markings to indicate the needed amounts.
- Finish urinating into the toilet.
- Return the sample container as instructed by your health-care provider.

WILL YOU NEED TO DO ANYTHING TO PREPARE FOR THE TEST?

You do not need any special preparations before getting a test for blood in your urine. If your health-care provider has ordered other urine or blood tests, you may need to fast (not eat or drink) for several hours before the test. Your health-care provider will let you know if there are any special instructions to follow.

ARE THERE ANY RISKS TO THE TEST?

There is no known risk to having a urinalysis or a blood in urine test.

WHAT DO THE RESULTS MEAN?

There are a variety of factors that can cause RBCs or WBCs to be present in the urine. Many are not cause for concern. Small amounts of blood in the urine may be due to certain medicines, intense exercise, sexual activity, or menstruation. If larger amounts of blood are found, your health-care provider may request further testing.

Increased RBCs in urine may indicate:

- A viral infection
- Inflammation of the kidney or bladder
- A blood disorder
- Bladder or kidney cancer

Increased WBCs in urine may indicate:

- A bacterial urinary tract infection. This is the most common cause of a high WBC count in urine.
- Inflammation of the urinary tract or kidneys

To learn what your results mean, talk to your health-care provider.

Section 12.5 | **Crystals in Urine Test**

This section includes text excerpted from "Crystals in Urine," MedlinePlus, National Institutes of Health (NIH), July 31, 2020.

WHAT IS A CRYSTALS IN URINE TEST?

Your urine contains many chemicals. Sometimes these chemicals form solids, called "crystals." A crystals in urine test looks at the amount, size, and type of crystals in your urine. It is normal to have a few small urine crystals. Larger crystals or specific types of crystals can become kidney stones. Kidney stones are hard, pebble-like substances that can get stuck in the kidneys. A stone can be as small as a grain of sand, as big as a pea, or even larger. While kidney stones rarely cause serious damage, they can be very painful.

Other names include urinalysis (crystals) microscopic urine analysis, and microscopic examination of urine.

WHAT IS IT USED FOR?

A crystals in urine test is often part of a urinalysis, a test that measures different substances in your urine. A urinalysis may include a visual check of your urine sample, tests for certain chemicals, and an examination of urine cells under a microscope. A crystals in urine test is part of a microscopic exam of urine. It may be used to help diagnose kidney stones or a problem with your metabolism, the process of how your body uses food and energy.

WHY DO YOU NEED A CRYSTALS IN URINE TEST?

A urinalysis is often part of a routine checkup. Your health-care provider may include a crystals in urine test in your urinalysis if you have symptoms of a kidney stone. These include:

- Sharp pains in your abdomen, side, or groin
- Back pain
- Blood in your urine
- Frequent urge to urinate
- Pain when urinating

- Cloudy or bad-smelling urine
- Nausea and vomiting

WHAT HAPPENS DURING A CRYSTALS IN URINE TEST

You will need to provide a sample of your urine. During your office visit, you will receive a container to collect the urine and special instructions to make sure the sample is sterile. These instructions are often called the "clean catch method." The clean catch method includes the following steps:

- Wash your hands.
- Clean your genital area with a cleansing pad. Men should wipe the tip of their penis. Women should open their labia and clean from front to back.
- Start to urinate into the toilet.
- Move the collection container under your urine stream.
- Collect at least an ounce or two of urine into the container, which should have markings to indicate the amount.
- Finish urinating into the toilet.
- Return the sample container as instructed by your health-care provider.

Your health-care provider may also request that you collect all urine during a 24-hour period. This is called a "24-hour urine sample test." It is used because the amounts of substances in urine, including crystals, can vary throughout the day. Your health-care provider or a laboratory professional will give you a container to collect your urine and instructions on how to collect and store your samples. A 24-hour urine sample test usually includes the following steps:

- Empty your bladder in the morning and flush that urine away. Record the time.
- For the next 24 hours, save all your urine passed in the container provided.
- Store your urine container in the refrigerator or a cooler with ice.
- Return the sample container to your health-care provider's office or the laboratory as instructed.

WILL YOU NEED TO DO ANYTHING TO PREPARE FOR THE TEST?

You do not need any special preparations for crystals in urine test. Be sure to carefully follow all the instructions for providing a 24-hour urine sample.

ARE THERE ANY RISKS TO THE TEST?

There is no known risk to having a crystals in urine test.

WHAT DO THE RESULTS MEAN?

If a large number, large size, or certain types of crystal are found in your urine, it may mean you have a kidney stone that requires medical treatment, but it does not always mean you need treatment. Sometimes a small kidney stone can pass through your urine on its own, and cause little or no pain. Also, certain medicines, your diet, and other factors can affect your results. If you have questions about your urine crystal results, talk to your health-care provider.

Chapter 13 | Stool Tests

Chapter Contents

Section 13.1 | **Stool Culture**

WHAT IS A STOOL CULTURE?

A stool culture is a diagnostic test to detect or rule out the presence of bacterial organisms in the stool that can cause gastrointestinal (GI) symptoms, infections, and diseases. The test helps the doctor understand if there are any digestive problems in the GI tract. The laboratory staff may examine the stool under a microscope to check for any signs of ova or parasites using a dye-staining method. The following bacteria are examined in the stool:

- *Campylobacter* species
- *Salmonella* species
- *Shigella* species

The following risk factors may be analyzed if you are considering traveling outside of the United States:

- *Plesiomonas*
- *Vibrio* species
- *Yersinia enterocolitica*
- *Escherichia coli* 0157:H7
- *Aeromonas*

Other tests include a test for *Clostridium difficile* (*C. difficile*) toxin or an ova and parasite examination to look for parasites in the intestine.

HOW IS A STOOL CULTURE PERFORMED?

A sample of your stool is collected by the doctor. A clean, dry, and airtight container is used to collect the sample. The sample is sent to the laboratory for culturing and examining under a microscope. Special dyes allow the laboratory to identify the type of bacteria in the sample. The lab technician uses a special dish to place the sample. A gel is added to the sample to identify bacterial growth. After examining it, the results of the stool culture is sent to the doctor.

WHEN IS A STOOL CULTURE PERFORMED?

A stool culture is performed when the following signs and symptoms are detected in the digestive tract:

- Diarrhea with blood or mucus
- Green-colored loose stools
- Abdominal pain and cramping
- Nausea and vomiting
- Fever

Other symptoms that require a stool culture are:

- Severe dehydration, electrolyte imbalance, or other complications
- Symptoms that persist for an extended period of time and require treatment
- When fluids or food are contaminated with pathogenic bacteria
- An outbreak of foodborne or waterborne diseases

WHAT DOES THE TEST RESULT MEAN?

Your doctor will recommend follow-up steps based on the results of your stool sample. For instance, the doctor might look for signs of irritable bowel syndrome (IBS), a parasitic infection, or other problems related to GI infection. Common bacteria that are known to cause infections in the United States are:

- *Salmonella* – found in raw eggs, raw poultry, uncooked vegetables, and reptiles. Some people may carry *Salmonella* in their intestines without being ill themselves. *Salmonella* is usually transmitted from person to person.
- *Campylobacter* – found in raw or undercooked poultry and unpasteurized milk, and is one of the most common causes of bacterial diarrhea in the United States. Long-term complications might result in arthritis and Guillain-Barre syndrome.
- *Shigella* – found in contaminated food and water, and it can also pass from one infected person to another when proper sanitation and hygiene are not observed.

Other bacterial infections can be identified with a stool culture. Some examples include:

- *Escherichia coli* 0157:H7 and other toxin-producing *E. coli* – found in raw or undercooked beef, spinach, and unpasteurized cider. It causes watery stools and may eventually lead to hemolytic uremic syndrome (HUS).
- *Clostridium difficile* – toxin-producing strains that can cause diarrhea and other serious intestinal complications. Tests to detect the presence of these strains are performed separately.

Examples of other less common causes include:

- *Vibrio cholerae* and other *Vibrio* species
- *Yersinia enterocolitica*
- *Aeromonas*
- *Plesiomonas*

References

1. Case-Lo, Christine. "Stool Culture," Healthline, July 21, 2016.
2. "Fecal Culture," MedlinePlus, National Institutes of Health (NIH), April 30, 2018.
3. "Stool Culture," Lab Tests Online, June 5, 2018.

Section 13.2 | **Detecting Parasite Antigens**

This section includes text excerpted from "Stool Specimens – Detection of Parasite Antigens," Centers for Disease Control and Prevention (CDC), November 2, 2020.

The diagnosis of human intestinal protozoa depends on microscopic detection of the various parasite stages in feces, duodenal fluid, or small intestine biopsy specimens. Since fecal examination is very labor-intensive and requires a skilled microscopist, antigen detection tests have been developed as alternatives using direct fluorescent antibody (DFA), enzyme immunoassay

(EIA), and rapid, dipstick-like tests. Antigen detection methods can be performed quickly and do not require an experienced and skilled morphologist. Much work has been accomplished on the development of antigen detection tests, resulting in commercially available reagents for the intestinal parasites *Cryptosporidium* spp., *Entamoeba histolytica*, *Giardia duodenalis*, and *Trichomonas vaginalis*. In addition, antigen detection tests using blood or serum are available for *Plasmodium* and *Wuchereria bancrofti*.

SPECIMENS FOR ANTIGEN DETECTION

Fresh or preserved stool samples are the appropriate specimen for antigen detection testing with most kits, but refer to the recommended collection procedures included with each specific kit.

AMEBIASIS

The EIA kits are commercially available for detection of fecal antigens for the diagnosis of intestinal amebiasis. Organisms of both the pathogenic *E. histolytica* and the nonpathogenic *Entamoeba dispar* strains are morphologically identical. These assays use monoclonal antibodies that detect the galactose-inhibitable adherence protein in the pathogenic *E. histolytica*. The primary drawback of these assays is the requirement for fresh, unpreserved stool specimens. Several EIA kits for antigen detection of the *E. histolytica/E. dispar* group are available in the United States, but only the TechLab kit is specific for *E. histolytica*.

CRYPTOSPORIDIOSIS

Immunodetection of antigens on the surface of organisms in stool specimens, using monoclonal antibody-based DFA assays, is the current test of choice for diagnosis of cryptosporidiosis and provides increased sensitivity over modified acid-fast staining techniques. There are commercial products (DFA, IFA, EIA, and rapid tests) available in the United States for the diagnosis of cryptosporidiosis. Several kits are combined tests for *Cryptosporidium*,

Giardia, and *E. histolytica*. Factors, such as ease of use, technical skill and time, single versus batch testing, and test cost must be considered when determining the test of choice for individual laboratories. The most sensitive (99%) and specific (100%) method is reported to be the DFA test, which identifies oocysts in concentrated or unconcentrated fecal samples by using a fluorescein isothiocyanate (FITC)-labeled monoclonal antibody. A combined DFA test for the simultaneous detection of *Cryptosporidium* oocysts and *Giardia* cysts is available.

Some commercial EIA tests are available in the microplate format for the detection of *Cryptosporidium* antigens in fresh or frozen stool samples and also in stool specimens preserved in formalin, or sodium acetate-acetic acid-formalin (SAF) fixed stool specimens. Concentrated or polyvinyl alcohol-treated (PVA) samples are unsuitable for testing with available antigen detection EIA kits. The kits are reportedly superior to microscopy, especially acid-fast staining, and show a good correlation with the DFA test. Kit sensitivities and specificities reportedly range from 93 to 100 percent when used in a clinical setting. Laboratories that use these EIA kits need to be aware of potential problems with false-positive results and take steps to monitor kit performance.

Rapid immunochromatographic assays are available for the combined antigen detection of either *Cryptosporidium* and *Giardia* or *Cryptosporidium*, *Giardia*, and *E. histolytica*. These offer the advantage of short test time and multiple results in one reaction device. Initial evaluations indicate comparable sensitivity and specificity to previously available tests.

The Meridian Merifluor DFA Kit for *Cryptosporidium*/*Giardia*, modified acid-fast stain for *Cryptosporidium* spp., or Wheatley's trichrome stain for *Giardia* spp. are used at the CDC for routine identification of these parasites. These techniques can be used to confirm suspicious or discrepant diagnostic results.

GIARDIASIS

Detection of antigens on the surface of organisms in stool specimens is the current test of choice for diagnosis of giardiasis and provides increased sensitivity over more common microscopy techniques. Commercial products (DFA, EIAs, and rapid tests) are available in the United States for the immunodiagnosis of giardiasis. The DFA assays may be purchased that employ FITC-labeled monoclonal antibody for detection of *Giardia* cysts alone or in a combined kit for the simultaneous detection of *Giardia* cysts and *Cryptosporidium* oocysts. The sensitivity and specificity of these kits were both 100 percent compared to those of microscopy. They may be used for quantitation of cysts and oocysts, and thus may be useful for epidemiologic and control studies.

Some commercial EIA tests are available in the microplate format for the detection of *Giardia* antigen in fresh or frozen stool samples and also in stool specimens preserved in formalin, MIF, or SAF fixatives. Concentrated or PVA samples are not suitable for testing with EIA kits. EIA kit sensitivity rates were recently reported as ranging from 94–100 percent while specificity rates were all 100 percent.

TRICHOMONIASIS

Trichomoniasis, an infection caused by *Trichomonas vaginalis*, is a common sexually transmitted disease (STD). Diagnosis is made by detection of trophozoites in vaginal secretions or urethral specimens by wet mount microscopic examination, DFA staining of specimens, or culture. The sensitivity of the assays were reported as 60 percent for wet mounts and 86 percent for DFA when compared to cultures. A kit that employs FITC- or enzyme-labeled monoclonal antibodies for use in a DFA or EIA procedure is available for detection of whole parasites in fluids. A latex agglutination test for antigen detection in vaginal swab specimens is available; the manufacturer's evaluation indicated good sensitivity and specificity.

Table 13.1. Latex Agglutination Test for Antigen Detection in Vaginal Swab Specimens

Organism	Kit Name	Manufacturer – Distributor	Type of Test
Cryptosporidium spp.	Crypto CELISA	Cellabs	EIA
	PARA-TECT™ *Cryptosporidium* Antigen 96	Medical Chemical Corporation	EIA
	ProSpecT Rapid	Remel	EIA
	ProSpecT	Remel	EIA
	Cryptosporidium	TechLab	EIA
	Cryptosporidium	Wampole	EIA
	Crypto CEL	Cellabs	IFA
	XPect Crypto	Remel	Rapid
Cryptosporidium spp./*Giardia duodenalis*	PARA-TECT™ *Cryptosporidium*/ Giardia DFA 75	Medical Chemical Corporation	DFA
	Merifluor	Meridian	DFA
	ProSpecT	Remel	EIA
	Crypto/Giardia CEL	Cellabs	IFA
	ColorPAC	Becton Dickinson	Rapid
	ImmunoCard STAT!	Meridian	Rapid
	XPect	Remel	Rapid
Cryptosporidium spp./*Giardia duodenalis/Entamoeba histolytica/dispar*	Triage	BioSite	Rapid
Entamoeba histolytica	Entamoeba CELISA	Cellabs	EIA
	E. histolytica	Wampole	EIA
	E. histolytica II	TechLab	EIA
Entamoeba histolytica/E. dispar	ProSpecT	Remel	EIA

Table 13.1. Continued

Organism	Kit Name	Manufacturer – Distributor	Type of Test
	Giardia CELISA	Cellabs	EIA
	PARA-TECT™ Giardia Antigen 96	Medical Chemical Corporation	EIA
	ProSpecT	Remel	EIA
	Giardia II	TechLab	EIA
	Giardia	Wampole	EIA
	GiardiaEIA	Antibodies, Inc.	EIA
	Giardia CEL	Cellabs	IFA
	ProSpecT	Remel	Rapid
Giardia duodenalis	Simple-Read Giardia	Medical Chemical Corporation	Rapid
Wuchereria bancrofti	Filariasis CELISA	Cellabs	EIA

EIA = enzyme immunoassay; Rapid = immunochromatographic cartridge; DFA = direct immunofluorescence assay; IFA = indirect immunofluorescence assay.

Section 13.3 | **Fecal Occult Blood Test**

This section includes text excerpted from "Fecal Occult Blood Test (FOBT)," MedlinePlus, National Institutes of Health (NIH), July 31, 2020.

A fecal occult blood test (FOBT) looks at a sample of your stool (feces) to check for blood. Occult blood means that you cannot see it with the naked eye. Blood in the stool means there is likely some kind of bleeding in the digestive tract. It may be caused by a variety of conditions, including:

- Polyps
- Hemorrhoids
- Diverticulosis

- Ulcers
- Colitis, a type of inflammatory bowel disease (IBD)

Blood in the stool may also be a sign of colorectal cancer, a type of cancer that starts in the colon or rectum. Colorectal cancer is the second leading cause of cancer-related deaths in the United States and the third most common cancer in men and in women. A fecal occult blood test is a screening test that may help find colorectal cancer early, when treatment is most effective.

Other names: FOBT, stool occult blood, occult blood test, Hemoccult test, guaiac smear test, gFOBT, immunochemical FOBT, iFOBT; and FIT

WHAT IS FECAL OCCULT BLOOD TEST USED FOR?

A FOBT is used as an early screening test for colorectal cancer. It may also be used to diagnose other conditions that cause bleeding in the digestive tract.

WHY DO YOU NEED A FECAL OCCULT BLOOD TEST?

The National Cancer Institute (NCI) recommends that people get regular screenings for colorectal cancer starting at age 50. The screening may be a fecal occult test or another type of screening test. These tests may include:

- **A stool deoxyribonucleic acid (DNA) test.** For this test, you can use an at-home test kit to take a sample of your stool and return it to a lab. It will be checked for blood and genetic changes that may be signs of cancer. If the test is positive, you will need a colonoscopy.
- **A colonoscopy.** This is a minor surgical procedure. You will first be given a mild sedative to help you relax. Then a health-care provider will use a thin tube to look inside your colon.

There are advantages and disadvantages to each type of test. Talk to your health-care provider about which test is right for you.

If your provider recommends an FOBT, you need to get it every year. A stool DNA test should be taken every three years, and a colonoscopy should be done every ten years.

You may need screening more often if you have certain risk factors. These include:

- A family history of colorectal cancer
- Cigarette smoking
- Obesity
- Excessive alcohol use

WHAT HAPPENS DURING A FECAL OCCULT BLOOD TEST

An FOBT is a noninvasive test that you can perform at home at your convenience. Your health-care provider will give you a kit that includes instructions on how to do the test. There are two main types of FOBTs: the guaiac smear method (gFOBT) and the immunochemical method (iFOBT or FIT). Below are typical instructions for each test. Your instructions may vary slightly depending on the manufacturer of the test kit.

For a guaiac smear test (gFOBT), you will most likely need to:

- Collect samples from three separate bowel movements.
- For each sample, collect the stool and store it in a clean container. Make sure the sample does not mix in with urine or water from the toilet.
- Use the applicator from your test kit to smear some of the stool on the test card or slide, also included in your kit.
- Label and seal all your samples as directed.
- Mail the samples to your health-care provider or lab.

For a fecal immunochemical test (FIT), you will most likely need to:

- Collect samples from two or three bowel movements.
- Collect the sample from the toilet using the special brush or other device that was included in your kit.
- For each sample, use the brush or device to take the sample from the surface of the stool.
- Brush the sample onto a test card.

- Label and seal all your samples as directed.
- Mail the samples to your health-care provider or lab.

Be sure to follow all the instructions provided in your kit, and talk to your health-care provider if you have any questions.

WILL YOU NEED TO DO ANYTHING TO PREPARE FOR THE TEST?

Certain foods and drugs may affect the results of a guaiac smear method (gFOBT) test. Your health-care provider may ask you to avoid the following:

- Nonsteroidal anti-inflammatory drugs (NSAIDs), such as ibuprofen, naproxen, or aspirin for seven days prior to your test. If you take aspirin for heart problems, talk to your health-care provider before stopping your medicine. Acetaminophen may be safe to use during this time, but check with your health-care provider before taking it.
- More than 250 mg of vitamin C daily from supplements, fruit juices, or fruit for seven days prior to your test. Vitamin C can affect the chemicals in the test and cause a negative result even if there is blood present.
- Red meat, such as beef, lamb, and pork, for three days prior to the test. Traces of blood in these meats may cause a false-positive result.

There are no special preparations or dietary restrictions for a fecal immunochemical test (FIT).

ARE THERE ANY RISKS TO THE TEST?

There is no known risk to having a FOBT.

WHAT DO THE RESULTS MEAN?

If your results are positive for either type of fecal occult blood test, it means you likely have bleeding somewhere in your digestive tract. But, it does not necessarily mean you have cancer. Other conditions that may produce a positive result on a FOBT include ulcers, hemorrhoids, polyps, and benign tumors. If your test results are positive for blood, your health-care provider will likely recommend additional testing, such as a colonoscopy, to figure out the exact location and cause of your bleeding. If you have questions about your results, talk to your health-care provider.

IS THERE ANYTHING ELSE YOU NEED TO KNOW ABOUT A FECAL OCCULT BLOOD TEST?

Regular colorectal cancer screenings, such as the FOBT, are an important tool in the fight against cancer. Studies show that screening tests can help find cancer early, and may reduce deaths from the disease.

Chapter 14 | Yeast Infection Test

WHAT IS A YEAST INFECTION TEST?

Yeast is a type of fungus that can live on the skin, mouth, digestive tract, and genitals. Some yeast in the body is normal, but if there is an overgrowth of yeast on your skin or other areas, it can cause an infection. A yeast test can help determine whether you have a yeast infection. Candidiasis is another name for a yeast infection.

Other names include potassium hydroxide preparation, fungal culture; fungal antigen and antibody tests, calcofluor white stain, and fungal smear.

WHAT IS YEAST INFECTION TEST USED FOR?

A yeast test is used to diagnose and detect yeast infections. There are different methods of yeast testing, depending on where you have symptoms.

WHY DO YOU NEED A YEAST INFECTION TEST?

Your health-care provider may order a test if you have symptoms of a yeast infection. Your symptoms will vary, depending on where the infection is on your body. Yeast infections tend to happen in moist areas of the skin and mucous membranes. Below are symptoms of some common types of yeast infections. Your individual symptoms may vary.

Yeast infections on the folds of the skin include conditions such as athlete's foot and diaper rash. Symptoms include:

This chapter includes text excerpted from "Yeast Infection Tests," MedlinePlus, National Institutes of Health (NIH), July 31, 2020.

- Bright red rash, often redness or ulcers in the skin
- Itching
- Burning sensation
- Pimples

Yeast infections on the vagina are common. Nearly 75 percent of women will get at least one yeast infection in their lifetime. Symptoms include:

- Genital itching and/or burning
- A white, cottage cheese-like discharge
- Painful urination
- Redness in the vagina

Yeast infection of the penis may cause:

- Redness
- Scaling
- Rash

Yeast infection of the mouth is called "thrush." It is common in young children. Thrush in adults may indicate a weakened immune system. Symptoms include:

- White patches on the tongue and inside of cheeks
- Soreness on the tongue and inside of cheeks

Yeast infection at the corners of the mouth may be caused by thumb sucking, ill-fitting dentures, or frequent licking of the lips. Symptoms include:

- Cracks and tiny cuts at the corners of the mouth

Yeast infection in the nail beds can happen in the fingers or toes, but are more common in toenails. Symptoms include:

- Pain and redness around the nail
- Discoloration of nail
- Cracks in the nail
- Swelling
- Pus
- White or yellow nail that separates from nail bed

WHAT HAPPENS DURING A YEAST INFECTION TEST

The type of test depends on the location of your symptoms:

- If a vaginal yeast infection is suspected, your health-care provider will perform a pelvic exam and take a sample of the discharge from your vagina.
- If thrush is suspected, your health-care provider will look at the infected area in the mouth and may also take a small scraping to examine under the microscope.
- If a yeast infection is suspected on the skin or nails, your health-care provider may use a blunt-edged instrument to scrape off a small bit of skin or part of a nail for examination. During this type of test, you may feel some pressure and a little discomfort.

Your health-care provider may be able to tell if you have a yeast infection just by examining the infected area and looking at the cells under a microscope. If there are not enough cells to detect an infection, you may need a culture test. During a culture test, the cells in your sample will be put in a special environment in a lab to encourage cell growth. Results are often available within a few days. But, some yeast infections grow slowly, and it may take weeks to get a result.

WILL YOU NEED TO DO ANYTHING TO PREPARE FOR THE YEAST INFECTION TEST?

You do not need any special preparations for a yeast test.

ARE THERE ANY RISKS TO THE YEAST INFECTION TEST?

There is no known risk to having a yeast test.

WHAT DO THE RESULTS MEAN?

If your results indicate a yeast infection, your health-care provider may recommend an over-the-counter (OTC) antifungal medicine or prescribe an antifungal medicine. Depending on where your infection is, you may need a vaginal suppository, a medicine applied directly to the skin, or a pill. Your health-care provider will tell you which treatment is best for you.

It is important to take all your medicine as prescribed, even if you feel better sooner. Many yeast infections get better after a few days or weeks of treatment, but certain fungal infections may need to be treated for several months or longer before they clear up.

IS THERE ANYTHING ELSE YOU NEED TO KNOW ABOUT A YEAST INFECTION TEST?

Certain antibiotics can also cause an overgrowth of yeast. Be sure to tell your health-care provider about any medicines you are taking.

Yeast infections of the blood, heart, and brain are less common, but more serious than yeast infections of the skin and genitals. Serious yeast infections occur more often in hospital patients and in people with weakened immune systems.

Chapter 15 | **Drug Testing**

WHAT IS A DRUG TEST?

A drug test looks for the presence of one or more illegal or prescription drugs in your urine, blood, saliva, hair, or sweat. Urine testing is the most common type of drug screening. The drugs most often tested for include:

- Marijuana
- Opioids, such as heroin, codeine, oxycodone, morphine, hydrocodone, and fentanyl
- Amphetamines, including methamphetamine
- Cocaine
- Steroids
- Barbiturates, such as phenobarbital and secobarbital
- Phencyclidine (PCP)

Other names include drug screen, drug test, drugs of abuse testing, substance abuse testing, toxicology screen, tox screen, and sports doping tests.

WHAT IS IT USED FOR?

Drug screening is used to find out whether or not a person has taken a certain drug or drugs. It may be used for:

- **Employment.** Employers may test you before hiring and/or after hiring to check for on-the-job drug use.
- **Sports organizations.** Professional and collegiate athletes usually need to take a test for performance-enhancing drugs or other substances.

This chapter includes text excerpted from "Drug Testing," MedlinePlus, National Institutes of Health (NIH), July 31, 2020.

- **Legal or forensic purposes.** Testing may be part of a criminal or motor vehicle accident investigation. Drug screening may also be ordered as part of a court case.
- **Monitoring opioid use.** If you have been prescribed an opioid for chronic pain, your health-care provider may order a drug test to make sure you are taking the right amount of your medicine.

WHY DO YOU NEED A DRUG TEST?

Your health-care provider may order drug screening if you have symptoms of drug abuse. These symptoms include:

- Slowed or slurred speech
- Dilated or small pupils
- Agitation
- Panic
- Paranoia
- Delirium
- Difficulty breathing
- Nausea
- Changes in blood pressure or heart rhythm

WHAT HAPPENS DURING A DRUG TEST

A drug test generally requires that you give a urine sample in a lab. You will be given instructions to provide a "clean catch" sample. The clean catch method includes the following steps:

- Wash your hands.
- Clean your genital area with a cleansing pad given to you by your provider. Men should wipe the tip of their penis. Women should open their labia and clean from front to back.
- Start to urinate into the toilet.
- Move the collection container under your urine stream.
- Collect at least an ounce or two of urine into the container, which should have markings to indicate the amounts.
- Finish urinating into the toilet.

- Return the sample container to the lab technician or health-care provider.

In certain instances, a medical technician or other staff member may need to be present while you provide your sample.

For a blood test for drugs, you will go to a lab to provide your sample. During the test, a health-care professional will take a blood sample from a vein in your arm, using a small needle. After the needle is inserted, a small amount of blood will be collected into a test tube or vial. You may feel a little sting when the needle goes in or out. This usually takes less than five minutes.

WILL YOU NEED TO DO ANYTHING TO PREPARE FOR THE TEST?

Be sure to tell the testing provider or your health-care provider if you are taking any prescription drugs, over-the-counter (OTC) medicines, or supplements because they may give you a positive result for certain illegal drugs. Also, you should avoid foods with poppy seeds, which can cause a positive result for opioids.

ARE THERE ANY RISKS TO THE TEST?

There are no known physical risks to having a drug test, but a positive result may affect other aspects of your life, including your job, your eligibility to play sports, and the outcome of a court case.

Before you take a drug test, you should be told what you are being tested for, why you are being tested, and how the results will be used. If you have questions or concerns about your test, talk to your health-care provider or contact the individual or organization that ordered the test.

WHAT DO THE RESULTS MEAN?

If your results are negative, it means no drugs were found in your body, or the level of drugs was below an established level, which differs depending on the drug. If your results are positive, it means one or more drugs were found in your body above an established level. However, false positives can happen. So if your first test shows that you have drugs in your system, you will have further testing to figure out whether or not you are actually taking a certain drug or drugs.

IS THERE ANYTHING ELSE YOU NEED TO KNOW ABOUT A DRUG TEST?

If you test positive for a legal drug prescribed by your doctor, your employer cannot penalize you for a positive result, unless the drug is affecting your ability to perform your job.

If you test positive for marijuana and live in state where it has been legalized, employers may be able penalize you. Many employers want to maintain a drug-free workplace. Also, marijuana is still illegal under federal law.

Part 3 | **Imaging Tests**

Chapter 16 | Medical Imaging: Benefits and Risks

Medical imaging tests are noninvasive procedures that allow doctors to diagnose diseases and injuries without being intrusive. Some of these tests involve exposure to ionizing radiation, which can present risks to patients. However, if patients understand the benefits and risks, they can make the best decisions about choosing a particular medical imaging procedure.

Most people have had one or more medical imaging tests. Imaging procedures are medical tests that allow doctors to see inside the body in order to diagnose, treat, and monitor health conditions. Doctors often use medical imaging procedures to determine the best treatment options for patients. The type of imaging procedure that your doctor may suggest will depend on your health concern and the part of the body that is being examined. Some common examples of imaging tests include:

- X-rays (including dental x-rays, chest x-rays, spine x-rays)
- Computed tomography (CT) or CAT scans
- Fluoroscopy

If your doctor suggests x-rays or other medical imaging tests, you should consider the following:

This chapter includes text excerpted from "Radiation in Medicine: Medical Imaging Procedures," Centers for Disease Control and Prevention (CDC), November 10, 2020.

- Medical imaging tests should be performed only when necessary.
- The U.S. Food and Drug Administration (FDA) recommends discussing the benefits and risks of medical imaging procedures with your doctor.

BENEFITS AND RISKS OF MEDICAL IMAGING PROCEDURES THAT USE IONIZING RADIATION

Medical imaging tests can help doctors:

- Obtain a better view of organs, blood vessels, tissues and bones
- Determine whether surgery is a good treatment option
- Guide medical procedures involving placement of catheters, stents, or other devices inside the body, locate tumors for treatment and locate blood clots or other blockages
- Guide joint replacement options and treatment of fractures

As in many areas of medicine, there are risks associated with the use of medical imaging which uses ionizing radiation to create images of the body. Risks from exposure to ionizing radiation include:

- A small increase in the likelihood that a person exposed to radiation will develop cancer later in life
- Health effects that could occur after a large acute exposure to ionizing radiation such as skin reddening and hair loss
- Possible allergic reactions associated with a contrast dye injected into the veins to better see body structures being examined

HOW CAN YOU REDUCE YOUR EXPOSURE TO DIAGNOSTIC IONIZING RADIATION?

In the case of x-rays or other tests involving exposure to ionizing radiation, doctors and radiation experts can help reduce your exposure to and risk of harm from diagnostic ionizing radiation by:

- Checking to see if you have had a similar test done recently that can provide them with the background information they need
- Checking to see if a test that does not use ionizing radiation can provide similar information
- Making certain the least possible amount of radiation needed to obtain a good quality image is used for your procedure
- Providing protective lead shielding to prevent exposing other areas of the body to radiation

WHAT ARE THE RISKS OF MEDICAL IMAGING PROCEDURES FOR PREGNANT WOMEN?

Talk to your physician about the potential risks and benefits from the medical procedures. In many cases, the risk of an x-ray procedure to the mother and the unborn child is very small compared to the benefit of finding out about the medical condition of the mother or the child.

However, small risks should not be taken if they are unnecessary. You can reduce risks from medical imaging procedures by telling your doctor if you are, or think you might be, pregnant whenever an abdominal x-ray is suggested by your doctor. Other options suggested by FDA that may be considered are as follows:

- If you are pregnant, the doctor may decide that it would be best to cancel the medical imaging procedure, to postpone it, or to modify it to reduce the amount of radiation.
- Depending on your medical needs, and realizing that the risk is very small, the doctor may feel that it is best to proceed with using a medical imaging procedure as planned.

In any case, you should feel free to discuss the decision with your doctor.

ARE THERE SPECIAL CONSIDERATIONS FOR CHILDREN?

It is important that x-rays and other imaging procedures performed on children use the lowest exposure setting needed to obtain a good clinical image. The Image Gently Alliance, part of the Alliance for Radiation in Pediatric Imaging, suggests the following for imaging of children:

- Use imaging examinations when the medical benefit outweighs the risk.
- Use the most appropriate imaging techniques, matched to the size of the child.
- Use alternative imaging methods (such as ultrasound or magnetic resonance imaging (MRI)) when possible.

Chapter 17 | **Medical X-rays**

Chapter Contents

Section 17.1 | **Medical X-rays – Basics**

This section contains text excerpted from the following sources: Text beginning with the heading "What Are Medical X-rays?" is excerpted from "X-rays," National Institute of Biomedical Imaging and Bioengineering (NIBIB), February 29, 2016. Reviewed October 2021; Text under the heading "Radiography" is excerpted from "Radiography," U.S. Food and Drug Administration (FDA), September 28, 2020.

WHAT ARE MEDICAL X-RAYS?

X-rays are a form of electromagnetic radiation, similar to visible light. Unlike light, however, x-rays have higher energy and can pass through most objects, including the body. Medical x-rays are used to generate images of tissues and structures inside the body. If x-rays traveling through the body also pass through an x-ray detector on the other side of the patient, an image will be formed that represents the "shadows" formed by the objects inside the body.

One type of x-ray detector is photographic film, but there are many other types of detectors that are used to produce digital images. The x-ray images that result from this process are called "radiographs."

HOW DO MEDICAL X-RAYS WORK?

To create a radiograph, a patient is positioned so that the part of the body being imaged is located between an x-ray source and an x-ray detector. When the machine is turned on, x-rays travel through the body and are absorbed in different amounts by different tissues, depending on the radiological density of the tissues they pass through. Radiological density is determined by both the density and the atomic number (the number of protons in an atom's nucleus) of the materials being imaged. For example, structures such as bone contain calcium, which has a higher atomic number than most tissues. Because of this property, bones readily absorb x-rays and, thus, produce high contrast on the x-ray detector. As a result, bony structures appear whiter than other tissues against the black background of a radiograph. Conversely, x-rays travel more easily through less radiologically dense tissues such as fat and muscle, as well as through air-filled cavities such as the lungs. These structures are displayed in shades of gray on a radiograph.

WHEN ARE MEDICAL X-RAYS USED?

Listed below are examples of examinations and procedures that use x-ray technology to either diagnose or treat disease:

Diagnostic Purposes

X-ray radiography. Detects bone fractures, certain tumors and other abnormal masses, pneumonia, some types of injuries, calcifications, foreign objects, dental problems, etc.

Mammography. A radiograph of the breast that is used for cancer detection and diagnosis. Tumors tend to appear as regular or irregular-shaped masses that are somewhat brighter than the background on the radiograph (i.e., whiter on a black background or blacker on a white background). Mammograms can also detect tiny bits of calcium, called "microcalcifications," which show up as very bright specks on a mammogram. While usually benign, microcalcifications may occasionally indicate the presence of a specific type of cancer.

Computed tomography (CT). Combines traditional x-ray technology with computer processing to generate a series of cross-sectional images of the body that can later be combined to form a three-dimensional x-ray image. CT images are more detailed than plain radiographs and give doctors the ability to view structures within the body from many different angles.

Fluoroscopy. Uses x-rays and a fluorescent screen to obtain real-time images of movement within the body or to view diagnostic processes, such as following the path of an injected or swallowed contrast agent. For example, fluoroscopy is used to view the movement of the beating heart, and, with the aid of radiographic contrast agents, to view blood flow to the heart muscle as well as through blood vessels and organs. This technology is also used with a radiographic contrast agent to guide an internally threaded catheter during cardiac angioplasty, which is a minimally invasive procedure for opening clogged arteries that supply blood to the heart.

Therapeutic Purposes

Radiation therapy in cancer treatment. X-rays and other types of high-energy radiation can be used to destroy cancerous tumors and cells by damaging their deoxyribonucleic acid (DNA). The radiation dose used for treating cancer is much higher than the radiation dose used for diagnostic imaging. Therapeutic radiation can come from a machine outside of the body or from a radioactive material that is placed in the body, inside or near tumor cells, or injected into the blood stream.

ARE THERE RISKS?

When used appropriately, the diagnostic benefits of x-ray scans significantly outweigh the risks. X-ray scans can diagnose possibly life-threatening conditions such as blocked blood vessels, bone cancer, and infections. However, x-rays produce ionizing radiation – a form of radiation that has the potential to harm living tissue. This is a risk that increases with the number of exposures added up over the life of the individual. However, the risk of developing cancer from radiation exposure is generally small.

An x-ray in a pregnant woman poses no known risks to the baby if the area of the body being imaged is not the abdomen or pelvis. In general, if imaging of the abdomen and pelvis is needed, doctors prefer to use exams that do not use radiation, such as magnetic resonance imaging (MRI) or ultrasound. However, if neither of those can provide the answers needed, or there is an emergency or other time constraint, an x-ray may be an acceptable alternative imaging option.

Children are more sensitive to ionizing radiation and have a longer life expectancy and, thus, a higher relative risk for developing cancer than adults. Parents may want to ask the technologist or doctor if their machine settings have been adjusted for children.

RADIOGRAPHY

Medical radiography is a broad term that covers several types of studies that require the visualization of the internal parts of the body using x-ray techniques. For the purposes of this page radiography means a technique for generating and recording an x-ray pattern for the purpose of providing the user with a static image(s) after termination of the exposure. It is differentiated from fluoroscopy, mammography, and computed tomography. Radiography may also be used during the planning of radiation therapy treatment.

It is used to diagnose or treat patients by recording images of the internal structure of the body to assess the presence or absence of disease, foreign objects, and structural damage or anomaly.

During a radiographic procedure, an x-ray beam is passed through the body. A portion of the x-rays are absorbed or scattered by the internal structure and the remaining x-ray pattern is transmitted to a detector so that an image may be recorded for later evaluation. The recoding of the pattern may occur on film or through electronic means.

Uses of Radiography

Radiography is used in many types of examinations and procedures where a record of a static image is desired. Some examples include:

- Dental examination
- Verification of correct placement of surgical markers prior to invasive procedures
- Mammography
- Orthopedic evaluations
- Spot film or static recording during fluoroscopy
- Chiropractic examinations

Risks or Benefits of Radiography

Radiography is a type of x-ray procedure, and it carries the same types of risks as other x-ray procedures. The radiation dose the patient receives varies depending on the individual procedure, but is generally less than that received during fluoroscopy and computed tomography procedures.

The major risks associated with radiography are the small possibilities of:

- Developing a radiation-induced cancer or cataracts some time later in life, and
- Causing a disturbance in the growth or development of an embryo or fetus (teratogenic defect) when

performed on a pregnant patient or one of childbearing age.

When an individual has a medical need, the benefit of radiography far exceeds the small cancer risk associated with the procedure. Even when radiography is medically necessary, it should use the lowest possible exposure and the minimum number of images. In most cases many of the possible risks can be reduced or eliminated with proper shielding.

Section 17.2 | **Chest X-ray**

This section includes text excerpted from the following sources. Text under the headings marked 1 are © 2022 Omnigraphics. Reviewed October 2021; Text under the headings marked 2 are excerpted from "Chest X-ray," National Heart, Lung, and Blood Institute (NHLBI), December 9, 2016. Reviewed October 2021.

WHAT IS A CHEST X-RAY?[1]

Chest x-ray, also known as "chest radiography," is a commonly performed diagnostic test that produces images of the heart, lungs, blood vessels, and bones of the chest with the help of a small dose of focused beams of radiation.

WHY IS A CHEST X-RAY DONE?[1]

A chest x-ray can help diagnose cause for symptoms such as:

- Chronic cough
- Chest pain
- Breathing difficulty
- Prolonged fever

A health-care provider may also use x-rays to monitor:

- **Heart-related lung problems.** Chest x-rays may help identify specific conditions of the lung that are a result of heart problems. For example, congestive heart failure can cause the lungs to fill with fluid.

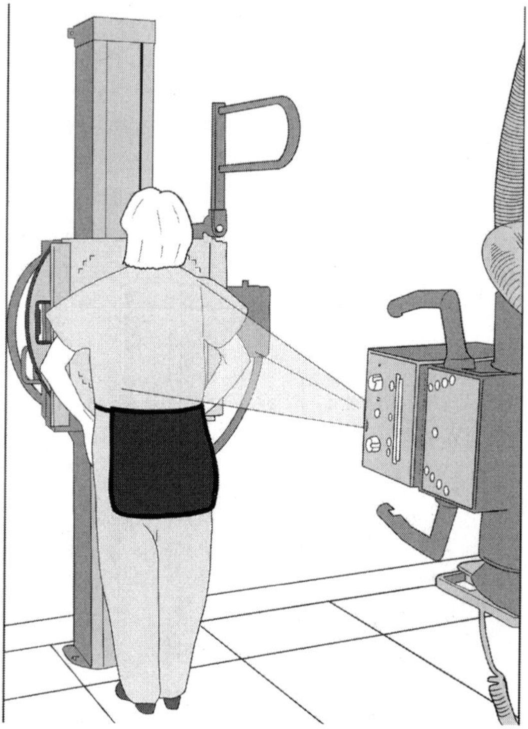

Figure 17.1. Chest X-ray Procedure

- **Size and outline of the heart.** Problems in the heart valves and fluid in the heart may change the size and shape of the heart and lead to heart failure.
- **Condition of the lungs.** Chest x-rays can help detect the presence of cancer, infection, or air collecting around the lungs that may lead to lung collapse. It can also detect chronic lung conditions such as cystic fibrosis, emphysema, and pneumonia.
- **Fractures.** A broken bone in the ribs or spine can be detected on an x-ray.
- **Blood vessels.** Large vessels such as the pulmonary artery, aorta, and veins are visible in an x-ray and may reveal conditions such as aortic aneurysms and other blood vessel problems.

- **Calcium deposits.** Calcium that has been accumulated in the heart or blood vessels can be detected via an x-ray. Its presence may also indicate damage to heart valves and muscles, coronary artery, the protective sac surrounding the heart, and presence of fats and other substances in your vessels.
- **Postoperative changes.** A doctor can monitor the heart, lungs, or esophagus' recovery after chest surgery.
- **A pacemaker, defibrillator, or catheter.** A chest x-ray helps to check the positions of these medical devices to make sure they are in their correct places.

HOW IS A CHEST X-RAY PERFORMED?[2]

The test may be done in the doctor's office, clinic, hospital, or other medical facility. Before having a chest x-ray, you will undress from the waist up, wear a gown, and remove jewelry and objects that could interfere with the test. You will stand, sit, or lie still for the test. A lead apron may be worn to protect your reproductive organs from the x-ray. The technician will operate the x-ray machine from behind a wall or in the next room. Usually, the technician takes two views, one from straight on and one from the side of your chest, but more views may be taken. A radiologist will analyze the images and send a report to your doctor.

LIMITATIONS OF CHEST X-RAYS[1]

Although chest x-rays are beneficial, some conditions such as blood clots in the lungs, cancers, and pulmonary embolism cannot be detected on a conventional x-ray image. Therefore, additional imaging studies may be required to investigate abnormalities not visible in a chest x-ray.

RISKS OF CHEST X-RAYS[2]

Chest x-rays have few risks. The amount of radiation used in a chest x-ray is very small. Talk to your doctor and the technicians performing the test about whether you are or could be pregnant. If the procedure is not urgent, they may have you wait to do the test until after your pregnancy. If it is urgent, the technicians will take extra steps to protect your baby during this test.

References

1. "Chest X-ray," National Heart, Lung, and Blood Institute (NHLBI), December 9, 2016.
2. "X-ray (Radiography) – Chest," RadiologyInfo.org, June 15, 2020.
3. "Chest X-rays," Mayo Clinic, May 2, 2020.

Section 17.3 | **Dental Imaging**

WHAT IS DENTAL IMAGING?

Dental imaging refers to the practice of creating pictures of a person's mouth and teeth using x-rays. X-rays, also known as "radiographs," are electromagnetic waves of energy that can pass through many materials including bones and teeth. Because different materials absorb x-rays to varying degrees, x-rays are used to show the internal composition of things that are not normally visible. X-rays provide dentists with a way to see inside a person's teeth and jawbone without surgery or other invasive procedures. X-rays are an important part of good dental care and are the most commonly used form of radiograph technology.

Dentists use x-rays to identify, diagnose, and monitor dental health issues for their patients. Dental x-rays allow dentists and other medical professionals to see details of teeth, bones, and mouth tissue. X-rays are used to examine the roots of teeth and their position within the jaw, locate cavities, diagnose dental diseases and other problems, and monitor the development of teeth.

DENTAL IMAGING PROCEDURES

Dental x-rays are classified in two groups: intraoral and extraoral. To create intraoral x-rays, technicians place x-ray film inside a person's mouth. Extraoral x-rays are created using film that is located outside the mouth.

Intraoral x-rays result in a highly detailed images and are the most common form of dental imaging. There are four main types of intraoral dental x-ray that are used to examine different aspects of the teeth and mouth. Intraoral x-ray procedures are painless and quick, usually taking only a few seconds to complete.

- Bite-wing x-rays are used to see examine the crowns of teeth in the back of the mouth, including the molars and bicuspids. To create bite-wing x-ray images, the technician asks the patient to bite down on a device that holds the x-ray film while the image is created.
- Periapical x-rays are used to examine one or two teeth in full, including the entire length of the tooth from crown to root. The procedure for periapical x-rays is similar to that of bite-wing x-rays.
- A full-mouth radiographic survey, or FMX, is a set of intraoral x-rays that includes images of every tooth from crown to root, including supporting tissue. An FMX survey is created using both bite-wing and periapical x-rays.
- Occlusal x-rays are used to produce images that are larger than other types of dental imaging, including the full arch of teeth in either the upper or lower jaw. Occlusal x-rays are most often used to monitor the dental health of children.

Extraoral x-rays provide fewer details than intraoral x-rays, and are generally used to create images that provide a broad view of a person's teeth, jaw, and skull. Dentists use extraoral x-rays to monitor the growth of teeth, the position of teeth in relation to the bones of the jaw and face, and the position of teeth relative to each other within the jaw bone. There are five main types of extraoral x-rays.

- Panoramic x-rays allow dentists and other medical professionals to create a single image of the entire mouth, including all the teeth and upper and lower jaws. Panoramic x-rays are created using a machine that directs x-rays forward from behind the head, while the film is gradually moved from one side of the face to the other. The panoramic x-ray machine holds a fixed position and the film moves on a fixed path. The procedure requires people to be positioned with attachments that hold the head and jaw in place for the duration of the x-ray. The procedure is safe, painless, and typically takes only a few minutes to complete.
- Cephalometric projections are extraoral x-rays that provide a view of the entire side of a person's head. These images are used to examine a person's profile and the location of their teeth in relation to the jaw. These x-rays are most often used by orthodontists in planning treatment strategies.
- Cone-beam computed tomography (CT) is a type of extraoral x-ray that is used to create three-dimensional images of a person's entire head. During this procedure, a person stands or sits without moving while the x-ray machine moves around their head. These images are most often used to determine treatment strategies for people who need dental implants.
- Standard computed tomography is a type of dental imaging procedure that is usually conducted at a hospital or a radiologist's office. The procedure usually requires a person to lie down while the image is created. These images are similar to cone-beam computed tomography and are used for similar purposes.
- Digital radiography is a type of dental imaging that replaces standard x-ray film with a tablet computer or other type of sensor. Digital x-ray images are created and stored as computer files. These images can then be viewed on screen or printed.

RADIATION AND RADIATION DOSE

X-ray images are created through the use of emitted radiation (electromagnetic energy waves). Radiation dose is the measurement of the amount of energy that is absorbed when a person is exposed to x-rays. Dental and medical x-rays emit extremely small doses of radiation. Excessive absorption of radiation can cause health problems, and people working with x-rays or those who are exposed to many x-rays over time should take precautions to protect themselves.

Modern x-ray machines are built to limit the amount of emitted radiation to the smallest possible effective dose. Dental x-ray machines generally emit radiation in a narrow beam that is less than three inches in diameter. Very little radiation is emitted outside of this beam. Modern x-ray film has also been engineered to produce images using the smallest possible amount of radiation. Film holders keep x-ray films in place without the need for people to directly handle the film. Digital radiography further reduces the emitted radiation dose by as much as 80 percent. X-ray procedures commonly include the use of lead shields or aprons that cover patients from the neck to the knees. A lead collar is also sometimes used for further protection of people with thyroid disease or other specific health concerns. Lead blocks emitted radiation and therefore protects the body from harm. To limit exposure to x-ray radiation over time, x-ray technicians typically leave the procedure room and operate x-ray machines remotely.

DENTAL RADIOLOGY AND PREGNANCY

Pregnant women and their fetuses are considered to be at a higher risk of physical damage from excessive radiation exposure over time. Although dental x-rays expose people to extremely small doses of radiation, it is common practice to protect pregnant women with lead aprons when creating dental x-rays.

References

1. "Radiation Protection of Patients: Dental Radiology – X-rays," International Atomic Energy Agency, 2013.

2. "Treatments and Procedures: Types of Dental X-rays," Cleveland Clinic Foundation, 2015.
3. "Types of X-rays," Aetna, 2013.

Section 17.4 | Bone Density Scan

This section includes text excerpted from "Bone Density Scan," MedlinePlus, National Institutes of Health (NIH), September 16, 2021.

WHAT IS A BONE DENSITY SCAN?

A bone density scan, also known as a "DEXA scan," is a type of low-dose x-ray test that measures calcium and other minerals in your bones. The measurement helps show the strength and thickness (known as "bone density" or "mass") of your bones. Most people's bones become thinner as they get older. When bones become thinner than normal, it is known as "osteopenia." Osteopenia puts you at risk for a more serious condition called "osteoporosis." Osteoporosis is a progressive disease that causes bones to become very thin and brittle. Osteoporosis usually affects older people and is most common in women over the age of 65. People with osteoporosis are at higher risk for fractures (broken bones), especially in their hips, spine, and wrists. Other names include bone mineral density test, BMD test, DEXA scan, DXA; dual-energy x-ray absorptiometry.

WHAT IS IT USED FOR?

A bone density scan is used to:

- Diagnose osteopenia (low bone mass)
- Diagnose osteoporosis
- Predict risk of future fractures
- See if treatment for osteoporosis is working

WHY DO YOU NEED A BONE DENSITY SCAN?

Most women age 65 or older should have a bone density scan. Women in this age group are at high risk for losing bone density, which can lead to fractures. You may also be at risk for low bone density if you:

- Have a very low body weight
- Have had one or more fractures after the age of 50
- Have lost a half inch or more in height within one year
- Are a man over the age of 70
- Have a family history of osteoporosis

Other risk factors include:

- Lack of physical activity
- Smoking cigarettes
- Heavy drinking
- Not getting enough calcium and in your diet

WHAT HAPPENS DURING A BONE DENSITY SCAN

There are different ways to measure bone density. The most common and accurate way uses a procedure called "dual-energy x-ray absorptiometry," also known as a "DEXA scan." The scan is usually done in a radiologist's office.

During a DEXA Scan

- You will lie on your back on a padded table. You will probably be able to leave your clothes on.
- You may need to lie with your legs straight, or you may be asked to rest your legs on a padded platform.
- A scanning machine will pass over your lower spine and hip. At the same time, another scanning machine called a "photon generator" will pass beneath you. The images from the two machines will be combined and sent to a computer. A health-care provider will view the images on the computer screen.
- While the machines are scanning, you will need to stay very still. You may be asked to hold your breath.

To measure bone density in the forearm, finger, hand, or foot, a provider may use a portable scanner known as a "peripheral DEXA" (p-DEXA) scan.

WILL YOU NEED TO DO ANYTHING TO PREPARE FOR THE TEST?

You may be told to stop taking calcium supplements 24 to 48 hours before your test. Also, you should avoid wearing metal jewelry or clothes with metal parts, such as buttons or buckles.

ARE THERE ANY RISKS TO THE TEST?

A bone density scan uses very low doses of radiation. It is safe for most people. But, it is not recommended for pregnant woman. Even low doses of radiation could harm an unborn baby. Be sure to tell your provider if you are pregnant or think you may be pregnant.

WHAT DO THE RESULTS MEAN?

Bone density results are often given in the form of a T score. A T score is a measurement that compares your bone density measurement with the bone density of a healthy 30-year-old. A low T score means you probably have some bone loss.

Your results may show one of the following:

- **A T score of -1.0 or higher.** This is considered normal bone density.
- **A T score between -1.0 and -2.5.** This means you have low bone density (osteopenia) and may be at risk for developing osteoporosis.
- **A T score of -2.5 or less.** This means you probably have osteoporosis.

If your results show you have low bone density, your health-care provider will recommend steps to prevent further bone loss. These may include:

- Getting more exercise, with activities such walking, dancing, and using weight machines.
- Adding calcium and vitamin D to your diet
- Taking prescription medicines to increase bone density

If you have questions about your results and/or treatments for bone loss, talk to your health-care provider.

Section 17.5 | **Fluoroscopy**

This section includes text excerpted from "Radiation in Medicine – Fluoroscopy," Centers for Disease Control and Prevention (CDC), November 8, 2016. Reviewed October 2021.

Fluoroscopy is a medical imaging test that uses an x-ray beam that passes continuously through the body to create an image. The image is projected on a monitor which allows doctors to see the movement of internal organs in real-time.

Medical imaging procedures such as fluoroscopy play a valuable role in preventing health problems and diagnosing diseases. During a hospital stay or outpatient procedures your doctor may request that you undergo fluoroscopy to determine treatment procedures for a particular health concern. Fluoroscopy procedures involve exposure to ionizing radiation, which can present risks. However, if patients understand the benefits and risks they can make the best decisions about their healthcare.

WHAT ARE SOME COMMON MEDICAL IMAGING TESTS THAT USE IONIZING RADIATION?

Most people have had one or more medical imaging tests that use ionizing radiation. The type of imaging procedure that your doctor may suggest will depend on your health concern and the part of the body that is being examined. Some other common examples of imaging tests include:

- X-rays (including dental x-rays, chest x-rays, spine x-rays)
- CT or CAT (computed tomography) scan

If your doctor suggests x-rays or other medical imaging procedures you should consider the following:

- Medical imaging tests should be performed only when necessary.
- The U.S. Food and Drug Administration (FDA) recommends discussing the benefits and risks of fluoroscopy with your doctor.

WHAT HAPPENS DURING A FLUOROSCOPY PROCEDURE

Before the Procedure

Ask your health-care provider to explain the procedure and make sure you ask her or him if you still have additional questions. Some fluoroscopy procedures may use a "contrast dye" which allows doctors to see specific organ(s). The dye may be administered by swallowing, an intravenous (IV) line in your hand or arm, or an enema.

Make sure to let the doctor know if:

- You have ever had a reaction to any contrast dye.
- You are pregnant or suspect that you may be pregnant.

During the Procedure

- You will be asked to remove any clothing and jewelry that may interfere with the procedure.
- You will be positioned on the x-ray table, and depending on the type of procedure, you may be asked to do the following: assume different positions, move a specific body part, or hold your breath at intervals while the fluoroscopy is being performed.
- A special x-ray machine will produce fluoroscopic views of the body structure being examined or treated.

WHAT ARE THE BENEFITS AND RISKS OF FLUOROSCOPY?

Medical imaging tests such as fluoroscopy are noninvasive procedures that allow doctors to diagnose diseases and injuries.

These tests can help doctors:

- Obtain a better view of organs, blood vessels, tissues and bones
- Determine whether surgery is a good treatment option
- Guide medical procedures involving placement of catheters, stents, or other devices inside the body, locate tumors for treatment and locate blood clots or other blockages
- Guide joint replacement options and treatment for fractures

As in many areas of medicine, there are risks associated with the use of fluoroscopy, which uses ionizing radiation to generate images of the body. Risks from exposure to ionizing radiation include:

- A small increase in the likelihood that a person exposed to radiation will develop cancer later in life.
- Health effects that could occur after a large exposure to ionizing radiation such as acute skin reddening, and hair loss.
- Possible allergic reactions associated with a contrast dye injected intravenously into the veins to better see body structures being examined.

While fluoroscopy itself is not painful, the particular procedure being performed may be painful, such as the injection into a joint or accessing of an artery or vein for angiography. In these cases, the radiologist will take all comfort measures possible, which could include local anesthesia, conscious sedation, or general anesthesia, depending on the particular procedure.

HOW CAN YOU REDUCE YOUR EXPOSURE TO DIAGNOSTIC IONIZING RADIATION?

In the case of x-rays or other tests involving exposure to ionizing radiation, doctors and radiation experts can help reduce your exposure to and risk of harm from diagnostic ionizing radiation by:

- Checking to see if you have had a similar test done recently that can provide them with the background information they need.
- Checking to see if a test that does not use ionizing radiation can provide similar information.
- Making certain the least possible amount of radiation needed to obtain a good quality image is used for your procedure.
- Providing protective lead shielding to prevent exposing other areas of the body to radiation.

Radiation experts include the following:

- Hospital radiation safety officer
- Medical physicist

- Radiation physicist
- Diagnostic medical physicist

WHAT ARE THE RISKS OF MEDICAL IMAGING PROCEDURES FOR PREGNANT WOMEN?

Talk to your physician about the potential risks and benefits from the medical procedures. In many cases, the risk of an x-ray procedure to the mother and the unborn child is very small compared to the benefit of finding out about the medical condition of the mother or the child.

Many doctors use ultrasound to examine the abdomen, pelvic area, or heart. Ultrasound does not use ionizing radiation, so it does not expose women of childbearing age to radiation in the pelvic area. This is particularly important in pregnancy.

Risks that are considered small should not be taken if they are unnecessary. You can reduce risks from medical imaging procedures by telling your doctor if you are, or think you might be, pregnant whenever an abdominal x-ray is suggested by your doctor. Other options suggested by the FDA that may be considered are as follows:

- If you are pregnant, the doctor may decide that it would be best to cancel the medical imaging procedure, to postpone it, or to modify it to reduce the amount of radiation.
- Depending on your medical needs, and realizing that the risk is very small, the doctor may feel that it is best to proceed with using a medical imaging procedure as planned.

In any case, you should feel free to discuss the decision with your doctor.

ARE THERE SPECIAL CONSIDERATIONS FOR CHILDREN?

It is important that x-rays and other medical imaging procedures performed on children use the lowest exposure setting needed to obtain a good quality image. The Image Gently Alliance (www.

imagegently.org), part of the Alliance for Radiation in Pediatric Imaging, suggests the following for imaging of children:

- Use imaging examinations when the medical benefit outweighs the risk.
- Use the most appropriate imaging techniques, matched to the size of the child.
- Use alternative imaging methods (such as ultrasound or MRI) when possible.

The FDA also provides information for parents, patients and health-care providers to address concerns about the benefits and risks of medical imaging procedures for children.

ARE THERE MEDICAL IMAGING TESTS THAT DO NOT USE IONIZING RADIATION?

There are also medical imaging procedures such as magnetic resonance imaging (MRI) or ultrasound that do not use ionizing radiation to diagnose illnesses or injuries.

What Is Magnetic Resonance Imaging?

MRI procedures, which can lasts from 30 to 60 minutes, use magnetic fields and radio waves to produce images of specific parts of the body. MRI scans are often performed along with other medical imaging procedures to provide a more detailed view of the area of the body that is being examined.

What Is an Ultrasound?

Ultrasound imaging uses high-frequency sound waves to see inside the body. There is no ionizing radiation used and in most ultrasound examinations, no contrast is given.

Section 17.6 | **Pediatric X-ray Imaging**

This section includes text excerpted from "Pediatric X-ray Imaging," U.S. Food and Drug Administration (FDA), January 18, 2018. Reviewed October 2021.

X-RAY IMAGING FOR PEDIATRICS

Medical x-ray imaging has led to improvements in the diagnosis and treatment of numerous medical conditions in pediatric patients. The Federal Food, Drug, and Cosmetic Act (FD&C Act) defines pediatric patients as persons aged 21 or younger at the time of their diagnosis or treatment. Typically these are broken down into different groups based on age ranges (neonates, infants, children, and adolescents). For medical x-ray imaging, the pediatric patient's size is even more important to consider than age, because patient size determines how much radiation is needed to produce a quality medical image.

The individual risk from x-ray imaging is small when compared to the benefits that it can provide through helping with accurate diagnosis. Still, efforts should be made to minimize risk by reducing unnecessary exposure to ionizing radiation. This is important because:

- Pediatric patients are more radiosensitive than adults (i.e., the cancer risk per unit dose of ionizing radiation is higher)
- Use of equipment and exposure settings designed for adults may result in excessive radiation exposure if used on smaller patients
- Pediatric patients have a longer expected lifetime, putting them at higher risk of cancer from the effects of radiation exposure.

The U.S. Food and Drug Administration (FDA) recommends that medical x-ray imaging exams, which include computed tomography (CT), fluoroscopy, and conventional x-rays, use the lowest radiation dose necessary, taking into account the size and age of the patient. Whether grouped by age or by size, an x-ray image should always be adjusted to meet the needs of the specific type of pediatric patient receiving the exam.

X-ray exams should be performed for children only when the child's physician believes they are necessary to answer the clinical question or to guide treatment. Medical imaging professionals should use techniques that are adjusted to administer the lowest radiation dose that yields an image quality adequate for diagnosis or intervention (i.e., radiation doses should be "As Low as Reasonably Achievable"). The technique factors used should be chosen based on the clinical indication, patient size, and anatomical area scanned, and the equipment should be properly maintained and tested.

THE FDA'S ROLE IN X-RAY SAFETY

The FDA collaborates with stakeholders across the imaging community to protect children's health by helping prevent unnecessary radiation exposure from x-ray exams, which includes:

- Encouraging manufacturers to address pediatric safety issues in current x-ray imaging devices and consider radiation safety of pediatric populations in the design of new x-ray imaging devices
- Publishing guidelines and other tools and resources to help enable imaging professionals to safely use imaging equipment on pediatric patients
- Fostering and strengthening relationships between manufacturers and health-care professionals to improve device design and instructions for use
- Engaging in broad outreach efforts to incorporate radiation protection principles into facility quality assurance and personnel credentialing and training requirements

Section 17.7 | Mammograms

This section contains text excerpted from the following sources: Text beginning with the heading "What Is a Mammogram?" is excerpted from "Mammograms," Office on Women's Health (OWH), U.S. Department of Health and Human Services (HHS), April 1, 2019; Text under the heading "Digital Mammography" is excerpted from "Frequently Asked Questions about Digital Mammography," U.S. Food and Drug Administration (FDA), November 14, 2017. Reviewed October 2021.

WHAT IS A MAMMOGRAM?

A mammogram is a low-dose x-ray exam of the breasts to look for changes that are not normal. The results are recorded on x-ray film or directly into a computer for a doctor called a "radiologist" to examine.

A mammogram allows the doctor to have a closer look for changes in breast tissue that cannot be felt during a breast exam. It is used for women who have no breast complaints and for women who have breast symptoms, such as a change in the shape or size of a breast, a lump, nipple discharge, or pain. Breast changes occur in almost all women. In fact, most of these changes are not cancer and are called "benign," but only a doctor can know for sure.

WHAT IS THE BEST METHOD OF DETECTING BREAST CANCER AS EARLY AS POSSIBLE?

A high-quality mammogram plus a clinical breast exam, an exam done by your doctor, is the most effective way to detect breast cancer early. Finding breast cancer early greatly improves a woman's chances for successful treatment.

Like any test, mammograms have both benefits and limitations. For example, some cancers cannot be found by a mammogram, but they may be found in a clinical breast exam.

Checking your own breasts for lumps or other changes is called a "breast self-exam" (BSE). Studies so far have not shown that BSE alone helps reduce the number of deaths from breast cancer. BSE should not take the place of routine clinical breast exams and mammograms.

If you choose to do BSE, remember that breast changes can occur because of pregnancy, aging, menopause, menstrual cycles, or from taking birth control pills or other hormones. It is normal for breasts to feel a little lumpy and uneven. Also, it is common for breasts to be swollen and tender right before or during a menstrual period. If you notice any unusual changes in your breasts, contact your doctor.

HOW IS A MAMMOGRAM DONE?

You stand in front of a special x-ray machine. The person who takes the x-rays, called a "radiologic technician," places your breasts, one at a time, between an x-ray plate and a plastic plate. These plates are attached to the x-ray machine and compress the breasts to flatten them. This spreads the breast tissue out to obtain a clearer picture.

You will feel pressure on your breast for a few seconds. It may cause you some discomfort; you might feel squeezed or pinched. This feeling only lasts for a few seconds, and the flatter your breast, the better the picture. Most often, two pictures are taken of each breast – one from the side and one from above. A screening mammogram takes about 20 minutes from start to finish.

ARE THERE DIFFERENT TYPES OF MAMMOGRAMS?

- Screening mammograms are done for women who have no symptoms of breast cancer. It usually involves two x-rays of each breast. Screening mammograms can detect lumps or tumors that cannot be felt. They can also find microcalcifications or tiny deposits of calcium in the breast, which sometimes mean that breast cancer is present.
- Diagnostic mammograms are used to check for breast cancer after a lump or other symptom or sign of breast cancer has been found. Signs of breast cancer may include pain, thickened skin on the breast, nipple discharge, or a change in breast size or shape. This type of mammogram also can be used to find out more about breast changes found on a screening mammogram, or to view breast tissue that is hard to see on a screening mammogram. A diagnostic mammogram takes longer than a screening mammogram because it involves more x-rays in order to obtain views of

the breast from several angles. The technician can magnify a problem area to make a more detailed picture, which helps the doctor make a correct diagnosis.

A digital mammogram also uses x-rays to produce an image of the breast, but instead of storing the image directly on film, the image is stored directly on a computer. This allows the recorded image to be magnified for the doctor to take a closer look. Current research has not shown that digital images are better at showing cancer than x-ray film images in general. But, women with dense breasts who are pre- or perimenopausal, or who are younger than age 50, may benefit from having a digital rather than a film mammogram.

Digital mammography may offer these benefits:

- Long-distance consultations with other doctors may be easier because the images can be shared by computer.
- Slight differences between normal and abnormal tissues may be more easily noted.
- The number of follow-up tests needed may be fewer.
- Fewer repeat images may be needed, reducing exposure to radiation.

WHAT CAN MAMMOGRAMS SHOW?

The radiologist will look at your x-rays for breast changes that do not look normal and for differences in each breast. She or he will compare your past mammograms with your most recent one to check for changes. The doctor will also look for lumps and calcifications.

- **Lump or mass.** The size, shape, and edges of a lump sometimes can give doctors information about whether or not it may be cancer. On a mammogram, a growth that is benign often looks smooth and round with a clear, defined edge. Breast cancer often has a jagged outline and an irregular shape.
- **Calcification.** A calcification is a deposit of the mineral calcium in the breast tissue. Calcifications appear as small white spots on a mammogram. There are two types:

- Macrocalcifications are large calcium deposits often caused by aging. These usually are not a sign of cancer.
- Microcalcifications are tiny specks of calcium that may be found in an area of rapidly dividing cells.

If calcifications are grouped together in a certain way, it may be a sign of cancer. Depending on how many calcium specks you have, how big they are, and what they look like, your doctor may suggest that you have other tests. Calcium in the diet does not create calcium deposits, or calcifications, in the breast.

WHAT IF YOUR SCREENING MAMMOGRAM SHOWS A PROBLEM?

If you have a screening test result that suggests cancer, your doctor must find out whether it is due to cancer or to some other cause. Your doctor may ask about your personal and family medical history. You may have a physical exam. Your doctor also may order some of these tests:

- Diagnostic mammogram, to focus on a specific area of the breast
- Ultrasound, an imaging test that uses sound waves to create a picture of your breast. The pictures may show whether a lump is solid or filled with fluid. A cyst is a fluid-filled sac. Cysts are not cancer. But, a solid mass may be cancer. After the test, your doctor can store the pictures on video or print them out. This exam may be used along with a mammogram.
- Magnetic resonance imaging (MRI), which uses a powerful magnet linked to a computer. MRI makes detailed pictures of breast tissue. Your doctor can view these pictures on a monitor or print them on film. MRI may be used along with a mammogram.
- Biopsy, a test in which fluid or tissue is removed from your breast to help find out if there is cancer. Your doctor may refer you to a surgeon or to a doctor who is an expert in breast disease for a biopsy.

WHERE CAN YOU GET A HIGH-QUALITY MAMMOGRAM?

Women can get high-quality mammograms in breast clinics, hospital radiology departments, mobile vans, private radiology offices, and doctor's offices. The U.S. Food and Drug Administration (FDA) certifies mammography facilities that meet strict quality standards for their x-ray machines and staff and are inspected every year. You can ask your doctor or the staff at the mammography center about FDA certification before making your appointment. A list of FDA-certified facilities can be found on the Internet.

Your doctor, local medical clinic, or local or state health department can tell you where to get no-cost or low-cost mammograms. You can also call the National Cancer Institute's (NCI) Cancer Information Service (CIS) at toll-free: (800-422-6237).

WHAT IF YOU HAVE BREAST IMPLANTS?

Women with breast implants should also have mammograms. A woman who had an implant after breast cancer surgery in which the entire breast was removed (mastectomy) should ask her doctor whether she needs a mammogram of the reconstructed breast.

If you have breast implants, be sure to tell your mammography facility that you have them when you make your appointment. The technician and radiologist must be experienced in x-raying patients with breast implants. Implants can hide some breast tissue, making it harder for the radiologist to see a problem when looking at your mammogram. To see as much breast tissue as possible, the x-ray technician will gently lift the breast tissue slightly away from the implant and take extra pictures of the breasts.

HOW DO YOU GET READY FOR YOUR MAMMOGRAM?

First, check with the place you are having the mammogram for any special instructions you may need to follow before you go. Here are some general guidelines to follow:

- If you are still having menstrual periods, try to avoid making your mammogram appointment during the week before your period. Your breasts will be less tender and swollen. The mammogram will hurt less and the picture will be better.

- If you have breast implants, be sure to tell your mammography facility that you have them when you make your appointment.
- Wear a shirt with shorts, pants, or a skirt. This way, you can undress from the waist up and leave your shorts, pants, or skirt on when you get your mammogram.
- Do not wear any deodorant, perfume, lotion, or powder under your arms or on your breasts on the day of your mammogram appointment. These things can make shadows show up on your mammogram.
- If you have had mammograms at another facility, have those x-ray films sent to the new facility so that they can be compared to the new films.

LIMITATIONS OF MAMMOGRAMS

Although they are not perfect, mammograms are the best method to find breast changes that cannot be felt. If your mammogram shows a breast change, sometimes other tests are needed to better understand it. Even if the doctor sees something on the mammogram, it does not mean it is cancer.

As with any medical test, mammograms have limits. These limits include:

- **They are only part of a complete breast exam.** Your doctor also should do a clinical breast exam. If your mammogram finds something abnormal, your doctor will order other tests.
- **Finding cancer does not always mean saving lives.** Even though mammography can detect tumors that cannot be felt, finding a small tumor does not always mean that a woman's life will be saved. Mammography may not help a woman with a fast-growing cancer that has already spread to other parts of her body before being found.
- **False negatives can happen.** This means everything may look normal, but cancer is actually present. False negatives do not happen often. Younger women are more likely to have a false negative mammogram than

are older women. The dense breasts of younger women make breast cancers harder to find in mammograms.
- **False positives can happen.** This is when the mammogram results look like cancer is present, even though it is not. False positives are more common in younger women, women who have had breast biopsies, women with a family history of breast cancer, and women who are taking estrogen, such as menopausal hormone therapy (MHT).
- **Mammograms (as well as dental x-rays and other routine x-rays) use very small doses of radiation.** The risk of any harm is very slight, but repeated x-rays could cause cancer. The benefits nearly always outweigh the risk. Talk to your doctor about the need for each x-ray. Ask about shielding to protect parts of the body that are not in the picture. You should always let your doctor and the technician know if there is any chance that you are pregnant.

DIGITAL MAMMOGRAPHY

What Is Digital Mammography?

Full field digital mammography (FFDM, also known simply as "digital mammography") is a mammography system where the x-ray film used in screen-film mammography is replaced by solid-state detectors, similar to those found in digital cameras, which convert x-rays into electrical signals. The electrical signals are used to produce images of the breast that can be seen on a computer screen, or printed on special films to look like screen-film mammograms. Types of digital mammography include direct radiography (the most common type, which captures the image directly onto a flat-panel detector), computed radiography (which involves the use of a cassette that contains an imaging plate), or digital breast tomosynthesis (DBT).

What Is Digital Breast Tomosynthesis?

Digital breast tomosynthesis is a relatively new technology. In DBT, the x-ray tube moves in an arc around the breast and takes multiple images from different angles. Similar to computed tomography (CT scan), these images are then reconstructed into parallel "slices" through the breast. This allows interpreting physicians to see through layers of overlapping tissue.

How Can Women Find an FDA-Certified Digital Mammography Facility?

Digital mammography has been in use since 2001. Ninety-six percent of all certified mammography facilities in the U.S. use digital units of some type. You can find a list of certified facilities, searchable by state or ZIP Code, at the website: www.fda.gov/findmammography.

Do Private Insurance Companies, Medicare and Medicaid Pay for Digital Mammography Exams, Such as Digital Breast Tomosynthesis?

Contact your insurance provider before the procedure to determine what procedures are covered by your insurance plan. The telephone number for questions about Medicare reimbursement is toll-free: 800-MEDICARE (800-633-4227).

Chapter 18 | **Contrast Radiography**

Chapter Contents

Section 18.1 | Coronary Angiography

This section includes text excerpted from the following sources. Text under the headings marked 1 are © 2022 Omnigraphics. Reviewed October 2021; Text under the heading marked 2 is excerpted from "Coronary Angiography," National Heart, Lung, and Blood Institute (NHLBI), January 31, 2013. Reviewed October 2021.

WHAT IS CORONARY ANGIOGRAPHY?[1]

Coronary angiography is a procedure that uses x-ray imaging to identify blockages in the heart's blood vessels and is also called "cardiac angiogram," "catheter arteriography," or "cardiac catheterization." With the help of a contrast dye injected into the arteries through a catheter, a doctor can observe the flow of blood through the blood vessels of the heart on an x-ray screen. Blockages in the arteries prevent the heart from getting oxygen and important nutrients.

WHY IS A CORONARY ANGIOGRAPHY DONE?[1]

Coronary angiography is done if you show the following symptoms:

- Chest pain (angina)
- Pain in the jaw, neck, chest, or arm that other tests cannot explain
- Increasing chest pain (unstable angina)
- Born with congenital heart disease
- Chest injury
- A problem in other blood vessels
- A heart valve problem

HOW TO PREPARE FOR THE PROCEDURE[1]

Unless it is done on an emergency basis, the doctor will give you specific guidelines and time to prepare for the procedure. General instructions include not eating or drinking anything after midnight before the angiogram, carrying all medications in their original containers, asking the doctor if you can take your morning medications, and checking with your doctor if you can take insulin or other medicines if you have diabetes.

BEFORE THE PROCEDURE[1]

The health-care team will check your vital signs, review your medical history, and ask questions regarding any medications you take and any allergies. You will also be given a hospital gown to change into and asked to empty the bladder, remove glasses or contact lenses, any jewelry, and hairpins.

DURING THE PROCEDURE[1]

The procedure is performed on an x-ray table, and x-ray cameras will take pictures of your head and chest. Safety straps across your chest and legs may be required if the table is titled for the procedure. Then, with the help of an intravenous (IV) line in your arm, you will be given sedatives, medications, and fluids. The sedative will help you relax, and you may doze off during the procedure, but you will be able to easily wake up to follow any instructions that the doctor gives. Throughout the procedure, electrodes on the chest will monitor your heart, blood pressure cuffs will monitor your blood pressure, and an oximeter will measure the amount of oxygen in the blood.

A small area in your arm, neck, upper thigh, or groin will be cleaned and numbed using local anesthesia. A small incision will be made at the entry site, and a small plastic tube called a "sheath" will be inserted into the blood vessel. A catheter is placed through the sheath into the blood vessel and threaded to the coronary arteries. Once the catheter is in place, the doctor will inject a contrast dye to identify any blockages. The contrast dye is easily seen on x-ray images. Based on what the doctor discovers, additional procedures such as stent placement (to open narrow arteries) or balloon angioplasty may be done.

AFTER THE PROCEDURE[1]

Once the angiogram is over, the catheter is removed, and the blood vessel is closed with a small plug, a clamp, or manual pressure. You will then be sent to a recovery room for observation and then to your room to be monitored regularly. You would have to lie on your back for several hours to avoid bleeding if the catheter was inserted near the groin. Depending on your case, you may be allowed to go home the same day or stay overnight at the hospital. Drink plenty of water to flush out the dye from your body and check with the health-care team before resuming any medications. Avoid lifting heavy objects or any strenuous activities for the next few days.

RECOVERY AND FOLLOW-UP[1]

- Relax and drink plenty of water.
- Do not consume alcohol or smoke.
- Remove bandages only after 24 hours. If any minor oozing occurs at the incision site, apply a clean bandage for another 12 hours.
- Do not engage in heavy exercises or sex for at least two days.
- You may take a sponge bath; however, avoid taking any other forms of baths for a minimum of three days.
- Do not apply any lotion on or near the incision site for three days.

COMPLICATIONS OF CORONARY ANGIOGRAPHY[2]

Coronary angiography is a common procedure that rarely causes serious problems. However, possible complications may include bleeding, allergic reactions to the contrast dye, infection, blood vessel damage, arrhythmias, blood clots that can trigger a heart attack or stroke, kidney damage, and fluid buildup around the heart. The risk of complications is higher in people who are older or who have certain conditions such as chronic kidney disease or diabetes. An imaging test called "coronary computed tomography angiography," or "coronary CTA," may be preferred over coronary angiography to detect blockages in the heart. Although coronary CTA still uses contrast dye, it does not require the invasive cardiac catheterization procedure that causes many of the complications of coronary angiography.

RESULTS[1]

Coronary angiography can show doctors:

- Number of coronary arteries blocked or narrowed by fatty plaques (atherosclerosis)

- The amount of blood flow that is blocked through the blood vessels
- The exact location of the blockage in the blood vessels
- The result of any previous coronary bypass surgery

References

1. "Coronary Angiography," National Heart, Lung, and Blood Institute (NHLBI), January 31, 2013.
2. "Coronary Angiogram," Mayo Clinic, December 22, 2020.
3. Smith, Charlene. "Coronary Angiography," Healthline, September 16, 2018.

Section 18.2 | **Cystogram**

WHAT IS A CYSTOGRAM?

A cystogram is a study of the urinary tract, which is located in the pelvic region. Cystograms employ fluoroscopic imaging to show how the bladder fills up. This imaging allows the radiologist to monitor a patient's internal organs. A cystogram is used to diagnose a condition called "urinary reflux," which causes urine to move back up the ureter from the bladder to the kidneys. Usually, a cystogram is performed when a patient has experienced pelvic injury or in case of a torn bladder. It is also used to detect polyps or tumors in the bladder.

WHY SHOULD YOU HAVE A CYSTOGRAM?

The cystogram helps your doctor diagnose a problem in the urinary tract. In the case of urinary tract infections or urinary incontinence, a follow-up examination detects any structural problems in the bladder. After the cystogram, further questions can be taken up with the doctor.

A cystogram helps determine the following conditions:

- Urinary reflux, when urine flows back into the ureter and, in some cases, to one or both kidneys
- Urinary tract infections that keep coming back
- Problems emptying your bladder, a bladder tear, or trauma to the bladder
- Problems with nerve supply
- Blood clots in the bladder
- Blockages in the ureters
- Urinary incontinence
- Foreign bodies
- Bladder fistulae
- Tumors

WHAT ARE THE RISK FACTORS?

It is important to consider the following risk factors before a cystogram:

- Radiation exposure might lead to birth defects during pregnancy.
- Check with your doctor if you are allergic or sensitive to medicines, contrast dyes, local anesthesia, iodine, or latex, or you have kidney failure or other kidney problems.

You are at risk in the case of bleeding or hematuria. It is important to consider the following conditions in case the test results are less accurate. These include:

- If you have gas or stool in your intestines
- If you have had a barium enema

You may not be able to have a cystogram if you:

- Are allergic to contrast dyes
- Are pregnant
- Had recent bladder surgery
- Have a blocked or damaged urethra
- Have a urinary tract infection

In the case of a specific health condition, be sure to talk with your health provider about any concerns you have before the procedure.

WHAT HAPPENS BEFORE A CYSTOGRAM?

A cystogram examination does not require any specific preparation. Your physician will ask you to take your medicines promptly and to follow up on appointments. The physician will also make sure to keep you involved in decisions concerning your care and treatment. With your consent, the physician will proceed with the treatment. It is important to consider the following before proceeding with a cystogram:

- Ask your health-care provider if you have any concerns about the procedure and read the instructions in the consent form before proceeding with the treatment.
- Your health-care provider will give you specific instructions regarding your dietary plan before the procedure.
- Tell your provider if you are pregnant or think you may be pregnant.
- If you have had a reaction to any contrast dye, it is important to keep your health-care provider informed.
- If you are allergic to any medicines, latex, tape, or anesthetic medicines, inform your health provider prior to any procedures or treatment.
- If you have a bleeding disorder or if you are taking blood-thinning medicines (anticoagulants), aspirin, or other medicines that affect blood clotting, your physician might ask you to stop these medicines before the test.

The physician will give you an enema or medicine to make you have a bowel movement before the test.

WHAT HAPPENS DURING A CYSTOGRAM?

- The physician will ask you to remove your clothing and put on a gown.
- You will be asked to empty your bladder before the test.
- After placing a thin tube (catheter) into your bladder, the physician will inject the contrast dye.

- The physician will take an x-ray of your kidneys, ureters, and bladder (KUB) to make sure that she or he can monitor the urinary tract system.
- After injecting the contrast dye into your bladder through the catheter, the physician will clamp the catheter tubing to keep the dye from draining out of your bladder.
- Your health-care provider will take x-rays while the dye is in your bladder.

WHAT HAPPENS AFTER A CYSTOGRAM?

The radiologist will monitor the radiographs before handing over the report to your physician. After discussing the results and further courses of action with you, the physician will ask you to resume your normal diet (unless your health-care provider informs you differently). It is important to drink additional fluids for the next few days. This will help to prevent any bladder infection. It is important to keep your health-care provider informed if you observe any of the following conditions:

- Pain when you urinate that gets worse or lasts more than two days
- Less urine than usual
- Pain in your belly
- Fever or chills
- Blood in your urine

WHEN WILL YOU GET THE RESULTS?

The cystogram report is studied by the radiologist and sent to a physician. The referred physician will discuss the results with you. Follow up on the treatment by visiting your physician.

References

1. "What You Need to Know about Cystogram," American Society of Radiologic Technologists (ASRT), 2009.
2. "Cystogram," Guy's and St. Thomas' NHS Foundation Trust, April 2017.

3. "Cystogram," University of Washington Medicine, 2018.
4. "Cystography," Johns Hopkins Medicine, May 5, 2016.

Section 18.3 | **Upper Gastrointestinal Series**

This section includes text excerpted from "Upper GI Series," National Institute of Diabetes and Digestive and Kidney Diseases (NIDDK), August 2016. Reviewed October 2021.

WHAT IS AN UPPER GASTROINTESTINAL SERIES?

An upper gastrointestinal (GI) series is a procedure in which a doctor uses x-rays, fluoroscopy, and a chalky liquid called "barium" to view your upper GI tract. The barium will make your upper GI tract more visible on an x-ray.

The two types of upper GI series are:

- A standard barium upper GI series, which uses only barium
- A double-contrast upper GI series, which uses both air and barium for a clearer view of your stomach lining

WHY DO DOCTORS USE UPPER GASTROINTESTINAL SERIES?

An upper GI series can help a doctor find the cause of:

- Nausea and vomiting
- Pain in the abdomen
- Problems swallowing
- Unexplained weight loss

An upper GI series can also show:

- Abnormal growths such as cancer
- Esophageal varices
- Gastroesophageal reflux
- A hiatal hernia
- Scars or strictures
- Ulcers

HOW DO YOU PREPARE FOR AN UPPER GASTROINTESTINAL SERIES?

To prepare for an upper GI series, do not eat, drink, smoke, or chew gum. You also will need to talk with your doctor.

Do Not Eat, Drink, Smoke, or Chew Gum

In order to see your upper GI tract clearly, your doctor will most likely ask you not to eat, drink, smoke, or chew gum during the 8 hours before the upper GI series.

Talk with Your Doctor

You should talk with your doctor about any medical conditions you have and all prescribed and over-the-counter medicines, vitamins, and supplements you take.

Talk with your doctor about any medical conditions you have and all prescribed and over-the-counter medicines, vitamins, and supplements you take.

Doctors do not recommend x-rays for pregnant women because x-rays may harm the fetus. Tell your doctor if you are, or may be, pregnant. Your doctor may suggest a different procedure.

A doctor may recommend an upper GI series for your child when the benefits of the procedure outweigh the relatively small risk of x-rays. Talk with your child's doctor about safety measures used to lower your child's exposure to x-rays during the procedure.

HOW DO DOCTORS PERFORM AN UPPER GASTROINTESTINAL SERIES?

An x-ray technician and a radiologist perform an upper GI series at a hospital or an outpatient center. You do not need anesthesia. The procedure usually takes about 2 hours. The procedure can take up to 5 hours if the barium moves slowly through your small intestine.

For the procedure, you will be asked to stand or sit in front of an x-ray machine and drink barium, which coats the lining of your upper GI tract. You will then lie on the x-ray table, and the radiologist will watch the barium move through your GI tract on the x-ray and fluoroscopy. The technician may press on your abdomen or ask you to change position several times to evenly coat your upper GI tract with the barium.

If you are having a double-contrast study, you will swallow gas-forming crystals that mix with the barium coating your stomach. Gas forms when the crystals and barium mix. The gas expands your stomach, which lets the radiologist see more details of your upper GI tract lining. The technician will then take additional x-rays.

WHAT SHOULD YOU EXPECT AFTER AN UPPER GASTROINTESTINAL SERIES?

After an upper GI series, you can expect the following:

- You may have cramping in your abdomen and bloating during the first hour after the procedure.
- You may resume most normal activities after leaving the hospital or outpatient center.
- For several days, your stools may be white or light colored from the barium in your GI tract.
- A health-care professional will give you instructions on how to care for yourself after the procedure. The instructions will explain how to flush the remaining barium from your GI tract. You should follow all instructions.

A specialist will read the x-rays and send a report of the findings to your doctor.

WHAT ARE THE RISKS OF AN UPPER GASTROINTESTINAL SERIES?

The risks of an upper GI series include:

- Constipation from the barium – the most common complication of an upper GI series
- An allergic reaction to the barium or flavoring in the barium
- Intestinal obstruction

SEEK CARE RIGHT AWAY

If you have any of the following symptoms after an upper GI series, seek medical attention right away:

- Fever
- No bowel movement within 2 days after the procedure
- Inability to pass gas
- Severe pain in your abdomen

Section 18.4 | Lower Gastrointestinal Series (Barium Enema)

This section includes text excerpted from "Lower GI Series," National Institute of Diabetes and Digestive and Kidney Diseases (NIDDK), June 2016. Reviewed October 2021.

WHAT IS LOWER GASTROINTESTINAL SERIES?

A lower gastrointestinal (GI) series is a procedure in which a doctor uses x-rays and a chalky liquid called "barium" to view your large intestine. The barium will make your large intestine more visible on an x-ray.

The two types of lower GI series are:

- A single-contrast lower GI series, which uses only barium
- A double-contrast or air-contrast lower GI series, which uses both barium and air for a clearer view of your large intestine

Does Lower Gastrointestinal Series Have Another Name?

A lower GI series is also called a "barium enema."

WHY DO DOCTORS USE LOWER GASTROINTESTINAL SERIES?

A lower GI series can help a doctor find the cause of:

- Bleeding from your anus
- Changes in your bowel activity
- Chronic diarrhea

- Pain in your abdomen
- Unexplained weight loss

A lower GI series can also show:
- Cancerous growths
- Diverticula
- Fistula
- Polyps
- Ulcers

HOW DO YOU PREPARE FOR A LOWER GASTROINTESTINAL SERIES?

To prepare for a lower GI series, you will need to talk with your doctor, change your diet, and clean out your bowel.

Talk with Your Doctor

You should talk with your doctor about any medical conditions you have and all prescribed and over-the-counter medicines, vitamins, and supplements you take.

Also tell your doctor whether you have had a colonoscopy with a biopsy or polyp removal in the last 4 weeks.

Doctors do not recommend x-rays for pregnant women because x-rays may harm the fetus. Tell your doctor if you are, or may be, pregnant. Your doctor may suggest a different procedure.

Change Your Diet and Clean Out Your Bowel

A health-care professional will give you written bowel prep instructions to follow at home before the procedure. A health-care professional orders a bowel prep so that little to no stool is present in your intestine. A complete bowel prep lets you pass stool that is clear and liquid. Stool inside your colon can prevent the x-ray machine from taking clear images of your intestine.

You may need to follow a clear liquid diet for 1 to 3 days before the procedure. The instructions will provide specific direction about when to start and stop the clear liquid diet. In most cases, you may drink or eat the following:

- Fat-free bouillon or broth
- Gelatin in flavors such as lemon, lime, or orange
- Plain coffee or tea, without cream or milk
- Sports drinks in flavors such as lemon, lime, or orange
- Strained fruit juice, such as apple or white grape – doctors recommend avoiding orange juice
- Water

You may need to follow a clear liquid diet for 1 to 3 days before a lower gastrointestinal (GI) series.

Your doctor will tell you how long before the procedure you should have nothing by mouth.

A health-care professional will ask you to follow the directions for a bowel prep before the procedure. The bowel prep will cause diarrhea, so you should stay close to a bathroom.

Different bowel preps may contain different combinations of laxatives – pills that you swallow or powders that you dissolve in water and other clear liquids – and enemas. Some people will need to drink a large amount, often a gallon, of liquid laxative during a scheduled amount of time – most often the night before the procedure.

You may find this part of the bowel prep difficult; however, completing the prep is very important. Your doctor will not be able to see your large intestine clearly if the prep is incomplete.

Call a health-care professional if you have side effects that prevent you from finishing the prep.

HOW DO DOCTORS PERFORM A LOWER GASTROINTESTINAL SERIES?

An x-ray technician and a radiologist perform a lower GI series at a hospital or an outpatient center. You do not need anesthesia. The procedure usually takes 30 to 60 minutes.

For the procedure, you will be asked to lie on a table while the radiologist inserts a flexible tube into your anus and fills your large intestine with barium. The radiologist prevents barium from leaking from your anus by inflating a balloon on the end of the tube. You may be asked to change position several times to evenly coat the large intestine with the barium. If you are having a double-contrast lower GI series, the radiologist will inject air through the tube to inflate the large intestine.

During the procedure, you may have some discomfort and feel the urge to have a bowel movement. You will need to hold still in various positions while the radiologist and technician take x-ray images and possibly an x-ray video, called "fluoroscopy."

The radiologist or technician will deflate the balloon on the tube when the imaging is complete. Most of the barium will drain through the tube. You will push out the remaining barium into a bedpan or nearby toilet. A health-care professional may give you an enema to flush out the rest of the barium.

WHAT SHOULD YOU EXPECT AFTER A LOWER GASTROINTESTINAL SERIES?

After a lower GI series, you can expect the following:

- You may have cramping in your abdomen and bloating during the first hour after the procedure.
- You may resume most normal activities after leaving the hospital or outpatient center.
- For several days, your stools may be white or light colored from the barium in your large intestine.
- A health-care professional will give you instructions on how to care for yourself after the procedure. The instructions will explain how to flush the remaining barium from your large intestine. You should follow all instructions.

The radiologist will read the x-rays and send a report of the findings to your doctor.

WHAT ARE THE RISKS OF A LOWER GASTROINTESTINAL SERIES?

The risks of a lower GI series include

- Constipation from the barium enema – the most common complication of a lower GI series

- An allergic reaction to the barium
- Intestinal obstruction
- Leakage of barium into your abdomen through a tear or hole in the lining of the large intestine

SEEK CARE RIGHT AWAY

If you have any of the following symptoms after a lower GI series, seek medical care right away:

- Bloody bowel movements or bleeding from your anus
- Fever
- Inability to pass gas
- Severe constipation
- Severe pain in your abdomen

Section 18.5 | Lung Ventilation/Perfusion Scan

A lung ventilation/perfusion scan is often abbreviated as a lung VQ scan and is also known as a "pulmonary ventilation (V) and perfusion (Q) scan." It is primarily an imaging test comprising a ventilation scan to determine the airflow in the lungs and a perfusion scan to chart the direction of blood flow. The scan is a nuclear imaging test consisting of two scans administered together or separately by a technician and prescribed by a doctor. The V and Q together make up a math equation that permits doctors to calculate air and blood flow.

WHY IS A LUNG VQ SCAN PRESCRIBED?

The scans are prescribed primarily to check for a pulmonary embolism, which denotes a blood clot in the lungs. The embolism can present symptoms such as:

- Strained breathing
- Chest pain

- Reduced oxygen saturation levels
- Rapid heart rates
- Coughing blood
- Back pain
- Pain or swelling in the legs
- Excess perspiration
- Blue lips or nails
- Lightheadedness or having episodes of fainting

A VQ scan may also be prescribed before lung surgery to check for normal lung function. Before administering a VQ scan, a doctor will check the patient for risk factors that include smoking, reduced physical activity due to travel, surgery, or sedentary lifestyles.

A VQ scan can be prescribed to check regional lung function in patients with severe pulmonary disease such as chronic obstructive pulmonary disease (COPD). A VQ scan can also be used to detect abnormal shunts in the pulmonary vessels of the lungs.

HOW IS A VQ SCAN PERFORMED?

The lung VQ scan lasts for approximately 45 minutes, wherein the patient is asked to lie flat on an examination table. Since the VQ scan comprises two separate scans, there is a slight difference in the procedures, too.

For a perfusion scan, the patient will be given an intravenous (IV) line through which radionuclide dye is introduced into the patient's bloodstream. This dye generally contains small amounts of technetium. The IV line is given to help provide access to a vein on the inside of the elbow or the back of the hand. After the injection of the dye, the IV is removed, and the patient is placed under a specialized scanner that detects the dye and shows how it flows into the lungs through the bloodstream. The patient is required to stay still during the scan. Upon instructions from the scanning technician, they may need to change positions.

During a pulmonary ventilation scan, which is usually performed first, the patient is given a mouthpiece while they are under the scanner. The mouthpiece consists of oxygen mixed with radioactive substances such as radioactive xenon or technetium. The patient will be instructed to breathe through this mouthpiece while the scanner simultaneously captures images of the lungs during the procedure. The patient must avoid ingesting the gas as it can interfere with the results of the scan. Some scans may require the patient to hold their breath while it is underway. Once the scan is completed, the mouthpiece is removed, and if trace amounts of gas remains in the patient's body, it is likely to be expended by their normal breathing pattern.

HOW TO PREPARE FOR A VQ SCAN

Some tips to remember before going through a VQ scan include:

- A doctor will ensure that the patient understands the risks and procedures of the scan, after which they will be asked to sign a consent form. Patients can utilize this window to address any concerns regarding the scan they might have.
- Patients must reveal details of any allergies to latex or contrast dyes to their health-care provider. Pregnancy or breastfeeding information is also crucial and must be admitted to the doctor before the scan.
- Details of any recent nuclear scans must be provided to the doctor.
- Patients scheduled for a scan must avoid wearing clothes that have metal fasteners and opt for loose-fitting attire instead. Jewelry can also be avoided. There are no dietary restrictions before a VQ scan that involves fasting or other conditions.
- An x-ray taken 24 to 48 hours before the scan may be required depending on the preference of the referring physician.

AFTER THE VQ SCAN

Once the scans are complete, the health-care team monitors the patient for any allergic reactions for a small duration. The IV insertion point is also checked for redness and swelling. Long durations of lying flat can also cause spells of dizziness in some patients. It is recommended that patients consume plenty of fluids, mostly in the form of just water, to help flush out the remnant radioactive dye from the bloodstream. Any redness or soreness at the IV site after returning home must be immediately reported to the doctor. After that, the patient can return to regular diets and routines unless otherwise specified. It is best to avoid any nuclear procedures for the next 24 to 48 hours.

CONSIDERATIONS OF A VQ SCAN

Generally, VQ scans are risk- and pain-free but, in certain instances, a VQ scan can be unsuitable for patients who may have conditions such as:

- An allergic reaction to the injected radioactive isotope
- Pregnancy or lactation
- Contracting an infection at the injection site

WHAT DO THE RESULTS DENOTE?

The results of a VQ scan are usually available within a day of conducting the test. They are classified as either normal or abnormal. Normal results are denoted to lung scanning images where both lungs look the same and evenly take up the radioactive dye during perfusion and ventilation scans. Abnormal results are seen in scanning images where the lungs take up lower than usual quantities of the radioactive dye. These scans can be classified as:

- Scans where the ventilation scan is abnormal, but the perfusion scan is normal, are caused by abnormal airways in the entire lung or parts of it. This result can be indicative of chronic obstructive pulmonary disease (COPD) or asthma.
- Scans where the perfusion scan is abnormal but the ventilation scan is normal, which can result from a pulmonary embolism.
- Scans, where both are abnormal, indicate lung diseases such as pneumonia, COPD, or embolisms.

While reporting the results of a VQ scan, it can be categorized as:

- **Normal.** No problem with lungs.
- **Low probability.** Indicating a low likelihood of blood clots requiring further tests.
- **Indeterminate or intermediate probability.** An increased likelihood of blood clots in the lungs requiring further investigations.
- **High probability.** A high likelihood of the presence of a blood clot requiring medication or other medical interventions.

WHAT ARE THE RISKS OF A VQ SCAN?

A VQ scan does not present many risks except for pregnant and lactating women. The radioactive substances used in the scan are administered in restricted amounts and are excreted out from the body in a day, and allergic reactions are rare in these cases. Though minimal, the risks are similar to those for an x-ray or needle prick. The scanners used do not emit any radiation. On the contrary, they detect radiation within the body, which is then transferred onto an image. Radiation exposure can cause a certain degree of cell and tissue damage, but the chance of this damage occurring is lesser compared to the advantages of the test.

References

1. "Lung VQ Scan," National Heart, Lung, and Blood Institute (NHLBI), December 10, 2016.
2. "Pulmonary Ventilation/Perfusion Scan," MedlinePlus, National Institutes of Health (NIH), September 1, 2021.
3. Martel, Janelle. "What Is a VQ Scan?" Healthline, February 26, 2018.
4. "Lung Scan," University of Michigan Health, September 23, 2020.
5. "Ventilation Perfusion (VQ) Scan," Baptist Health, February 28, 2021.
6. "Pulmonary Ventilation/Perfusion Scan," SLUCare Physician Group, August 3, 2020.
7. "What to Know about a VQ Scan," WebMD, June 29, 2021.

Chapter 19 | **Ultrasound (Sonography) Exams**

Chapter Contents

Section 19.1 | **Ultrasound Overview**

This section includes text excerpted from "Ultrasound," National Institute of Biomedical Imaging and Bioengineering (NIBIB), July 2016. Reviewed October 2021.

WHAT IS MEDICAL ULTRASOUND?

Medical ultrasound falls into two distinct categories: diagnostic and therapeutic.

Diagnostic ultrasound is a noninvasive diagnostic technique used to image inside the body. Ultrasound probes, called "transducers," produce sound waves that have frequencies above the threshold of human hearing (above 20KHz), but most transducers in current use operate at much higher frequencies (in the megahertz (MHz) range). Most diagnostic ultrasound probes are placed on the skin. However, to optimize image quality, probes may be placed inside the body via the gastrointestinal tract, vagina, or blood vessels. In addition, ultrasound is sometimes used during surgery by placing a sterile probe into the area being operated on.

Diagnostic ultrasound can be further sub-divided into anatomical and functional ultrasound. Anatomical ultrasound produces images of internal organs or other structures. Functional ultrasound combines information such as the movement and velocity of tissue or blood, softness or hardness of tissue, and other physical characteristics, with anatomical images to create "information maps." These maps help doctors visualize changes/differences in function within a structure or organ.

Therapeutic ultrasound also uses sound waves above the range of human hearing but does not produce images. Its purpose is to interact with tissues in the body such that they are either modified or destroyed. Among the modifications possible are: moving or pushing tissue, heating tissue, dissolving blood clots, or delivering drugs to specific locations in the body. These destructive, or ablative, functions are made possible by use of very high-intensity beams that can destroy diseased or abnormal tissues such as tumors. The advantage of using ultrasound therapies is that, in most cases, they are noninvasive. No incisions or cuts need to be made to the skin, leaving no wounds or scars.

HOW DOES IT WORK

Ultrasound waves are produced by a transducer, which can both emit ultrasound waves, as well as detect the ultrasound echoes reflected back. In most cases, the active elements in ultrasound transducers are made of special ceramic crystal materials called "piezoelectrics." These materials are able to produce sound waves when an electric field is applied to them, but can also work in reverse, producing an electric field when a sound wave hits them. When used in an ultrasound scanner, the transducer sends out a beam of sound waves into the body. The sound waves are reflected back to the transducer by boundaries between tissues in the path of the beam (e.g., the boundary between fluid and soft tissue or tissue and bone). When these echoes hit the transducer, they generate electrical signals that are sent to the ultrasound scanner. Using the speed of sound and the time of each echo's return, the scanner calculates the distance from the transducer to the tissue boundary. These distances are then used to generate two-dimensional images of tissues and organs.

During an ultrasound exam, the technician will apply a gel to the skin. This keeps air pockets from forming between the transducer and the skin, which can block ultrasound waves from passing into the body.

WHAT IS ULTRASOUND USED FOR?

Diagnostic ultrasound. This type of ultrasound able to noninvasively image internal organs within the body. However, it is not good for imaging bones or any tissues that contain air, such as the lungs. Under some conditions, ultrasound can image bones (such as in a fetus or in small babies) or the lungs and lining around the lungs, when they are filled or partially filled with fluid. One of the most common uses of ultrasound is during pregnancy, to monitor the growth and development of the fetus, but there are many other uses, including imaging the heart, blood vessels, eyes, thyroid, brain, breast, abdominal organs, skin, and muscles. Ultrasound images are displayed in either 2D, 3D, or 4D (which is 3D in motion).

Functional ultrasound. This type of ultrasound applications include Doppler and color Doppler ultrasound for measuring and visualizing blood flow in vessels within the body or in the heart. It can also measure the speed of the blood flow and direction of movement. This is done using color-coded maps called "color Doppler imaging." Doppler ultrasound is commonly used to determine whether plaque buildup inside the carotid arteries is blocking blood flow to the brain.

Another functional form of ultrasound is elastography, a method for measuring and displaying the relative stiffness of tissues, which can be used to differentiate tumors from healthy tissue. This information can be displayed as either color-coded maps of the relative stiffness; black and white maps that display high-contrast images of tumors compared with anatomical images; or color-coded maps that are overlayed on the anatomical image. Elastography can be used to test for liver fibrosis, a condition in which excessive scar tissue builds up in the liver due to inflammation.

Ultrasound is also an important method for imaging interventions in the body. For example, ultrasound-guided needle biopsy helps physicians see the position of a needle while it is being guided to a selected target, such as a mass or a tumor in the breast. Also, ultrasound is used for real-time imaging of the location of the tip of a catheter as it is inserted in a blood vessel and guided along the length of the vessel. It can also be used for minimally invasive surgery to guide the surgeon with real-time images of the inside of the body.

Therapeutic or interventional ultrasound. This type of ultrasound produces high levels of acoustic output that can be focused on specific targets for the purpose of heating, ablating, or breaking up tissue. One type of therapeutic ultrasound uses high-intensity beams of sound that are highly targeted, and is called "high intensity focused ultrasound" (HIFU). HIFU is being investigated as a method for modifying or destroying diseased or abnormal tissues inside the body (e.g., tumors) without having to open or tear the skin or cause damage to the surrounding tissue. Either ultrasound or MRI is used to identify and target the tissue to be treated, guide and control the treatment in real time, and confirm the effectiveness of the treatment. HIFU is currently FDA approved for the treatment of uterine fibroids, to alleviate pain from bone metastases, and most recently for the ablation of prostate tissue.

HIFU is also being investigated as a way to close wounds and stop bleeding, to break up clots in blood vessels, and to temporarily open the blood brain barrier so that medications can pass through.

ARE THERE RISKS?

Diagnostic ultrasound is generally regarded as safe and does not produce ionizing radiation like that produced by x-rays. Still, ultrasound is capable of producing some biological effects in the body under specific settings and conditions. For this reason, the FDA requires that diagnostic ultrasound devices operate within acceptable limits. The FDA, as well as many professional societies, discourage the casual use of ultrasound (e.g., for keepsake videos) and recommend that it be used only when there is a true medical need.

Section 19.2 | Carotid Ultrasound

This section includes text excerpted from "Carotid Ultrasound," National Heart, Lung, and Blood Institute (NHLBI), March 20, 2007. Reviewed October 2021.

Carotid ultrasound test uses an ultrasound machine, which includes a computer, a screen, and a transducer. The transducer is a handheld device that sends and receives sound waves. If combined with Doppler ultrasound, this test also can show how blood is moving through your arteries. Carotid ultrasound is done to detect plaque buildup in one or both of the carotid arteries in the neck and to see whether the buildup is narrowing your carotid arteries and blocking blood flow to the brain. Test results will help your doctor plan treatment to remove the plaque and help prevent a stroke.

Carotid ultrasound usually is done in a doctor's office or hospital. You will lie on your back on an exam table for your test. The ultrasound technician will put gel on your neck where your carotid arteries are located. The gel helps the sound waves reach your arteries. The technician will move the transducer against different areas on your neck. The transducer will detect the sound waves after they have bounced off your artery walls and blood cells. A computer will use the sound waves to create and record pictures of the inside of your carotid arteries and to show how blood is flowing in your carotid arteries.

Carotid ultrasound has no risks because the test uses harmless sound waves. They are the same type of sound waves that doctors use to create and record pictures of a baby inside a pregnant woman.

Section 19.3 | Echocardiography (Heart)

This section includes text excerpted from "Echocardiography," National Heart, Lung, and Blood Institute (NHLBI), September 27, 2011. Reviewed October 2021.

WHAT IS ECHOCARDIOGRAPHY?

Echocardiography, or echo, is a painless test that uses sound waves to create moving pictures of your heart. The pictures show the size and shape of your heart. They also show how well your heart's chambers and valves are working.

Echo also can pinpoint areas of heart muscle that are not contracting well because of poor blood flow or injury from a previous heart attack. A type of echo called "Doppler ultrasound" shows how well blood flows through your heart's chambers and valves.

Echo can detect possible blood clots inside the heart, fluid buildup in the pericardium (the sac around the heart), and problems with the aorta. The aorta is the main artery that carries oxygen-rich blood from your heart to your body.

Doctors also use echo to detect heart problems in infants and children.

WHO NEEDS ECHOCARDIOGRAPHY

Your doctor may recommend echocardiography (echo) if you have signs or symptoms of heart problems.

For example, shortness of breath and swelling in the legs are possible signs of heart failure. Heart failure is a condition in which your heart cannot pump enough oxygen-rich blood to meet your body's needs. Echo can show how well your heart is pumping blood.

Echo also can help your doctor find the cause of abnormal heart sounds, such as heart murmurs. Heart murmurs are extra or unusual sounds heard during the heartbeat. Some heart murmurs are harmless, while others are signs of heart problems.

Your doctor also may use echo to learn about:

- **The size of your heart.** An enlarged heart might be the result of high blood pressure, leaky heart valves, or heart failure. Echo also can detect increased thickness of the ventricles (the heart's lower chambers). Increased thickness may be due to high blood pressure, heart valve disease, or congenital heart defects.
- **Heart muscles that are weak and are not pumping well.** Damage from a heart attack may cause weak areas of heart muscle. Weakening also might mean that the area is not getting enough blood supply, a sign of coronary heart disease.
- **Heart valve problems.** Echo can show whether any of your heart valves do not open normally or close tightly.
- **Problems with your heart's structure.** Echo can detect congenital heart defects, such as holes in the heart. Congenital heart defects are structural problems present at birth. Infants and children may have echo to detect these heart defects.
- **Blood clots or tumors.** If you have had a stroke, you may have echo to check for blood clots or tumors that could have caused the stroke.

Your doctor also might recommend echo to see how well your heart responds to certain heart treatments, such as those used for heart failure.

TYPES OF ECHOCARDIOGRAPHY

There are several types of echocardiography (echo) – all use sound waves to create moving pictures of your heart. This is the same technology that allows doctors to see an unborn baby inside a pregnant woman.

Unlike x-rays and some other tests, echo does not involve radiation.

Transthoracic Echocardiography

Transthoracic echo is the most common type of echocardiogram test. It is painless and noninvasive. "Noninvasive" means that no surgery is done and no instruments are inserted into your body.

This type of echo involves placing a device called a "transducer" on your chest. The device sends special sound waves, called "ultrasound," through your chest wall to your heart. The human ear cannot hear ultrasound waves.

As the ultrasound waves bounce off the structures of your heart, a computer in the echo machine converts them into pictures on a screen.

Stress Echocardiography

Stress echo is done as part of a stress test. During a stress test, you exercise or take medicine (given by your doctor) to make your heart work hard and beat fast. A technician will use echo to create pictures of your heart before you exercise and as soon as you finish.

Some heart problems, such as coronary heart disease, are easier to diagnose when the heart is working hard and beating fast.

Transesophageal Echocardiography

Your doctor may have a hard time seeing the aorta and other parts of your heart using a standard transthoracic echo. Thus, she or he may recommend transesophageal echo, or TEE.

During this test, the transducer is attached to the end of a flexible tube. The tube is guided down your throat and into your esophagus (the passage leading from your mouth to your stomach). This allows your doctor to get more detailed pictures of your heart.

Fetal Echocardiography

Fetal echo is used to look at an unborn baby's heart. A doctor may recommend this test to check a baby for heart problems. When recommended, the test is commonly done at about 18 to 22 weeks of pregnancy. For this test, the transducer is moved over the pregnant woman's belly.

Three-Dimensional Echocardiography

A three-dimensional (3D) echo creates 3D images of your heart. These detailed images show how your heart looks and works.

During transthoracic echo or TEE, 3D images can be taken as part of the process used to do these types of echo.

Doctors may use 3D echo to diagnose heart problems in children. They also may use 3D echo for planning and overseeing heart valve surgery.

Researchers continue to study new ways to use 3D echo.

WHAT TO EXPECT BEFORE ECHOCARDIOGRAPHY

Echocardiography (echo) is done in a doctor's office or a hospital. No special preparations are needed for most types of echo. You usually can eat, drink, and take any medicines as you normally would.

The exception is if you are having a transesophageal echo. This test usually requires that you do not eat or drink for 8 hours prior to the test.

If you are having a stress echo, you may need to take steps to prepare for the stress test. Your doctor will let you know what steps you need to take.

WHAT TO EXPECT DURING ECHOCARDIOGRAPHY

Echocardiography (echo) is painless; the test usually takes less than an hour to do. For some types of echo, your doctor will need to inject saline or a special dye into one of your veins. The substance makes your heart show up more clearly on the echo pictures.

The dye used for echo is different from the dye used during angiography (a test used to examine the body's blood vessels).

For most types of echo, you will remove your clothing from the waist up. Women will be given a gown to wear during the test. You will lie on your back or left side on an exam table or stretcher.

Soft, sticky patches called "electrodes" will be attached to your chest to allow an EKG (electrocardiogram) to be done. An EKG is a test that records the heart's electrical activity.

A doctor or sonographer (a person specially trained to do ultrasounds) will apply gel to your chest. The gel helps the sound waves reach your heart. A wand-like device called a "transducer" will then be moved around on your chest.

The transducer transmits ultrasound waves into your chest. A computer will convert echoes from the sound waves into pictures of your heart on a screen. During the test, the lights in the room will be dimmed so the computer screen is easier to see.

Echocardiography

The sonographer will record pictures of various parts of your heart. She or he will put the recordings on a computer disc for a cardiologist (heart specialist) to review.

During the test, you may be asked to change positions or hold your breath for a short time. This allows the sonographer to get better pictures of your heart.

At times, the sonographer may apply a bit of pressure to your chest with the transducer. You may find this pressure a little uncomfortable, but it helps get the best picture of your heart. You should let the sonographer know if you feel too uncomfortable.

The process described above is similar to the process for fetal echo. For that test, however, the transducer is placed over the pregnant woman's belly at the location of the baby's heart.

Transesophageal Echocardiography

Transesophageal echo (TEE) is used if your doctor needs a more detailed view of your heart. For example, your doctor may use TEE to look for blood clots in your heart. A doctor, not a sonographer, will perform this type of echo.

TEE uses the same technology as transthoracic echo, but the transducer is attached to the end of a flexible tube.

Your doctor will guide the tube down your throat and into your esophagus (the passage leading from your mouth to your stomach). From this angle, your doctor can get a more detailed image of the heart and major blood vessels leading to and from the heart.

For TEE, you will likely be given medicine to help you relax during the test. The medicine will be injected into one of your veins.

Your blood pressure, the oxygen content of your blood, and other vital signs will be checked during the test. You will be given oxygen through a tube in your nose. If you wear dentures or partials, you will have to remove them.

The back of your mouth will be numbed with gel or spray. Your doctor will gently place the tube with the transducer in your throat and guide it down until it is in place behind your heart.

The pictures of your heart are then recorded as your doctor moves the transducer around in your esophagus and stomach. You should not feel any discomfort as this happens.

Although the imaging usually takes less than an hour, you may be watched for a few hours at the doctor's office or hospital after the test.

Stress Echocardiography

Stress echo is a transthoracic echo combined with either an exercise or pharmacological stress test.

For an exercise stress test, you will walk or run on a treadmill or pedal a stationary bike to make your heart work hard and beat fast. For a pharmacological stress test, you will be given medicine to increase your heart rate.

A technician will take pictures of your heart using echo before you exercise and as soon as you finish. *The Health Topics Stress Testing* article provides more information about what to expect during a stress test.

WHAT YOU MAY SEE AND HEAR DURING ECHOCARDIOGRAPHY

As the doctor or sonographer moves the transducer around, you will see different views of your heart on the screen of the echo machine. The structures of your heart will appear as white objects, while any fluid or blood will appear black on the screen.

Doppler ultrasound often is used during echo tests. Doppler ultrasound is a special ultrasound that shows how blood is flowing through the blood vessels.

This test allows the sonographer to see blood flowing at different speeds and in different directions. The speed and direction of blood flow appear as different colors moving within the black and white images.

The human ear is unable to hear the sound waves used in echo. If you have a Doppler ultrasound, you may be able to hear "whooshing" sounds. Your doctor can use these sounds to learn about blood flow through your heart.

WHAT TO EXPECT AFTER ECHOCARDIOGRAPHY

You usually can go back to your normal activities right after having echocardiography (echo).

If you have a transesophageal echo (TEE), you may be watched for a few hours at the doctor's office or hospital after the test. Your throat might be sore for a few hours after the test.

You also may not be able to drive for a short time after having TEE. Your doctor will let you know whether you need to arrange for a ride home.

WHAT DOES ECHOCARDIOGRAPHY SHOW?

Echocardiography (echo) shows the size, structure, and movement of various parts of your heart. These parts include the heart valves, the septum (the wall separating the right and left heart chambers), and the walls of the heart chambers. Doppler ultrasound shows the movement of blood through your heart.

Your doctor may use echo to:

- Diagnose heart problems
- Guide or determine next steps for treatment

- Monitor changes and improvement
- Determine the need for more tests

Echo can detect many heart problems. Some might be minor and pose no risk to you. Others can be signs of serious heart disease or other heart conditions. Your doctor may use echo to learn about:

- **The size of your heart.** An enlarged heart might be the result of high blood pressure, leaky heart valves, or heart failure. Echo also can detect increased thickness of the ventricles (the heart's lower chambers). Increased thickness may be due to high blood pressure, heart valve disease, or congenital heart defects.
- **Heart muscles that are weak and are not pumping well.** Damage from a heart attack may cause weak areas of heart muscle. Weakening also might mean that the area is not getting enough blood supply, a sign of coronary heart disease.
- **Heart valve problems.** Echo can show whether any of your heart valves do not open normally or close tightly.
- **Problems with your heart's structure.** Echo can detect congenital heart defects, such as holes in the heart. Congenital heart defects are structural problems present at birth. Infants and children may have echo to detect these heart defects.
- **Blood clots or tumors.** If you have had a stroke, you may have echo to check for blood clots or tumors that could have caused the stroke.

WHAT ARE THE RISKS OF ECHOCARDIOGRAPHY?

Transthoracic and fetal echocardiography (echo) have no risks. These tests are safe for adults, children, and infants.

If you have a transesophageal echo (TEE), some risks are associated with the medicine given to help you relax. For example, you may have a bad reaction to the medicine, problems breathing, and nausea (feeling sick to your stomach).

Your throat also might be sore for a few hours after the test. Rarely, the tube used during TEE causes minor throat injuries.

Stress echo has some risks, but they are related to the exercise or medicine used to raise your heart rate, not the echo. Serious complications from stress tests are very uncommon.

Section 19.4 | **Pelvic Ultrasound**

"Pelvic Ultrasound," © 2018 Omnigraphics. Reviewed October 2021.

WHAT IS A PELVIC ULTRASOUND?

A pelvic ultrasound is a diagnostic procedure that uses ultrasound waves to generate images of the pelvic organs, including the uterus, cervix, vagina, fallopian tubes, and the ovaries. A transducer sends out ultrasound waves at a high frequency when placed over the skin. The sound waves reflected by the transducer are converted into images on the computer screen. The transducer translates the different types of tissues encountered in the process, depending on the speed of the sound waves. The pelvic ultrasound can be done either as a transabdominal ultrasound or transvaginal ultrasound. Other procedures related to problems of the pelvis include hysteroscopy, colposcopy, and laparoscopy.

WHY IS A PELVIC ULTRASOUND PERFORMED?

The pelvic ultrasound procedure may not offer all the answers to pelvic problems but it is important for diagnosis and treatment. A pelvic ultrasound is used for the treatment of the following conditions:

- Postmenopausal bleeding
- Monitoring fetal development during pregnancy
- Abnormalities in the uterine structure, including endometrial conditions
- Fibroid tumors, pelvic masses, ovarian cysts, and other types of tumors in the pelvic region
- Pelvic inflammatory disease (PID) and other types of inflammation

- Ectopic pregnancy (pregnancy occurring outside of the uterus, usually in the fallopian tube)
- Aspiration of follicle fluid and eggs from ovaries for in vitro fertilization
- Certain factors in a pelvic ultrasound may interfere with the results of the test, such as:
- Intestinal gas, barium in the intestines
- Severe obesity
- Inadequate filling of the bladder

Keep your doctor informed if any concern arises during the procedure.

HOW DO YOU PREPARE FOR A PELVIC ULTRASOUND?

It is important to ask for instructions from your doctor to help you prepare for a pelvic ultrasound.

No fasting is required for a pelvic ultrasound unless the procedure requires the use of general anesthesia.

Drink at least three cups (24 ounces) of clear fluid an hour before the procedure; but do not empty your bladder. A full bladder helps the physician look at the pelvic organs clearly.

You will be asked to empty your bladder before a transvaginal procedure.

Your doctor will explain the procedure to you if any other preparation is required because of your medical condition.

THE PROCEDURE

The procedure of a pelvic ultrasound may differ based on hospital practices and is usually carried out either in the doctor's office or at an outpatient clinic.

For a Transabdominal Ultrasound

The transabdominal ultrasound procedure is as follows:

- You will be given a gown to wear during the examination.

- You will be asked to lie down on the examination table, and then a gel-like substance will be applied to your abdomen.
- The transducer will be pressed against the skin of your abdomen and moved around over the area being studied.
- When blood flow is being assessed, you may hear a "whoosh, whoosh" sound if a Doppler probe is being used.
- Images of structures will be displayed on the computer screen for the doctor to analyze or detect any abnormalities.
- Once the procedure is completed, you can empty your bladder.

For a Transvaginal Ultrasound

The transvaginal ultrasound is as follows:

- You will be given a gown to wear during the examination.
- After your legs are placed into position for a pelvic examination, a transvaginal transducer will be lubricated and inserted into the vagina. Make sure to inform your doctor if you experience any discomfort during this procedure.
- The transducer will be angled and gently turned to bring the area of study into focus. You might feel some pressure when the transducer is being moved.
- Images of the organs and structures will be displayed on the computer screen for the doctor to analyze or detect any abnormalities.
- Once the procedure is completed, the transducer will be removed.
- Most pelvic ultrasounds are performed using both the transabdominal and transvaginal approaches.

RESULTS

A normal result indicates that there is no problem with the pelvic organs or structures. However, an abnormal result may be due to the following conditions:

- Adenomyosis (benign infiltration of the endometrium into the surrounding uterine muscle)
- Growths in or around the uterus and ovaries (such as cysts or fibroids, or benign muscular growths)
- Endometrial polyps as a result of abnormal vaginal bleeding
- Abscess in the ovaries, fallopian tubes, or pelvis
- Ectopic pregnancy and appendicitis
- Blockages in the fallopian tube
- Cancers of the bladder, cervix, uterus, ovaries, vagina, and other pelvic structures

References

1. "Pelvic/Gynaecologic Ultrasound," Advanced Women's Imaging, May 19, 2010.
2. "Pelvic Ultrasound – Abdominal," MedlinePlus, National Institutes of Health (NIH), April 30, 2018.
3. "Pelvic Ultrasound," Johns Hopkins Medicine, June 29, 2011.

Section 19.5 | **Abdominal Ultrasound**

An abdominal ultrasound is a quick and painless imaging test or scan that uses no radiation but high-frequency sound waves to provide detailed images of abdominal structures that include the liver, gallbladder, spleen, pancreas, and kidneys. Images of blood vessels opening into these organs can also be captured with an abdominal ultrasound scan. An abdominal ultrasound can also be prescribed to detect and diagnose conditions that may affect the uterus, fallopian tubes, ovaries, and cervix. An abdominal ultrasound procedure generally lasts for 30 minutes. However, it could be longer or shorter. It is one of the most prescribed diagnostic procedures to check the growth of the fetus during pregnancy and is often called a "prenatal ultrasound."

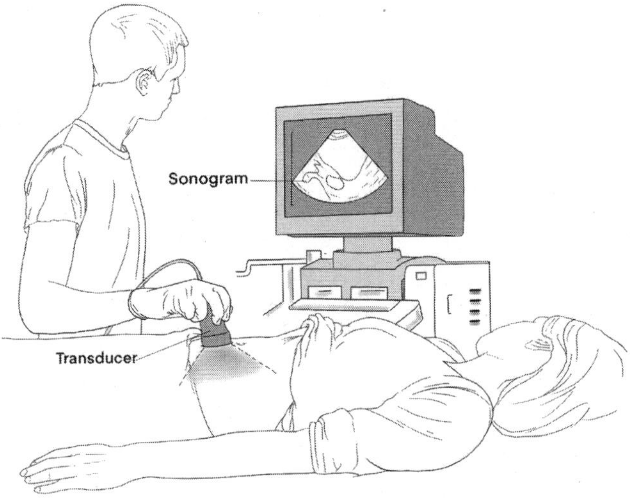

Figure 19.1. Abdominal Ultrasound Procedure

WHY DO YOU NEED AN ABDOMINAL SCAN?

Doctors will recommend an ultrasound of the abdomen to:

- Check for an abdominal aortic aneurysm (a weakened spot in the abdominal aorta)
- Evaluate abdominal organs as a routine examination or for abnormalities
- Diagnose abdominal pains
- Detect abnormal liver function
- Kidney stones and gallstones
- Guide doctors during biopsies

HOW IS AN ABDOMINAL ULTRASOUND PERFORMED?

An abdominal ultrasound examination will require the patient to lay flat on their back on the examination table, after which a gel is applied on the skin surface of the abdomen. The gel aids in accurate scanning. It is performed with a transducer, which is a handheld device that produces sound waves. The technician will move the transducer across the abdomen to capture the desired images. The sound waves pass through the body, and the transducer receives the sound waves that are reflected. This data is collected by a nearby computer and processed to form a detailed image of the targeted body structure. The accompanying technician will simultaneously capture still images from one or more frames or record a short video of the images.

BEFORE THE SCAN

In preparation for the scan, patients are advised to:

- Wear loose clothing and avoid any jewelry
- Avoid any fat-free meals from the previous evening and be asked to avoid food intake for 8 to 12 hours before the scan, if undergoing an ultrasound to study the liver, gallbladder, spleen, or pancreas
- Drink 4 to 6 glasses of water an hour before the scan to study the kidneys

AFTER THE SCAN

Once the scan is complete, the technician will wipe away the applied gel, and the patient will be asked to wait while the radiologist reviews the images and formulates the report for the referring doctor. If the results are abnormal, the doctor will ask for a follow-up ultrasound. The patient can return to regular routines and diets almost immediately after the scan.

BENEFITS AND RISKS

Benefits and Risks

- It is a safe, painless, and noninvasive procedure.
- It is less expensive.
- Soft tissues such as blood vessels are better detailed than they would in x-rays.
- The diagnostic procedure of ultrasound has not been found to cause any adverse effects and is one of the safest procedures in medical technology.

References

1. "Abdominal Ultrasound," MedlinePlus, National Institutes of Health (NIH), September 1, 2021.
2. "Abdominal Ultrasound," Mayo Clinic, March 30, 2021.
3. "Ultrasound – Abdomen," RadiologyInfo.org, January 16, 2020.
4. Sanyal, Shivani. "Abdominal Ultrasound," Healthline, September 17, 2018.
5. "Abdominal Ultrasound," Cleveland Clinic, October 28, 2020.

Chapter 20 | **Computed Tomography**

Chapter Contents

Section 20.1 | Introduction to Computed Tomography

This section includes text excerpted from "Computed Tomography (CT)," National Institute of Biomedical Imaging and Bioengineering (NIBIB), November 13, 2014. Reviewed October 2021.

WHAT IS A COMPUTED TOMOGRAPHY SCAN?

The term "computed tomography" (CT), refers to a computerized x-ray imaging procedure in which a narrow beam of x-rays is aimed at a patient and quickly rotated around the body, producing signals that are processed by the machine's computer to generate cross-sectional images – or "slices" – of the body. These slices are called "tomographic images" and contain more detailed information than conventional x-rays. Once a number of successive slices are collected by the machine's computer, they can be digitally "stacked" together to form a three-dimensional image of the patient that allows for easier identification and location of basic structures as well as possible tumors or abnormalities.

HOW DOES COMPUTED TOMOGRAPHY WORK?

Unlike a conventional x-ray – which uses a fixed x-ray tube – a CT scanner uses a motorized x-ray source that rotates around the circular opening of a donut-shaped structure called a "gantry." During a CT scan, the patient lies on a bed that slowly moves through the gantry while the x-ray tube rotates around the patient, shooting narrow beams of x-rays through the body. Instead of film, CT scanners use special digital x-ray detectors, which are located directly opposite the x-ray source. As the x-rays leave the patient, they are picked up by the detectors and transmitted to a computer.

Each time the x-ray source completes one full rotation, the CT computer uses sophisticated mathematical techniques to construct a 2D image slice of the patient. The thickness of the tissue represented in each image slice can vary depending on the CT machine used, but usually ranges from 1 to 10 millimeters. When a full slice is completed, the image is stored and the motorized bed is moved forward incrementally into the gantry. The x-ray scanning process is then repeated to produce another image slice. This process continues until the desired number of slices is collected.

Image slices can either be displayed individually or stacked together by the computer to generate a 3D image of the patient that shows the skeleton, organs, and tissues as well as any abnormalities the physician is trying to identify. This method has many advantages including the ability to rotate the 3D image in space or to view slices in succession, making it easier to find the exact place where a problem may be located.

WHEN WOULD YOU GET A COMPUTED TOMOGRAPHY SCAN?

Computed tomography scans can be used to identify disease or injury within various regions of the body. For example, CT has become a useful screening tool for detecting possible tumors or lesions within the abdomen. A CT scan of the heart may be ordered when various types of heart disease or abnormalities are suspected. CT can also be used to image the head in order to locate injuries, tumors, clots leading to stroke, hemorrhage, and other conditions. It can image the lungs in order to reveal the presence of tumors, pulmonary embolisms (blood clots), excess fluid, and other conditions such as emphysema or pneumonia. A CT scan is particularly useful when imaging complex bone fractures, severely eroded joints, or bone tumors since it usually produces more detail than would be possible with a conventional x-ray.

WHAT IS A COMPUTED TOMOGRAPHY CONTRAST AGENT?

As with all x-rays, dense structures within the body – such as bone – are easily imaged, whereas soft tissues vary in their ability to stop x-rays and, thus, may be faint or difficult to see. For this reason, intravenous contrast agents have been developed that are highly visible in an x-ray or CT scan and are safe to use in patients. Contrast agents contain substances that are better at stopping x-rays and, thus, are more visible on an x-ray image. For example, to examine the circulatory system, a contrast agent based on iodine is injected into the bloodstream to help illuminate blood vessels. This type of test is used to look for possible obstructions in blood vessels, including those in the heart. Oral contrast agents, such as barium-based compounds, are used for imaging the digestive system, including the esophagus, stomach, and GI tract.

ARE THERE RISKS?

Computed tomography scans can diagnose possibly life-threatening conditions such as hemorrhage, blood clots, or cancer. An early diagnosis of these conditions could potentially be life-saving. However, CT scans use x-rays, and all x-rays produce ionizing radiation. Ionizing radiation has the potential to cause biological effects in living tissue. This is a risk that increases with the number of exposures added up over the life of an individual. However, the risk of developing cancer from radiation exposure is generally small.

A CT scan in a pregnant woman poses no known risks to the baby if the area of the body being imaged is not the abdomen or pelvis. In general, if imaging of the abdomen and pelvis is needed, doctors prefer to use exams that do not use radiation, such as magnetic resonance imaging (MRI) or ultrasound. However, if neither of those can provide the answers needed, or there is an emergency or other time constraint, CT may be an acceptable alternative imaging option.

In some patients, contrast agents may cause allergic reactions, or in rare cases, temporary kidney failure. Contrast agents should not be administered to patients with abnormal kidney function since they may induce a further reduction of kidney function, which may sometimes become permanent.

Children are more sensitive to ionizing radiation and have a longer life expectancy and, thus, a higher relative risk for developing cancer than adults. Parents may want to ask the technologist or doctor if their machine settings have been adjusted for children.

WHAT ARE EXAMPLES OF NIBIB-FUNDED PROJECTS USING COMPUTED TOMOGRAPHY?

Customized Imaging

The amount of radiation required for a CT scan depends on a number of variables, including the size of the patient, the part of the body being scanned, and the diagnostic task at hand. For example, smaller patients require less radiation than larger patients, and scanning a denser part of the body, such as soft tissue near the pelvis, requires more radiation than scanning the lungs. In addition, diagnostic tasks that require high image clarity, such as locating a faint tumor, generally require more radiation. The goal of this project is to modify both the hardware and software of modern CT systems so that the device can adapt the shape, position, and intensity of the x-ray beam to the specific imaging scenario. The research leverages patient-specific anatomical models and mathematical models of imaging performance to direct x-rays where they are needed and, consequently, to avoid or to limit x-ray exposure where it is not needed. This will help maximize imaging performance for specific diagnostic tasks while minimizing radiation exposures.

Constructing Tools for Researchers

The goal of this work is to develop resources that enable the research community to easily create and compare new approaches to reducing radiation dose of routine CT scans without compromising diagnostic accuracy. So far, this has entailed creating a library of raw data from patient CT scans that researchers can manipulate to test new approaches, and developing computer-based methods for evaluating new approaches, so that researchers do not have to rely on radiologists, which can be costly and time consuming. Using these assets, researchers have demonstrated that there is considerable potential for radiation dose reduction in CT exams of the abdomen, which are among the highest dose CT exams in common clinical use.

Faster Processing

To reduce radiation yet still produce good quality CT images, more sophisticated methods are needed to process the raw data from the CT system. Those advanced methods, called "image reconstruction algorithms," can require undesirably long computing times, so they can be used only for some patients currently. The goal of this project is to develop algorithms that are fast enough to allow low-dose CT imaging to be used for every patient.

An Integrated Approach

At every stage in the design of CT scanners, there are opportunities to make changes that reduce radiation dose. Because these changes are inter-related, the goal of this project is to take an integrated approach, exploring approaches such as modifying the photon counting detector (the part of the CT scanner that detects x-rays), dynamic x-ray illumination (adjusting the amount of radiation used throughout the duration of a scan), and image reconstruction methods. These will be tested using a table top experimental system. The researchers believe that these combined strategies can lead to as much as 80 percent reduction in radiation dose compared to today's typical systems, and also enable higher resolution images.

SparseCT

Investigators at New York University School of Medicine, Brigham and Women's Hospital, and Siemens Healthineers are working together to develop a new ultra-low-dose CT technique called "SparseCT." The key idea behind SparseCT is to block most of the x-rays in a CT scan before they reach the patient, but to do so in a way that preserves all the essential image information. The approach combines a new x-ray blocking device with the mathematics of compressed sensing, which allows images to be reconstructed from reduced datasets. Compression sensing can be likened to filming a movie with a very fast, but low-pixel camera and then using math to convert the image to high-definition quality.

Section 20.2 | **Chest CT Scan**

A chest CT scan is a computed tomography scan that utilizes x-rays to provide detailed pictures of the structures in the chest. Sometimes a chest CT can include images of the upper abdomen. The scan utilizes a specialized machine that captures images of the chest in slices which are then overlaid to provide a complete picture of the lungs or chest for radiologists to observe. Chest CT scans can help doctors diagnose symptoms such as cough, breathlessness or chest pain, early-stage lung cancer, or other lung diseases.

WHY ARE CHEST CT SCANS PRESCRIBED?

Doctors may require a chest CT scan to look for conditions such as:

- Injuries
- Trauma
- Blockages
- Tumors and lesions
- Infections
- Bleeding in the chest
- Inflammation
- Undiagnosed chest pain
- Fluid accumulation in the lungs
- The progress of treatments on tumors
- Blood clots
- Tuberculosis
- Emphysema
- Pneumonia

Chest CT scans are crucial in providing doctors with an idea of the mucus lining and thickened regions of the lungs, which can be a cause for concern. A chest CT scan is also vital in helping doctors track the progress of cystic fibrosis in patients. A chest CT scan can help provide more detailed images compared to x-rays. In addition, the scan can help guide needles during biopsies in the chest and the removal of sample fluid from the lungs.

WHAT TO KNOW BEFORE THE SCAN

- Patients must reveal medical history information to the technician and the doctor before scheduling a chest CT scan.
- Any pregnancy-related information must be given to the health-care team.
- A consent form may be required if the scan involves the use of contrast dye. If the patient has reduced kidney

function, the dye may cause further renal damage. This kind of information must be given before the scan, along with accommodations.
- Claustrophobic patients may require additional medication to help them relax before entering the CT scanner.
- Loose-fitting clothes are preferred.
- Patients must avoid wearing jewelry, glasses, dentures, piercings, hearing aids, or clothing with metal wiring.
- If the scan requires a contrast dye, the patient will be advised not to eat or drink for a few hours before the scan appointment.
- Allergic reactions to contrast dyes, iodine, or shellfish must be communicated to the health-care team.
- If the patient is using metformin, they will be advised to stop the medication for at least 48 hours after the injection of the dye.

SCAN PROCEDURE

The general procedure for a chest CT scan lasts anywhere from 30 seconds to a few minutes and includes steps such as:

- The patient will be asked to change into a medical gown and remove any jewelry, belts, or other metal accessories that can interfere with the scan.
- Scans with a contrast dye will need an intravenous line (IV) placed on the patient's arm or hand. For oral contrast, the patient will need to drink a liquid contrast fluid.
- The patient must lie flat on a movable table with their arms above their head. The table is attached to a large circular machine with a tunnel in between to allow the table to move in and out.
- Pillows and straps may be used to keep the patient still during the scan.
- The technician will be in an adjacent room where the scanner's controls are located. The scanner will have

speakers that will let the patient hear the instructions of the technician. The patient is also provided with a call button to contact the technician if in discomfort or an emergency.
- The patient will be instructed to breathe in, out, or hold their breath during the scan to get precise images of the chest.
- Once the scanner moves around the patient, it will pass short durations of x-rays through the body, which are absorbed by the body's cells. The images are transmitted to a nearby computer to process and be displayed for the radiologist to interpret.
- If a contrast dye is injected, there will be two sets of scans, one before and the other after the injection. The dye may cause sensations such as a salty or metallic taste, nausea, and a flushing sensation which will last only for a few seconds.
- The patient must inform the technician of any discomfort during the scan. They will be asked to wait for some time before they can leave.

AFTER THE SCAN

Once the scan is completed, the patient can return to regular diets and routines unless otherwise specified. The images from the scan are reviewed by a radiologist, who will then send the report to the referring doctor.

ASSOCIATED RISKS

The risk of exposure to x-rays depends on the number of previous scans one has undergone. This information must be given to the doctor. Any questions regarding the dose of radiation are encouraged as well. Pregnancy is a significant risk factor for radiation exposure and must be revealed to the doctor. A kidney problem may also exacerbate the risk of radiation. Other risks may be present depending on the patient's overall health.

References

1. "Chest CT Scan," National Heart, Lung, and Blood Institute (NHLBI), July 25, 2012.
2. "Chest CT," MedlinePlus, National Institutes of Health (NIH), October 5, 2021.
3. "Chest CT Scan," St. Vincent's Hospital Lung Health, August 3, 2019.
4. "CT Scan of the Chest," UW Medicine, April 1, 2021.
5. "What to Expect at a Chest CT Scan," Health Union, September 23, 2019.
6. "CT Scan of the Chest: About This Test," Kaiser Permanente, June 17, 2021.

Section 20.3 | **Full Body CT Scans – What You Need to Know**

This section includes text excerpted from "Full-Body CT Scans – What You Need to Know," U.S. Food and Drug Administration (FDA), December 5, 2017. Reviewed October 2021.

Using a technology that "takes a look" at people's insides and promises early warnings of cancer, cardiac disease, and other abnormalities, clinics and medical imaging facilities nationwide are touting a new service for health-conscious people. A whole-body CT screening typically involves scanning the body from the chin to below the hips with a form of x-ray imaging that produces cross-sectional images.

The technology used is called "x-ray computed tomography" (CT), sometimes referred to as "computerized axial tomography" (CAT). A number of different types of x-ray CT systems are being promoted for various types of screening. For example, "multi-slice" CT (MSCT) and "electron beam" CT (EBCT) – also called "electron beam tomography" (EBT) – are x-ray CT systems that produce images rapidly and are often promoted for screening the buildup of calcium in arteries of the heart.

Computed tomography, MSCT and EBCT all use x-rays to produce images representing "slices" of the body – like the slices of a loaf of bread. Each image slice corresponds to a wafer-thin section which can be viewed to reveal body structures in great detail.

Computed tomography is recognized as an invaluable medical tool for the diagnosis of disease, trauma, or abnormality in patients with signs or symptoms of disease. It is also used for planning, guiding, and monitoring therapy. What is new is that CT is being marketed as a preventive or proactive health-care measure to healthy individuals who have no symptoms of disease.

NO PROVEN BENEFITS FOR HEALTHY PEOPLE

Taking preventive action, finding unsuspected disease, uncovering problems while they are treatable, these all sound great, almost too good to be true! In fact, at this time the U.S. Food and Drug Administration (FDA) knows of no scientific evidence demonstrating that whole-body scanning of individuals without symptoms provides more benefit than harm to people being screened. The FDA is responsible for assuring the safety and effectiveness of such medical devices, and it prohibits manufacturers of CT systems to promote their use for whole-body screening of asymptomatic people. The FDA, however, does not regulate practitioners and they may choose to use a device for any use they deem appropriate.

Compared to most other diagnostic x-ray procedures, CT scans result in relatively high radiation exposure. The risks associated with such exposure are greatly outweighed by the benefits of diagnostic and therapeutic CT. However, for whole-body CT screening of asymptomatic people, the benefits are questionable:

- Can it effectively differentiate between healthy people and those who have a hidden disease?
- Do suspicious findings lead to additional invasive testing or treatments that produce additional risk with little benefit?
- Does a "normal" finding guarantee good health?

Many people do not realize that getting a whole body CT screening exam would not necessarily give them the "peace of mind" they are hoping for, or the information that would allow them to prevent a health problem. An abnormal finding, for example, may not be a serious one, and a normal finding may be inaccurate. CT scans, like other medical procedures, will miss some conditions, and "false" leads can prompt further, unnecessary testing.

POINTS TO CONSIDER IF YOU ARE THINKING OF HAVING A WHOLE-BODY SCREENING

- Whole-body CT screening has not been demonstrated to meet generally accepted criteria for an effective screening procedure.
- Medical professional societies have not endorsed whole-body CT scanning for individuals without symptoms.
- Computed tomography screening of high-risk individuals for specific diseases such as lung cancer or colon cancer is currently being studied.
- The radiation from a CT scan may be associated with a very small increase in the possibility of developing cancer later in a person's life.

Chapter 21 | Magnetic Resonance Imaging

Magnetic resonance imaging (MRI) is a medical imaging procedure for making images of the internal structures of the body. MRI scanners use strong magnetic fields and radio waves (radiofrequency energy) to make images. The signal in an MR image comes mainly from the protons in fat and water molecules in the body.

During an MRI exam, an electric current is passed through coiled wires to create a temporary magnetic field in a patient's body. Radio waves are sent from and received by a transmitter/receiver in the machine, and these signals are used to make digital images of the scanned area of the body. A typical MRI scan last from 20–90 minutes, depending on the part of the body being imaged.

For some MRI exams, intravenous (IV) drugs, such as gadolinium-based contrast agents (GBCAs) are used to change the contrast of the MR image. GBCAs are rare earth metals that are usually given through an IV in the arm.

CHEST MRI

A chest MRI is a painless imaging test that uses radio waves, magnets, and a computer to create detailed pictures of the structures in your chest, including your chest wall, heart, and blood vessels.

Chest MRI can provide detailed information to help your doctor diagnose lung problems such as a tumor or pleural disorder, blood

This chapter contains text excerpted from the following sources: Text in this chapter begins with excerpts from "MRI (Magnetic Resonance Imaging)," U.S. Food and Drug Administration (FDA), August 29, 2018. Reviewed October 2021; Text under the heading "Chest MRI" is excerpted from "Chest MRI," National Heart, Lung, and Blood Institute (NHLBI), December 10, 2016. Reviewed October 2021; Text under the heading "What Is Magnetic Resonance Imaging of the Spine?" is © 2018 Omnigraphics. Reviewed October 2021.

vessel problems, or abnormal lymph nodes. Chest MRI can help explain the results of other imaging tests such as chest x-rays and chest CT scans.

Chest MRI may be done in a medical imaging facility or hospital. You may feel some discomfort from the needle or have a cool feeling as the contrast dye is injected. The MRI machine is a large, tunnel-like machine that has a table. You will lie still on the table, and the table will slide into the machine. You will hear loud humming, tapping, and buzzing sounds when you are inside the machine as pictures of your chest are being taken. You will be able to hear from and talk to the technician performing the test while you are inside the machine. The technician may ask you to hold your breath for a few seconds during the test.

Chest MRI has few risks. In rare instances, the contrast dye may harm people who have kidney disease, or it may cause an allergic reaction. Researchers are studying whether multiple contrast dye injections, defined as four or more, may cause other adverse effects. Talk to your doctor and the technicians performing the test about whether you are or could be pregnant. Let your doctor know if you are breastfeeding because the contrast dye can pass into your breast milk. If you must have the contrast dye injected, you may want to pump and save enough breast milk for one to two days after your test or you may bottle-feed your baby for that time. Tell your doctor if you have:

- A pacemaker or other implanted device because the MRI machine can damage these devices.
- Metal inside your body from previous surgeries because it can interfere with the MRI machine.
- Metal on your body from piercings, jewelry, or some transdermal skin patches because they can interfere with the MRI machine or cause skin burns. Tattoos may cause a problem because older tattoo inks may contain small amounts of metal.

WHAT IS MAGNETIC RESONANCE IMAGING OF THE SPINE?

Magnetic resonance imaging is a medical test that helps physicians diagnose the medical condition of the body using a large magnet, radio frequencies, and a computer to produce images of organs and structures within the body. The anatomy of the vertebrae, the ligaments, disks, spinal cord, and the spaces between the vertebrae can be examined in an MRI scan. MRI machines usually look like narrow tunnels, although some are more spacious or wider. Typically, an MRI scan can last from 30 minutes to two hours.

What Are Some Common Uses of MRI Scan?

- Explore the causes of back pain, compression fracture or bone swelling, such as edema
- Detect congenital anomalies of the vertebrae or the spinal cord
- Assess spinal anatomy, alignment, compression, and inflammation of spinal cord and nerves
- Help plan spinal surgical procedures, decompression of a pinched nerve, spinal fusion, or injection of steroids to relieve spinal pain
- Monitor changes after spinal surgery

How Does an MRI Scan Work?

The MRI scan utilizes radio frequencies to realign hydrogen atoms in your body without causing any chemical change in the tissues. When the hydrogen atoms return to their usual alignment, energy is emitted from different tissues of the body, which is captured by the MRI scanner. A radiologist interprets the signals processed by the computer. The MRI scan also helps differentiate between abnormal and normal tissue and is better than viewing the images by x-ray, computed tomography (CT), or ultrasound.

What Are the Risk Factors of MRI Scan?

The following risk factors may prohibit some patients from having an MRI scan:

- Cochlear implants or pacemakers
- Internal metal objects such as clips, plates, screws, or wire mesh

- Claustrophobic patients, or those taking anti-anxiety medications
- Patients allergic or sensitive to contrast dye or iodine
- Pregnant patients

The Procedure

An MRI scan is usually painless. However, patients who experience anxiety or feel claustrophobic may opt to be sedated. Make sure to inform the radiologist of any concerns. It is normal for the body to feel warm during an MRI scan, and important that a patient remain still while the images are being obtained. Each MRI scan usually takes a few seconds to a few minutes and the radiologist informs the patient before the scan begins and when it ends.

Occasionally a contrast dye is administered intravenously in order to obtain certain images. On such occasions, you may experience irritation at the injection site or a metallic taste in your mouth after the contrast injection is administered. Some patients may experience allergic reactions to the contrast dye. It is important to keep the radiologist or the physician informed on such occasions.

After an MRI scan, you may be required to rest for a period of time if you have been sedated. You will be under supervision for a period of time if a contrast dye was used as well. Inform your physician immediately if side effects such as itching, swelling, rashes, or breathing difficulties develop. Before leaving the medical center, the physician may give you additional instructions depending on your situation.

Who Does Interpret the Results and How Do You Get Them?

The radiologist will analyze the images, sign the report, and refer you to your physician. The physician will evaluate the results, explain your results, and prescribe medications as required. In case of any abnormalities, a follow-up exam may be recommended. Sometimes, follow-up examinations are the best way to determine if a treatment is working or discover any changes that have occurred as a result of your treatment.

References

1. "Magnetic Resonance Imaging (MRI) – Spine," *Radiologyinfo*, 2018.
2. "Magnetic Resonance Imaging (MRI) of the Spine and Brain," Johns Hopkins Medicine, June 29, 2011.

Chapter 22 | Nuclear Imaging

Molecular and nuclear imaging use low doses of radioactive substances linked to compounds used by the body's cells or compounds that attach to tumor cells. Using special detection equipment, the radioactive substances can be traced in the body to see where and when they concentrate.

PET SCAN

The positron emission tomography (PET) scan creates computerized images of chemical changes, such as sugar metabolism, that take place in tissue. Typically, the patient is given an injection of a substance that consists of a combination of a sugar and a small amount of radioactively labeled sugar. The radioactive sugar can help in locating a tumor, because cancer cells take up or absorb sugar more avidly than other tissues in the body.

After receiving the radioactive sugar, the patient lies still for about 60 minutes while the radioactively labeled sugar circulates throughout the body. If a tumor is present, the radioactive sugar will accumulate in the tumor. The patient then lies on a table, which gradually moves through the PET scanner incrementally several times during a 15-60-minute period. The PET scanner is used to detect the distribution of the sugar in the tumor and in the body.

This chapter contains text excerpted from the following sources: Text in this chapter begins with excerpts from "Molecular and Nuclear Imaging (PET and SPECT)," Cancer Imaging Program (CIP), National Cancer Institute (NCI), December 22, 2016. Reviewed October 2021; Text under the heading "Nuclear Heart Scan" is excerpted from "Nuclear Heart Scan," National Heart, Lung, and Blood Institute (NHLBI), December 10, 2016. Reviewed October 2021.

By the combined matching of a CT scan with PET images, there is an improved capacity to discriminate normal from abnormal tissues. A computer translates this information into the images that are interpreted by a radiologist.

PET scans may play a role in determining whether a mass is cancerous. However, PET scans are more accurate in detecting larger and more aggressive tumors than they are in locating tumors that are smaller than 8 mm a pinky nail (or half of a thumb nail) and/or less aggressive cancers. The size of smallest tumor mass that can be found at PET is constantly improving. They may also detect cancer when other imaging techniques show normal results. PET scans may be helpful in evaluating and staging recurrent disease (cancer that has come back). PET scans are beginning to be also commonly used to check if a treatment is working - if a tumor cells are dying and thus using less sugar.

SPECT SCAN

Similar to PET, single photon emission computed tomography (SPECT) uses radioactive tracers and a scanner to record data that a computer constructs into two- or three-dimensional images. A small amount of a radioactive drug is injected into a vein and a scanner is used to make detailed images of areas inside the body where the radioactive material is taken up by the cells. SPECT can give information about blood flow to tissues and chemical reactions (metabolism) in the body.

In this procedure, antibodies (proteins that recognize and stick to tumor cells) can be linked to a radioactive substance. If a tumor is present, the antibodies will stick to it. Then a SPECT scan can be done to detect the radioactive substance and reveal where the tumor is located.

NUCLEAR HEART SCAN

Also known as "nuclear stress test" and "radionuclide scan."

A nuclear heart scan is an imaging test that uses special cameras and a radioactive substance called a "tracer" to create pictures of your heart.

The tracer is injected into your blood and travels to your heart. Nuclear heart scans use single photon emission computed tomography (SPECT) or cardiac positron emission tomography (PET) to detect the energy from the tracer to make pictures of your heart. This imaging test can detect if blood is not flowing to parts of the heart and can diagnose coronary heart disease. It also can check for damaged or dead heart muscle tissue, possibly from a previous heart attack, and assess how well your heart pumps blood to your body. Compared to SPECT, PET takes clearer pictures; however, either option may be used.

A nuclear heart scan may be performed in a medical imaging facility or hospital. Your heart will be monitored during this test with an electrocardiogram (EKG). Two sets of pictures will be taken, each taking 15 to 30 minutes. The first set of pictures is taken right after an exercise or medicine stress test because some problems can be detected only when the heart is working hard or beating fast. If you are not able to exercise, your doctor may give you medicine to increase your heart rate. Shortly after the stress test, the tracer will be injected into a vein in your arm. You may bruise at the injection site. You will lie still on a table that slides through a tunnel-like machine as the first set of pictures is taken. The second set of pictures will be taken on either the same day or the next day after your heartbeat has returned to a normal rate.

Nuclear heart scans have few risks. The amount of radiation in this test is small. In rare instances, some people have a treatable allergic reaction to the tracer. If you have coronary heart disease, you may have chest pain during the stress test. Medicine can help relieve your chest pain. Talk to your doctor and the technicians performing the test about whether you are or could be pregnant. If the test is not urgent, they may have you wait to do the test until after your pregnancy. Let your doctor know if you are breastfeeding because radiation can pass into your breast milk. If the test is urgent, you may want to pump and save enough breast milk for one to two days after your test, or you may bottle-feed your baby for that time.

Chapter 23 | Neurological Imaging

A neurological examination assesses motor and sensory skills, hearing and speech, vision, coordination, and balance. It may also test mental status, mood, and behavior. The examination uses tools such as a tuning fork, flashlight, reflex hammer, and a tool for examining the eye. The results of the neurological examination and the patient's history are used to determine a list of possibilities, known as the "differential diagnosis," that help determine which additional diagnostic tests and procedures are needed.

The following list of procedures – in alphabetical order – describes some of the other tests used to help diagnose a neurological condition.

Angiography is a test that involves injecting dye into the arteries or veins to detect blockage or narrowing. A cerebral angiogram can show narrowing or obstruction of an artery or blood vessel in the brain, head, or neck. It can determine the location and size of an aneurysm or vascular malformation. Angiograms are used in certain strokes where there is a possibility of unblocking the artery using a clot retriever. Angiograms can also show the blood supply of a tumor prior to surgery or embolectomy (surgical removal of a blood clot or other material that is blocking a blood vessel).

Angiograms are usually performed in a hospital outpatient or inpatient setting and may take up to 3 hours, followed by a 6- to 8-hour resting period. The person, wearing a hospital or imaging gown, lies on a table that is wheeled into the imaging area. A physician anesthetizes a small area of the leg near the groin and then

This chapter includes text excerpted from "Neurological Diagnostic Tests and Procedures Fact Sheet," National Institute of Neurological Disorders and Stroke (NINDS), April 10, 2019.

inserts a catheter into a major artery located there. The catheter is threaded through the body and into an artery in the neck. Dye is injected and travels through the bloodstream into the head and neck. A series of x-rays is taken. The person may feel a warm to hot sensation or slight discomfort as the dye is released. In many situations, cerebral angiograms have been replaced by specialized magnetic resonance imaging (MRI) scans, called "MR angiograms" (MRA), or "CT angiograms." A spinal angiogram is used to detect blockage of arteries or blood vessels malformations in the vessels to the spinal cord.

Biopsy involves the removal and examination of a small piece of tissue from the body. Muscle or nerve biopsies are used to diagnose neuromuscular disorders. A small sample of muscle or nerve is removed under local anesthetic (pain-relieving medication) and studied under a microscope. The muscle sample may be removed either surgically, through a slit made in the skin, or by needle biopsy, in which a thin hollow needle is inserted through the skin and into the muscle. A piece of the nerve may be removed through a small surgical incision near the ankle, or occasionally near the wrist. Muscle and nerve biopsies are usually performed in an outpatient testing facility. A skin biopsy can be used to measure small nerve fibers or to test for certain metabolic disorders. A small piece of skin is removed under local anesthesia, usually in an office setting. A brain biopsy, used to determine tumor type or certain infections, requires surgery to remove a small piece of the brain or tumor. A brain biopsy is an invasive procedure that carries its own risks.

Cerebrospinal fluid analysis involves the removal of a small amount of the fluid that surrounds the brain and spinal cord. The procedure is commonly called a "lumbar puncture" or "spinal tap." The fluid is tested to detect evidence of brain hemorrhage, infection, multiple sclerosis, metabolic diseases, or other neurological conditions Pressure inside the skull can be measured to detect conditions such as a false brain tumor. The lumbar puncture may be done as an inpatient or as an outpatient procedure. During the lumbar puncture the person will either lie on one side, with knees close to the chest, or lean forward while sitting on a table, bed, or massage chair. The person's back will be cleaned and injected with a local anesthetic. The injection may cause a slight stinging sensation. Once the anesthetic has taken effect, a special needle is inserted between the vertebrae into the spinal sac and a small amount of fluid (usually about three teaspoons) is withdrawn for testing. Most people will only feel a sensation of pressure as the needle is inserted. Generally, people are asked to lie flat for an hour or two to reduce the after-effect of headache. There is a small risk of nerve root injury or infection from a lumbar puncture. The procedure takes about 45 minutes.

Electroencephalography (EEG) monitors the brain's electrical activity through the skull. EEG is used to help diagnose seizure disorders and metabolic, infectious, or inflammatory disorders that affect the brain's activity. EEGs are also used to evaluate sleep disorders, monitor brain activity when a person has been fully anesthetized or loses consciousness, and may be used to confirm brain death.

This painless, risk-free test can be performed in a doctor's office or at a hospital or testing facility. A person being tested usually reclines in a chair or on a bed during the test. A series of cup-like electrodes are attached to the scalp with a special conducting paste. The electrodes are attached to wires (also called "leads") that carry the electrical signals of the brain to a machine. During an EEG recording session, a variety of external stimuli, including bright or flashing lights, noise or certain drugs may be given.

Individuals may be asked to open and close their eyes, or to change their breathing patterns. Changes in brain wave patterns are transmitted to an EEG machine or computer. An EEG test usually takes about an hour. Testing for certain disorders requires performing an EEG during sleep, which takes at least 3 hours.

In people undergoing evaluation for epilepsy surgery, electrodes may be inserted through a surgical opening in the skull to reduce signal interference. This is called an "intracranial EEG." People typically remain in a hospital epilepsy monitoring unit while implanted electrodes are in place. During this time, the brain is monitored for seizures in order to determine where the seizures originate. People may also be asked to perform certain types of tasks (e.g., reading, speaking, or certain limited motor activities) so that the EEG can be used to identify brain regions that are important for normal function.

Electromyography (EMG) is used to diagnose nerve and muscle disorders, spinal nerve root compression, and motor neuron disorders such as amyotrophic lateral sclerosis. EMG records the electrical activity in the muscles. Muscles develop abnormal electrical signals when there is nerve or muscle damage. During an EMG, very fine needles or wires are inserted into a muscle to assess changes in electrical signals at rest and during movement. The needles are attached through wires to an EMG machine. Testing may take place in a doctor's office or clinic and lasts an hour or longer, depending on the number of muscles and nerves to be tested. Because of a slight risk of bruising or bleeding, people will be asked if they are on aspirin or blood thinners. Most people find this test to be somewhat uncomfortable.

An EMG is usually done in conjunction with a nerve conduction study (NCS). An NCS measures the nerve's ability to send a signal, as well as the speed (nerve conduction velocity) and size of the nerve signal. A set of recording electrodes is taped to the skin over the muscles or skin. Wires connect the electrodes to an EMG machine. A small electrical pulse (similar to the sensation of static electricity) is given on the skin a short distance away to stimulate the nerve to the muscle or skin. The electrical signal is viewed on the EMG machine. The physician then reviews the response to verify any nerve damage or muscle disease. There is minimal discomfort and no risk associated with this test.

Electronystagmography (ENG) describes a group of tests used to diagnose involuntary eye movement, dizziness, and balance disorders. The test is performed at a clinic or imaging center. Small electrodes are taped on the skin around the eyes to record eye movements. If infrared photography is used in place of electrodes, the person being tested wears special goggles that help record the information. Both versions of the test are painless and risk-free.

Evoked potentials, also called "evoked response," measure the electrical signals to the brain generated by hearing, touch, or sight. Evoked potentials are used to test sight and hearing (especially in infants and young children) and can help diagnose such neurological conditions as multiple sclerosis, spinal cord injury, and acoustic neuroma (small tumors of the acoustic nerve). Evoked potentials are also used to monitor brain activity among coma patients, and confirm brain death.

Testing may take place in a doctor's office or hospital setting. One set of electrodes is attached to the person's scalp with conducting paste. The electrodes measure the brain's electrical response to stimuli. A machine records the amount of time it takes for impulses generated by stimuli to reach the brain.

- Auditory evoked potentials (also called "brain stem auditory evoked response") can assess hearing loss and damage to the acoustic nerve and auditory pathways in the brainstem, and detect acoustic neuromas. The person being tested sits in a soundproof room and wears headphones. Clicking sounds are delivered one at a time to one ear while a masking sound is sent to the other ear. Each ear is usually tested twice, and the entire procedure takes about 45 minutes.
- Visual evoked potentials detect loss of vision from optic nerve damage (e.g., from multiple sclerosis). The person sits close to a screen and is asked to focus on the center of a shifting checkerboard pattern. One eye is tested at a time. Each eye is usually tested twice. Testing takes 30 to 45 minutes.
- Somatosensory evoked potentials (SSEPs) measure responses from electrical stimuli to the nerves. In addition to electrodes on the scalp, electrodes are pasted to the arms, leg, and back to measure the signal as it travels from the peripheral nerves to the brain. Tiny electrical shocks are delivered by electrodes pasted to the skin over a nerve in an arm or leg. SSEPs may be used to help diagnose multiple sclerosis, spinal cord compression or injury, and certain metabolic or degenerative diseases. SSEP tests usually take longer than an hour.

Myelography involves the injection of contrast dye into the spinal canal to enhance imaging of the spine, by computerized tomography (CT) or by x-ray. Myelograms have mostly been replaced by MRI, but may be used in special situations. For example, myelograms may be used to diagnose tumors of the spine or spinal cord or spinal cord compression from herniated discs or fractures. The procedure takes about 60 minutes and can be performed as an outpatient procedure. Following an injection of anesthesia to a site between two vertebrae in the lower back, a small amount of the cerebrospinal fluid is removed by spinal tap. Contrast dye is injected into the spinal canal and a CT scan or a series of x-rays is taken. People may experience some pain during the spinal tap as well as headache following the spinal tap. There is a slight risk of fluid leakage or allergic reaction to the dye.

A polysomnogram measures brain and body activity during sleep. It is performed over one or more nights at a sleep center. Electrodes are pasted or taped to the person's scalp, eyelids, and/or chin. Throughout the night and during the various wake/sleep cycles, the electrodes record brain waves, eye movement, breathing, leg and skeletal muscle activity, blood pressure, and heart rate. The person may be videotaped to note any movement during sleep. Results are then used to identify any characteristic patterns of sleep disorders, including restless legs syndrome, periodic limb movement disorder, insomnia, and breathing disorders such as sleep apnea. Polysomnograms are noninvasive, painless, and risk-free.

Thermography (also known as "digital infrared thermal imaging") uses infrared sensing devices to measure small temperature changes and thermal abnormalities between the two sides of the body or within a specific organ. Some scientists question its use in diagnosing neurological disorders. It may be used to evaluate complex regional pain syndromes and certain peripheral nerve disorders, and nerve root compression. It is performed at a specialized imaging center, using infrared light recorders to take pictures of the body. The information is converted into a computer-generated two-dimensional picture of abnormally cold or hot areas indicated by color or shades of black and white. Thermography does not use radiation and is safe, risk-free, and noninvasive.

Ultrasound imaging, also called "ultrasonography," uses high-frequency sound waves to obtain images inside the body.

During an ultrasound examination, the person lies on a table or reclines in an examination chair. A jellylike lubricant is applied to the bare skin and a transducer, which both sends and receives high-frequency sound waves, is passed over the body. The sound wave echoes are recorded and displayed as a computer-generated real-time visual image of the structure or tissue being examined. Ultrasound is painless, noninvasive, and risk-free. The test is performed on an outpatient basis and takes between 15 and 30 minutes to complete.

Ultrasound can be used to assess changes in the anatomy of soft tissues, including muscle and nerve. It is more effective than an x-ray in displaying soft tissue changes, such as tears in ligaments or soft tissue masses. In pregnant women, ultrasound can suggest the diagnosis of conditions such as chromosomal disorders in the fetus. The ultrasound creates a picture of the fetus and the placenta. Ultrasound also may be used in newborns to diagnose hydrocephalus (build-up of cerebrospinal fluid in the brain) or hemorrhage.

- Carotid doppler ultrasound is used to measure flow in arteries and blood vessels in the neck.
- Transcranial doppler ultrasound is used to view blood flow in certain arteries and blood vessels inside the skull. Carotid dopplers and transcranial dopplers are used to assess the risk of stroke.
- Duplex ultrasound refers to ultrasound studies that are combined with anatomical ultrasound.

X-rays of a person's chest and skull may be taken as part of a neurological work-up. X-rays can be used to view any part of the body, such as a joint or major organ system. In a conventional x-ray, a concentrated burst of low-dose ionized radiation passes through the body and onto a photographic plate. Since calcium in bones absorbs x-rays more easily than soft tissue or muscle, the bony structure appears white on the film. Any vertebral misalignment or fractures can be seen within minutes. Tissue masses such as injured ligaments or a bulging disc are not visible on conventional x-rays. This fast, noninvasive, painless procedure is usually performed in a doctor's office or at a clinic.

Fluoroscopy is a type of x-ray that uses a continuous or pulsed beam of low-dose radiation to produce continuous images of a body part in motion. The fluoroscope (x-ray tube) is focused on the area of interest and pictures are either videotaped or sent to a monitor for viewing. Fluoroscopy is used to evaluate swallowing and can be used for other procedures, such as a lumbar puncture, angiogram for clot removal, or myelogram.

Chapter 24 | Optical Imaging

WHAT IS OPTICAL IMAGING?

Optical imaging is a technique for noninvasively looking inside the body, as is done with x-rays. Unlike x-rays, which use ionizing radiation, optical imaging uses visible light and the special properties of photons to obtain detailed images of organs and tissues as well as smaller structures including cells and even molecules. These images are used by scientists for research and by clinicians for disease diagnosis and treatment.

WHAT ARE THE ADVANTAGES OF OPTICAL IMAGING?

Optical imaging offers a number of advantages over other radiological imaging techniques:

- Optical imaging significantly reduces patient exposure to harmful radiation by using nonionizing radiation, which includes visible, ultraviolet, and infrared light. These types of light generate images by exciting electrons without causing the damage that can occur with ionizing radiation used in some other imaging techniques. Because it is much safer for patients, and significantly faster, optical imaging can be used for lengthy and repeated procedures over time to monitor the progression of disease or the results of treatment.
- Optical imaging is particularly useful for visualizing soft tissues. Soft tissues can be easily distinguished

This chapter includes text excerpted from "Optical Imaging," National Institute of Biomedical Imaging and Bioengineering (NIBIB), May 2016. Reviewed October 2021.

from one another due to the wide variety of ways different tissues absorb and scatter light.

- Because it can obtain images of structures across a wide range of sizes and types, optical imaging can be combined with other imaging techniques, such as MRI or x-rays, to provide enhanced information for doctors monitoring complex diseases or researchers working on intricate experiments.
- Optical imaging takes advantage of the various colors of light in order to see and measure many different properties of an organ or tissue at the same time. Other imaging techniques are limited to just one or two measurements.

WHAT TYPES OF OPTICAL IMAGING ARE THERE AND WHAT ARE THEY USED FOR?

Optical imaging includes a variety of techniques that use light to obtain images from inside the body, tissues or cells.

- **Endoscopy.** The simplest and most widely recognized type of optical imaging is endoscopy. An endoscope consists of a flexible tube with a system to deliver light to illuminate an organ or tissue. For example, a physician can insert an endoscope through a patient's mouth to see the digestive cavity to find the cause of symptoms such as abdominal pain, difficulty swallowing, or gastrointestinal bleeding. Endoscopes are also used for minimally invasive robotic surgery to allow a surgeon to see inside the patient's body while remotely manipulating the thin robotic arms that perform the procedure.
- **Optical coherence tomography (OCT).** Optical coherence tomography is a technique for obtaining sub-surface images such as diseased tissue just below the skin. OCT is a well-developed technology with commercially available systems now in use in a variety of applications, including art conservation and diagnostic medicine. For example, ophthalmologists

use OCT to obtain detailed images from within the retina. Cardiologists also use it to help diagnose coronary artery disease.

- **Photoacoustic imaging.** During photoacoustic imaging, laser pulses are delivered to a patient's tissues; the pulses generate heat, expanding the tissues and enabling their structure to be imaged. The technique can be used for a number of clinical applications including monitoring blood vessel growth in tumors, detecting skin melanomas, and tracking blood oxygenation in tissues.
- **Diffuse optical tomography (DOT).** DOT can be used to obtain information about brain activity. A laser that uses near-infrared light is positioned on the scalp. The light goes through the scalp and harmlessly traverses the brain. The absorption of light reveals information about chemical concentrations in the brain. The scattering of the light reflects physiological characteristics such as the swelling of a neuron upon activation to pass on a neural signal.
- **Raman spectroscopy.** This technique relies on what is known as "Raman scattering" of visible, near infrared, or near-ultraviolet light that is delivered by a laser. The laser light interacts with molecular vibrations in the material being examined, and shifts in energy are measured that reveal information about the properties of the material. The technique has a wide variety of applications including identifying chemical compounds and characterizing the structure of materials and crystals. In medicine, Raman gas analyzers are used to monitor anesthetic gas mixtures during surgery.
- **Super-resolution microscopy.** This form of light microscopy encompasses a number of techniques used in research to obtain very high resolution images of individual cells, at a level of detail not feasible using normal microscopy. One example is a technique called "photoactivated localization microscopy" (PALM), which uses fluorescent markers to pinpoint single

molecules. PALM can be performed sequentially to create a super-resolution image from the series of molecules isolated in the sample tissue.

- **Terahertz tomography.** This relatively new, experimental technique involves sectional imaging using terahertz radiation. Terahertz radiation consists of electromagnetic waves, which are found on the spectrum between microwaves and infrared light waves. They are of great interest to scientists because terahertz radiation can "see" what visible and infrared light cannot, and holds great promise for detecting unique information unavailable via other optical imaging methods.

Part 4 | Endoscopic, Catheterization, and Electrical Tests and Assessments

Chapter 25 | **Endoscopy**

Chapter Contents

Section 25.1 | **Endoscopy Overview**

This section includes text excerpted from "Endoscopy," Surveillance, Epidemiology, and End Results (SEER) Program, National Cancer Institute (NCI), September 30, 2002. Reviewed October 2021.

An endoscopic exam involves using an instrument, inserted into natural openings or human-made openings, to examine internal passages or the inside of hollow organs or viscera. This can be effective in the nasopharynx, larynx, esophagus, stomach, large bowel, bladder and parts of the lungs. The common endoscopic procedures used in cancer diagnosis are listed in the table below.

A bronchoscopy is the examination of the bronchi in the lungs. The scope can be inserted through the oral or nasal cavity. The pharynx, larynx, and trachea can be seen as the bronchoscope goes through to the bronchi. Using the flexible bronchoscope, the interior segmental and subsegmental bronchi can be visualized. The endoscopist looks for irregular bronchial folds, mucosal thickening, stenosis, friable tissue, and many other abnormalities such a tumor mass. Normally, biopsies bronchial washings are obtained during a bronchoscopic exam. A proctoscopy is often done using a rigid scope.

A sigmoidoscope is more flexible and can be used to observe the colon, up into the descending colon at greater than 30 cm. In the past, rigid sigmoidoscopes were often used but they have been replaced with flexible sigmoidoscopes. Flexible scopes allow greater visualization of the sigmoid colon. A fiberoptic colonoscope is a flexible instrument that examines the colon to the cecum. Often, the physician will photograph and biopsy any abnormalities or suspicious areas seen during colonoscopy.

A cystoscope is used to examine the interior of the bladder. It is inserted through the urethra, so the urethra can also be examined. Abnormalities can be surgically removed or electrocauterized during the cystoscopic procedure.

The entire endoscopic procedure report must be read to obtain pertinent information. Endoscopic reports define certain observations, tumor location, pertinent findings, diagnosis, or the impressions of cancer. For example, colonoscopy reports should state the

Table 25.1. Common Endoscopic Examinations

Examination	Site Examined
Esophagoscopy	Bronchi
Colonoscopy	Colon and rectum
Cystoscopy	Urinary bladder
Esophagoscopy	Esophagus
Gastroscopy	Stomach
Laryngoscopy	Larynx
Nasopharyngoscopy	Nasopharynx, pharynx
Ophthalmoscopy	Interior of the eye
Panendoscopy	Urinary bladder and urethra
Proctoscopy	Rectum
Sigmoidoscopy	Colon up to sigmoid flexure

distance of the abnormality from the anal verge. Esophagoscopy reports should state the distance of the abnormality from the incisors to help determine the exact location of the tumor. Any biopsies or washings sent for microscopic examination should be noted. It is important to locate copies of the pathology and cytology reports to confirm the diagnosis of cancer.

Some endoscopic procedures can be accomplished through natural openings in the body. Others must be performed through incisions into the body. For example, thoracoscopy is used to examine the pleural cavity. The instrument is inserted through an intercostal space. Mediastinoscopy is performed through an incision in the neck and allows visualization of the area between the lungs. The mediastinal lymph nodes that are examined for potential involvement by metastatic cancer can determine the unresectability of a lung cancer.

Laparoscopy, performed through an incision in the abdominal wall, allows the visualization of intra-abdominal structures. Laparoscopy is useful in gastrointestinal and gynecologic malignancies to diagnose both the primary organ and metastatic involvement. Needle biopsies of the liver are often done under the direct visualization of the laparoscope. Some surgeries can be completed as laparoscopic or lapraroscope-aided procedures. A culdoscopy incision is made through posterior vaginal wall and allows visualization of the cul-de-sac.

The endoscopic retrograde cholangiopancreatogram (ERCP) allows direct visualization and contrast x-rays of the ampulla of Vater and the duodenal mucosal ERCP is helpful in diagnosing both pancreatic and bile duct cancers.

Section 25.2 | **Bronchoscopy**

A bronchoscopy is a technique that enables a doctor to investigate the lungs, especially the bronchi, which are the primary entrances to the lungs. Bronchoscopy is used by doctors to diagnose the source of breathing problems and lung disorders, such as tumors, infection, and bleeding. A thin tube that holds a light and a camera is inserted through the nose or mouth into the lungs, during the process. A doctor may place stents in the airways or perform a biopsy, which includes extracting a small sample of tissue for testing, during the surgery. Usually, the flexible bronchoscope, rather than the rigid bronchoscope, is utilized. This is because the flexible bronchoscope is less likely to cause tissue damage. It also allows for easier access to smaller regions of lung tissue.

WHY BRONCHOSCOPY IS DONE

A bronchoscopy may be recommended by a doctor to:

- Follow up on a scan that revealed a lung infection, malignancy, or lung collapse
- Find out why someone is coughing blood and the cause of a persistent cough

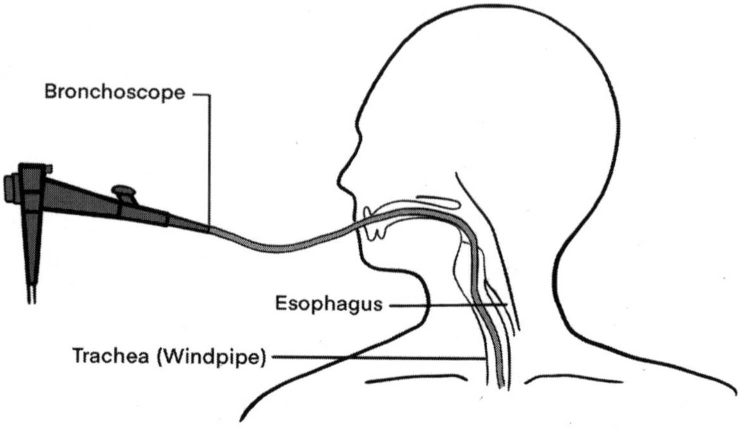

Figure 25.1. Bronchoscopy Procedure

- Look for obstructions in the airways and check for lung rejection after a transplant to figure out the cause of shortness of breath
- Assess any injury or damage to the airway after someone has inhaled chemicals or harmful fumes
- Perform a biopsy

Bronchoscopies are also used to treat specific disorders, such as:

- Remove fluid, mucus plugs, or foreign objects from the airways
- Enlarging a blocked or restricted airway

HOW BRONCHOSCOPY IS DONE

Before the surgery, a local anesthetic is injected into the nose and throat to numb the area. The doctor will generally introduce a flexible bronchoscope via the nose and mouth into the bronchi once the anesthesia has taken effect. The bronchoscope's light and camera allow the doctor to see the airways clearly.

Brushes, needles, and other tools can be passed via a tube in the bronchoscope if a clinician must implant a stent or take a sample for biopsy. A stent is a thin tube that aids in the opening of obstructed or narrowed airways.

A clinician may spray a saline solution into the airways to collect fluids or cells. This process is known as "lavage," or "bronchial washing."

The doctor may then use ultrasonography during the bronchoscopy to gain a better image of the lymph nodes and tissues in and around the bronchi. The bronchoscope will be removed once they have completed their examination of the airways. The procedure takes 20–30 minutes on average; however, it may take longer or shorter depending on the underlying issues.

PREPARING FOR A BRONCHOSCOPY

Your health-care practitioner will frequently advise you to refrain from eating or drinking, a few hours before the process.

Talk to your doctor about any current drugs you are taking, especially blood thinners, such as aspirin or warfarin. It is critical to follow all instructions, especially when it comes to medicine. Driving back home might not be feasible, due to the sedatives used during the procedure, and it is better to plan for a ride to and from the hospital.

RECOVERY PERIOD AFTER A BRONCHOSCOPY

A bronchoscopy is a painless and generally short operation. Following that, a person must stay in the hospital for a few hours until the anesthesia wears off. During this period, blood pressure and breathing are checked to rule out any problems.

The cough reflex, or the capacity to cough, should return within 2 hours. The person should not drive, operate equipment, or consume alcohol for 24 hours after undergoing the procedure. Most patients may resume normal activities after 24 hours, but a painful throat and hoarseness are common for a few days.

RISK FACTORS OF A BRONCHOSCOPY

Every operation entails some level of risk. The following are some of the hazards associated with this procedure:

- Bleeding due to damage of the airway
- Infection in the lung or trachea

- A hole in the airway (bronchial perforation)
- A condition known as "bronchospasm" in which the airways become irritated
- The voice chords are irritated (laryngospasm)
- The pleural space (the gap between the lung coverings) is filled with air, which causes the lung to collapse (pneumothorax)
- The trachea is severely narrowed or blocked (tracheal stenosis)
- The blood arteries in the lungs have high blood pressure (pulmonary hypertension)
- Coughing or gagging

References

1. "Bronchoscopy," Johns Hopkins Medicine, June 29, 2011.
2. "Bronchoscopy," MedlinePlus, National Institutes of Health (NIH), October 5, 2021.
3. Roth, Erica. "Bronchoscopy," Healthline, August 29, 2018.
4. Leonard, Jayne. "What to Expect from a Bronchoscopy," *Medical News Today*, June 18, 2018.

Section 25.3 | **Capsule Endoscopy**

WHAT IS CAPSULE ENDOSCOPY?

Capsule endoscopy is a tested method for screening polyps. The procedure allows physicians to examine a patient's gastrointestinal (GI) tract through the use of a wireless, pill-sized camera, also known as "capsule enteroscopy." The camera has a light source of its own and captures images of the intestines, which are then passed to a small recording device attached to your waist.

WHY IS CAPSULE ENDOSCOPY DONE?

Capsule endoscopy is recommended by your doctor in the following cases:

- Follow-up testing after x-rays or other imaging tests
- Gastrointestinal bleeding
- Ulcers
- Screening for polyps
- Inflammatory bowel disease, such as Crohn disease
- Celiac disease
- Tumors or cancer

RISK FACTORS FOR CAPSULE ENDOSCOPY

Capsule endoscopy is considered a safe procedure although complications are possible:

- If the capsule gets stuck in the digestive tract
- In the case of Crohn disease or a previous surgery in the digestive tract

If the following problems arise after swallowing the capsule, call your health provider immediately:

- Chest pain, cramping, or abdominal pain
- Trouble swallowing
- Vomiting or indigestion
- Fever

HOW TO PREPARE FOR A CAPSULE ENDOSCOPY

Your doctor will give you specific instructions on how to prepare for a capsule endoscopy:

- **Avoid consumption of food or beverages for 12 hours before the procedure.** This will ensure quality images of your digestive tract.
- **Stop taking certain medications.** Your doctor may instruct you to specifically stop taking certain medicines that may interfere with the procedure.
- **Plan to take it easy for the day.** In most cases, you will be allowed to resume regular activities after you have

swallowed the camera capsule. However, heavy lifting and strenuous exercises must be avoided.

THE PROCEDURE

The pill-sized capsule is about an inch long and less than half inch wide. The capsule has a slippery coating that makes it easier to swallow. A recorder is placed on your waist or shoulder and adhesive patches are attached to your abdomen. Each patch has an antenna that receives signals from the capsule and connects to the recorder. The recorder collects and stores the images that a physician uses later to examine your GI tract.

Generally, a physician will permit you to drink fluids after two hours and to consume food after four hours. The procedure is, however, completed only after eight hours when the physician removes the patches and the recorder from your body. The capsule will leave your body later during a bowel movement; however, it is important to inform your physician if this has not happened within two weeks.

Following the procedure, your doctor will give you specific instructions (such as avoiding strenuous physical activities). In most cases, the results of the test will be given to you a week after the procedure, although some tests may take a little longer.

RESULTS

The images saved on the recorder are transferred to your physician via software and made available to your physician as individual images and as images that have been strung together to create a video. Your physician may take a week or more to analyze these results, and will share them with you once analysis is complete.

Normal Result

If no problems were revealed during your test, then your result is normal.

Abnormal Result

If a problem with your digestive tract was discovered during the test, then your physician will discuss this result and further courses of treatment with you.

References

1. "Capsule Endoscopy," Mayo Clinic, 2018.
2. "Understanding Capsule Endoscopy," American Society for Gastrointestinal Endoscopy (ASGE), June 15, 2007.
3. "Capsule Endoscopy," MedlinePlus, National Institutes of Health (NIH), July 13, 2019.

Section 25.4 | **Colonoscopy**

This section includes text excerpted from "Colonoscopy," National Institute of Diabetes and Digestive and Kidney Diseases (NIDDK), July 2017. Reviewed October 2021.

WHAT IS COLONOSCOPY?

Colonoscopy is a procedure in which a doctor uses a colonoscope or scope, to look inside your rectum and colon. Colonoscopy can show irritated and swollen tissue, ulcers, polyps, and cancer.

HOW IS VIRTUAL COLONOSCOPY DIFFERENT FROM COLONOSCOPY?

Virtual colonoscopy and colonoscopy are different in several ways:

- Virtual colonoscopy is an x-ray test, takes less time, and you do not need anesthesia.
- With virtual colonoscopy, your doctor does not view the entire length of your colon.
- Virtual colonoscopy may not find certain polyps as easily as a colonoscopy can.
- Doctors cannot remove polyps or treat certain other problems during a virtual colonoscopy.
- Your health insurance coverage may be different for the two procedures.

WHY DO DOCTORS USE COLONOSCOPY?

A colonoscopy can help a doctor find the cause of symptoms, such as:

- Bleeding from your anus
- Changes in your bowel activity, such as diarrhea
- Pain in your abdomen
- Unexplained weight loss

Doctors also use colonoscopy as a screening tool for colon polyps and cancer. Screening is testing for diseases when you have no symptoms. Screening may find diseases at an early stage, when a doctor has a better chance of curing the disease.

SCREENING FOR COLON AND RECTAL CANCER

Your doctor will recommend screening for colon and rectal cancer – also called "colorectal cancer" – starting at age 45 if you do not have health problems or risk factors that make you more likely to develop colon cancer.

You have risk factors for colorectal cancer if you:

- Are male
- Are African American
- Or someone in your family has had polyps or colorectal cancer
- Have a personal history of inflammatory bowel disease, such as ulcerative colitis and Crohn disease
- Have Lynch syndrome, or another genetic disorder that increases the risk of colorectal cancer
- Have other factors, such as that you weigh too much or smoke cigarettes

If you are more likely to develop colorectal cancer, your doctor may recommend screening at a younger age, and more often.

If you are older than age 75, talk with your doctor about whether you should be screened.

Government health insurance plans, such as Medicare, and private insurance plans sometimes change whether and how often they pay for cancer screening tests. Check with your insurance plan to find out how often your plan will cover a screening colonoscopy.

HOW DO YOU PREPARE FOR A COLONOSCOPY?

To prepare for a colonoscopy, you will need to talk with your doctor, change your diet for a few days, clean out your bowel, and arrange for a ride home after the procedure.

Talk with Your Doctor

You should talk with your doctor about any health problems you have and all prescribed and over-the-counter medicines, vitamins, and supplements you take, including:

- Arthritis medicines
- Aspirin or medicines that contain aspirin
- Blood thinners
- Diabetes medicines
- Nonsteroidal anti-inflammatory drugs such as ibuprofen or naproxen
- Vitamins that contain iron or iron supplements

Change Your Diet and Clean Out Your Bowel

A health-care professional will give you written bowel prep instructions to follow at home before the procedure so that little or no stool remains in your intestine. A complete bowel prep lets you pass stool that is clear and liquid. Stool inside your intestine can prevent your doctor from clearly seeing the lining.

You may need to follow a clear liquid diet for 1 to 3 days before the procedure. You should avoid red and purple-colored drinks or gelatin. The instructions will include details about when to start and stop the clear liquid diet. In most cases, you may drink or eat the following:

- Fat-free bouillon or broth
- Gelatin in flavors such as lemon, lime, or orange
- Plain coffee or tea, without cream or milk
- Sports drinks in flavors such as lemon, lime, or orange
- Strained fruit juice, such as apple or white grape – avoid orange juice
- Water

Different bowel preps may contain different combinations of laxatives – pills that you swallow or powders that you dissolve in water or clear liquids. Some people will need to drink a large amount, often a gallon, of liquid laxative over a scheduled amount of time – most often the night before and the morning of the procedure. Your doctor may also prescribe an enema.

The bowel prep will cause diarrhea, so you should stay close to a bathroom. You may find this part of the bowel prep hard; however, finishing the prep is very important. Call a health-care professional if you have side effects that keep you from finishing the prep.

Your doctor will tell you how long before the procedure you should have nothing by mouth.

Arrange for a Ride Home

For safety reasons, you cannot drive for 24 hours after the procedure, as the sedatives or anesthesia need time to wear off. You will need to make plans for getting a ride home after the procedure.

HOW DO DOCTORS PERFORM A COLONOSCOPY?

A doctor performs a colonoscopy in a hospital or an outpatient center. A colonoscopy usually takes 30 to 60 minutes.

A health-care professional will place an intravenous (IV) needle in a vein in your arm or hand to give you sedatives, anesthesia, or pain medicine, so you would not be aware or feel pain during the procedure. The health-care staff will check your vital signs and keep you as comfortable as possible.

For the procedure, you will lie on a table while the doctor inserts a colonoscope through your anus and into your rectum and colon. The scope inflates your large intestine with air for a better view. The camera sends a video image to a monitor, allowing the doctor to examine your large intestine.

The doctor may move you several times on the table to adjust the scope for better viewing. Once the scope reaches the opening to your small intestine, the doctor slowly removes the scope and examines the lining of your large intestine again.

During the procedure, the doctor may remove polyps and will send them to a lab for testing. You will not feel the polyp removal.

Colon polyps are common in adults and are harmless in most cases. However, most colon cancer begins as a polyp, so removing polyps early helps to prevent cancer.

If your doctor finds abnormal tissue, she or he may perform a biopsy. You would not feel the biopsy.

WHAT SHOULD YOU EXPECT AFTER A COLONOSCOPY?

After a colonoscopy, you can expect the following:

- The anesthesia takes time to wear off completely. You will stay at the hospital or outpatient center for 1 to 2 hours after the procedure.
- You may feel cramping in your abdomen or bloating during the first hour after the procedure.
- After the procedure, you – or a friend or family member – will receive instructions on how to care for yourself after the procedure. You should follow all instructions.
- You will need your prearranged ride home, since you would not be able to drive after the procedure.
- You should expect a full recovery and return to your normal diet by the next day.

After the sedatives or anesthesia wear off, your doctor may share what was found during the procedure with you or, if you choose, with a friend or family member.

If the doctor removed polyps or performed a biopsy, you may have light bleeding from your anus. This bleeding is normal. A pathologist will examine the biopsy tissue, and results take a few days or longer to come back. A health-care professional will call you or schedule an appointment to go over the results.

WHAT ARE THE RISKS OF COLONOSCOPY?

The risks of colonoscopy include:

- Bleeding
- Perforation of the colon
- A reaction to the sedative, including breathing or heart problems

- Severe pain in your abdomen
- Death, although this risk is rare

A study of screening colonoscopies found roughly 4 to 8 serious complications for every 10,000 procedures.

Bleeding and perforation are the most common complications from colonoscopy. Most cases of bleeding occur in patients who have polyps removed. The doctor can treat bleeding that happens during the colonoscopy right away.

You may have delayed bleeding up to 2 weeks after the procedure. The doctor can diagnose and treat delayed bleeding with a repeat colonoscopy. The doctor may need to treat perforation with surgery.

Seek Care Right Away

If you have any of the following symptoms after a colonoscopy, seek medical care right away:

- Severe pain in your abdomen
- Fever
- Bloody bowel movements that do not get better
- Bleeding from the anus that does not stop
- Dizziness
- Weakness

Section 25.5 | **Virtual Colonoscopy**

This section includes text excerpted from "Virtual Colonoscopy," National Institute of Diabetes and Digestive and Kidney Diseases (NIDDK), August 2016. Reviewed October 2021.

WHAT IS VIRTUAL COLONOSCOPY?

Virtual colonoscopy is a procedure in which a radiologist uses x-rays and a computer to create images of your rectum and colon from outside the body. Virtual colonoscopy can show ulcers, polyps, and cancer. Virtual colonoscopy is also called "computerized tomography" (CT) colonography.

HOW IS VIRTUAL COLONOSCOPY DIFFERENT FROM COLONOSCOPY?

Colonoscopy and virtual colonoscopy are different in several ways. Colonoscopy is a procedure in which a trained specialist uses a long, flexible, narrow tube with a light and tiny camera on one end, called a "colonoscope" or "scope," to look inside your rectum and colon. Virtual colonoscopy is an x-ray test, takes less time, and does not require a doctor to insert a scope into the entire length of your colon. Unlike colonoscopy, virtual colonoscopy does not require sedation or anesthesia.

However, virtual colonoscopy may not be as effective as colonoscopy at finding certain polyps. Also, doctors cannot remove polyps or treat certain other problems during virtual colonoscopy, as they can during colonoscopy. Your health insurance coverage for virtual colonoscopy and colonoscopy also may be different.

WHY DO DOCTORS USE VIRTUAL COLONOSCOPY?

Doctors mainly use virtual colonoscopy to screen for polyps or cancer. Screening may find diseases at an early stage, when a doctor has a better chance of curing the disease.

Occasionally, doctors may use virtual colonoscopy when colonoscopy is incomplete or not possible due to other medical reasons.

Screening for Colon and Rectal Cancer

Your doctor will recommend screening for colon and rectal cancer at age 45 if you do not have health problems or other factors that make you more likely to develop colon cancer.

Factors that make you more likely to develop colorectal cancer include:

- Someone in your family has had polyps or cancer of the colon or rectum
- A personal history of inflammatory bowel disease, such as ulcerative colitis or Crohn disease
- Other factors, such as if you weigh too much or smoke cigarettes

If you are more likely to develop colorectal cancer, your doctor may recommend screening at a younger age, and you may need to be tested more often.

If you are older than age 75, talk with your doctor about whether you should be screened.

HOW CAN YOU PREPARE FOR A VIRTUAL COLONOSCOPY?

To prepare for a virtual colonoscopy, you will need to talk with your doctor, change your diet, clean out your bowel, and drink a special liquid called "contrast medium." The contrast medium makes your rectum and colon easier to see in the x-rays.

Talk with Your Doctor

You should talk with your doctor about any medical conditions you have and all prescribed and over-the-counter (OTC) medicines, vitamins, and supplements you take, including:

- Arthritis medicines
- Aspirin or medicines that contain aspirin
- Blood thinners
- Diabetes medicines
- Nonsteroidal anti-inflammatory drugs, such as ibuprofen or naproxen
- Vitamins that contain iron or iron supplements

X-rays may interfere with personal medical devices. Tell your doctor if you have any implanted medical devices, such as a pacemaker.

Doctors do not recommend x-rays for pregnant women because x-rays may harm the fetus. Tell your doctor if you are, or may be, pregnant. Your doctor may suggest a different procedure, such as a colonoscopy.

Change Your Diet and Clean Out Your Bowel

As in colonoscopy, a health-care professional will give you written bowel prep instructions to follow at home before the procedure. A health-care professional orders a bowel prep so that little or no stool is present in your intestine. A complete bowel prep lets you pass stool that is clear and liquid. Stool inside your colon can prevent the x-ray machine from taking clear images of the lining of your intestine.

You may need to follow a clear liquid diet the day before the procedure. The instructions will provide specific direction about when to start and stop the clear liquid diet. In most cases, you may drink or eat the following:

- Fat-free bouillon or broth
- Gelatin in flavors such as lemon, lime, or orange
- Plain coffee or tea, without cream or milk
- Sports drinks in such flavors as lemon, lime, or orange
- Strained fruit juice, such as apple or white grape – doctors recommend avoiding orange juice and red or purple beverages
- Water

Your doctor will tell you how long before the procedure you should have nothing by mouth.

A health-care professional will ask you to follow the directions for a bowel prep before the procedure. The bowel prep will cause diarrhea.

Different bowel preps may contain different combinations of laxatives – pills that you swallow or powders that you dissolve in water and other clear liquids, and enemas. Some people will need to drink a large amount, often a gallon, of liquid laxative over a scheduled amount of time – most often the night before the procedure.

You may find this part of the bowel prep difficult; however, completing the prep is very important. The images will not be clear if the prep is incomplete.

Drink Contrast Medium

The night before the procedure, you will drink a contrast medium. Contrast medium is visible on x-rays and can help your doctor tell the difference between stool and polyps.

HOW DO HEALTH-CARE PROFESSIONALS PERFORM A VIRTUAL COLONOSCOPY?

A specially trained x-ray technician performs a virtual colonoscopy at an outpatient center or a hospital. You do not need anesthesia.

For the procedure, you will lie on a table while the technician inserts a thin tube through your anus and into your rectum. The tube inflates your large intestine with air for a better view. The table slides into a tunnel-shaped device where the technician takes the x-ray images. The technician may ask you to hold your breath several times during the procedure to steady the images. The technician will ask you to turn over on your side or stomach so she or he can take different images of the large intestine. The procedure lasts about 10 to 15 minutes.

WHAT SHOULD YOU EXPECT AFTER A VIRTUAL COLONOSCOPY?

After a virtual colonoscopy, you can expect to:

- Feel cramping or bloating during the first hour after the test
- Resume your regular activities right after the test
- Return to a normal diet

After the test, a radiologist looks at the images to find any problems and sends a report to your doctor. If the radiologist finds problems, your doctor may perform a colonoscopy the same day or at a later time.

WHAT ARE THE RISKS OF A VIRTUAL COLONOSCOPY?

Inflating the colon with air has a small risk of perforating the lining of the large intestine. The doctor may need to treat perforation with surgery.

Seek Care Right Away

If you have any of the following symptoms after a virtual colonoscopy, you should seek medical attention right away:

- Severe pain in your abdomen
- Fever

- Bloody bowel movements or bleeding from your anus
- Dizziness
- Weakness

Section 25.6 | **Cystoscopy and Ureteroscopy**

This section includes text excerpted from "Cystoscopy and Ureteroscopy," National Institute of Diabetes and Digestive and Kidney Diseases (NIDDK), July 2021.

WHAT ARE CYSTOSCOPY AND URETEROSCOPY?

Cystoscopy and ureteroscopy are common procedures performed by a urologist to look inside the urinary tract.

Cystoscopy is a procedure that uses a cystoscope to look inside the urethra and bladder. A cystoscope is a long, thin optical instrument with an eyepiece at one end, a rigid or flexible tube in the middle, and a tiny lens and light at the other end of the tube. A urologist fills the bladder with fluid and looks at detailed images of the urethra and bladder linings on a computer monitor.

Ureteroscopy is a procedure that uses a ureteroscope to look inside the ureters and kidneys. Like a cystoscope, a ureteroscope has an eyepiece at one end, a rigid or flexible tube in the middle, and a tiny lens and light at the other end of the tube. However, a ureteroscope is longer and thinner than a cystoscope so the urologist can see detailed images of the lining of the ureters and kidneys.

WHY DO HEALTH-CARE PROFESSIONALS PERFORM CYSTOSCOPY?

A urologist performs a cystoscopy to find the cause of, and sometimes treat, urinary tract problems such as:

- Frequent urinary tract infections (UTIs)
- Blood in the urine, called "hematuria"
- Urinary frequency, urinary urgency, or urinary incontinence
- Urinary retention
- Pain or burning before, during, or after urination

- Trouble starting urination, completing urination, or both
- Abnormal cells, such as cancer cells, found in a urine sample

During a cystoscopy, a urologist can see:

- Stones – solid pieces of material in the bladder formed by high concentrations of minerals in the urine
- Abnormal tissue, tumors, or cancer in the urethra or bladder
- Stricture, a narrowing of the urethra – a possible sign of an enlarged prostate in men or of scar tissue in the urethra
- Secondary signs of obstruction (or blockage), such as an enlarged prostate gland
- Other congenital or acquired abnormalities such as duplicated ureters, ureterocele, or diverticulum

During a cystoscopy, a urologist can sometimes treat problems, such as bleeding in the bladder and blockage in the urethra. A urologist may also use a cystoscopy to

- Remove a stone in the bladder or urethra
- Remove or treat abnormal tissue and tumors
- Take a sample of the urethra or bladder tissue for a biopsy
- Inject material into the wall of the urethra to treat urinary leakage or prevent vesicoureteral reflux
- Inject medicines into the bladder to treat urinary leakage
- Obtain urine samples from the ureters
- Perform retrograde pyelography – an x-ray procedure in which a urologist injects a special dye into the urinary tract to create images of urinary flow, to show obstructions such as kidney stones and tumors
- Remove a stent that was placed in the ureter after a ureteroscopy with biopsy or stone removal

WHY DO HEALTH-CARE PROFESSIONALS PERFORM URETEROSCOPY?

A urologist performs a ureteroscopy to find the cause of urine blockage in a ureter or to evaluate other problems inside the ureters or kidneys. During a ureteroscopy, a urologist can see:

- A stone in a ureter or kidney
- Problematic tissue, tumors, or cancer in a ureter or in the lining of a kidney

During a ureteroscopy, a urologist can treat problems such as urine blockage in a ureter. The urologist can also:

- Remove a stone from a ureter or kidney
- Remove or treat abnormal tissue and tumors
- Take a sample of ureter or kidney tissue for a biopsy

HOW DO YOU PREPARE FOR A CYSTOSCOPY OR URETEROSCOPY?

Your urologist will ask about your medical history to determine whether you need a cystoscopy or ureteroscopy. You may need to give a urine sample to test for a UTI (urinary tract infection). If you have a UTI, you may need to take antibiotics before either procedure.

Your urologist will also ask about any medicines you are taking, ask if you have any allergies, talk about anesthesia, give instructions for what to do before the procedure, and discuss what to expect afterward. In some cases, you would not need special preparations for a cystoscopy. In other cases, your instructions may include

- When to stop certain medicines, such as blood thinners
- When to stop eating and drinking or, conversely, when to drink plenty of liquids
- When to empty your bladder before the procedure
- Whether to arrange for a ride home after the procedure

HOW DO HEALTH-CARE PROFESSIONALS PERFORM CYSTOSCOPY OR URETEROSCOPY?

A urologist can perform your cystoscopy during an office visit, in an outpatient center, or at a hospital. Ureteroscopies are usually performed in an operating room under anesthesia. A simple exploratory procedure takes about 15 to 30 minutes, including preparation. The procedure can be longer if your urologist performs additional work like taking a biopsy or removing stones from the bladder or ureters.

An anesthetic gel may be applied around the urethral opening, or a local anesthetic may be injected into the urethra.

Sedatives and general anesthesia are often given for a:

- Ureteroscopy
- Cystoscopy with biopsy
- Cystoscopy to inject material into the wall of the urethra or ureters
- Cystoscopy to inject medicine into the bladder

Sedation helps you relax and be comfortable. General anesthesia puts you into a deep sleep during the procedure.

The health-care team will monitor your vital signs and make you as comfortable as possible.

The urologist will position you and make sure the anesthesia is working. The urologist will then gently insert the cystoscope into your urethra and slowly guide it to the bladder. A sterile liquid called "saline" will be used to slowly fill the bladder, so the urologist has a better view of the bladder wall. As the bladder fills with liquid, you may feel some discomfort and the urge to urinate. The urologist may remove some of the liquid from the bladder during the procedure.

During a cystoscopy, the urologist will examine the lining of the urethra and bladder and may insert small instruments through the cystoscope to treat problems in the urethra and bladder or perform a biopsy.

During a ureteroscopy, the urologist will focus on viewing the ureter and lining of the kidney, known as the "renal pelvis." The urologist may also insert small instruments through the ureteroscope to treat problems in the ureter or kidney, perform a biopsy, or cauterize a bleeding area.

After either procedure, the urologist may remove the liquid from the bladder, or you may empty your bladder.

WHAT SHOULD YOU EXPECT AFTER A CYSTOSCOPY OR URETEROSCOPY?

You will be able to go home after almost any cystoscopy performed in an outpatient office setting. If it is performed in an operating room, you will most likely go home the same day as the procedure, depending on what type of anesthesia you receive. If you receive general anesthesia, you may have to wait 1 to 4 hours before going home. In some cases, you may need to stay overnight in the hospital.

Before leaving, try to use the restroom to make sure you can urinate. You will be given discharge instructions for rest, driving, and physical activities after the procedure.

Depending on your procedure and what was done, you may:

- Have a mild burning feeling when urinating
- See small amounts of blood in the urine
- Have mild discomfort in the bladder area or kidney area when urinating
- Need to urinate more frequently or urgently

These problems should not last more than 24 hours. Tell a health-care professional right away if bleeding or pain is severe, if you cannot urinate, or if problems last more than a day.

Once you are at home, your health-care professional may recommend you:

- Drink 16 ounces of water each hour for a few hours after the procedure
- Take a warm bath to relieve any burning feeling
- Hold a warm, damp washcloth over the urethral opening to relieve discomfort
- Take an over-the-counter pain reliever
- Take an antibiotic for 1 or 2 days to prevent an infection

If you had a ureteroscopy and needed a temporary stent placed in the ureter to drain urine while swelling goes away, the stent may cause some pain, discomfort in the kidney or bladder area, or the need to urinate frequently and urgently. The discomfort is generally mild. However, these sensations may be present during the entire time you have the stent. The stent may be left in the ureter for a few days to a week or more. Your urologist may need to perform a cystoscopy to remove the stent in the ureter.

WHAT ARE THE RISKS OF CYSTOSCOPY AND URETEROSCOPY?

The risks of cystoscopy and ureteroscopy include:

- UTIs
- Abnormal bleeding
- Abdominal pain or a burning feeling or pain while urinating
- The inability to urinate swelling
- Injury to the urethra, bladder, or ureters
- Urethral narrowing due to scar tissue formation
- Complications from anesthesia

Seek Care Right Away

After a cystoscopy or ureteroscopy, call or see a health-care professional right away if you:

- Cannot urinate and feel like your bladder is full
- Have burning or painful urination that lasts more than two days
- See bright red urine or blood clots in the urine
- Have a fever, with or without chills
- Feel severe discomfort

Section 25.7 | **Upper Endoscopy**

This section includes text excerpted from "Upper GI Endoscopy," National Institute of Diabetes and Digestive and Kidney Diseases (NIDDK), July 2017. Reviewed October 2021.

WHAT IS UPPER GASTROINTESTINAL ENDOSCOPY?

Upper gastrointestinal (GI) endoscopy is a procedure in which a doctor uses an endoscope – a flexible tube with a camera – to see the lining of your upper GI tract. A gastroenterologist, surgeon, or other trained health-care professional performs the procedure, most often while you receive light sedation to help you relax.

DOES UPPER GASTROINTESTINAL ENDOSCOPY HAVE ANOTHER NAME?

Health-care professionals may also call the procedure endoscopy, upper endoscopy, EGD or esophagogastroduodenoscopy.

WHY DO DOCTORS USE UPPER GASTROINTESTINAL ENDOSCOPY?

Doctors use upper GI endoscopy to help diagnose and treat symptoms and conditions that affect the esophagus, stomach, and upper intestine or duodenum.

Upper GI endoscopy can help find the cause of unexplained symptoms, such as:

- Persistent heartburn
- Bleeding
- Nausea and vomiting
- Pain
- Problems swallowing
- Unexplained weight loss

Upper GI endoscopy can be used to identify many different diseases:

- Gastroesophageal reflux disease
- Ulcers
- Cancer
- Inflammation, or swelling
- Precancerous abnormalities such as Barrett esophagus
- Celiac disease
- Strictures or narrowing of the esophagus
- Blockages

Upper GI endoscopy can check for damage after a person eats or drinks harmful chemicals.

During upper GI endoscopy, a doctor obtains biopsies by passing an instrument through the endoscope to obtain a small piece of tissue for testing. Biopsies are needed to diagnose conditions such as:

- Cancer
- Celiac disease
- Gastritis

Doctors also use upper GI endoscopy to

- Treat conditions such as bleeding from ulcers, esophageal varices, or other conditions
- Dilate or open up strictures with a small balloon passed through the endoscope
- Remove objects, including food, that may be stuck in the upper GI tract
- Remove polyps or other growths
- Place feeding tubes or drainage tubes

Doctors are also starting to use upper GI endoscopy to perform weight loss procedures for some people with obesity.

HOW DO YOU PREPARE FOR AN UPPER GASTROINTESTINAL ENDOSCOPY?

Talk with Your Doctor

You should talk with your doctor about your medical history, including medical conditions and symptoms you have, allergies, and all prescribed and over-the-counter medicines, vitamins, and supplements you take, including:

- Aspirin or medicines that contain aspirin
- Arthritis medicines
- Blood thinners
- Blood pressure medicines
- Diabetes medicines
- Nonsteroidal anti-inflammatory drugs such as ibuprofen and naproxen

You can take most medicines as usual, but you may need to adjust or stop some medicines for a short time before your upper GI endoscopy. Your doctor will tell you about any necessary changes to your medicines before the procedure.

Arrange for a Ride Home

For safety reasons, you cannot drive for 24 hours after the procedure, as the sedatives used during the procedure need time to wear off. You will need to make plans for getting a ride home after the procedure.

Do Not Eat or Drink before the Procedure

To see your upper GI tract clearly, your doctor will most likely ask you not to eat or drink up to 8 hours before the procedure.

HOW DO DOCTORS PERFORM AN UPPER GASTROINTESTINAL ENDOSCOPY?

A doctor performs an upper GI endoscopy in a hospital or an outpatient center. Before the procedure, you will likely get a sedative or a medicine to help you stay relaxed and comfortable during the procedure. The sedative will be given to you through an intravenous (IV) needle in your arm. In some cases, the procedure can be done without getting a sedative. You may also be given a liquid medicine to gargle or a spray to numb your throat and help prevent you from gagging during the procedure. The health-care staff will monitor your vital signs and keep you as comfortable as possible.

You will be asked to lie on your side on an exam table. The doctor will carefully pass the endoscope down your esophagus and into your stomach and duodenum. A small camera mounted on the endoscope will send a video image to a monitor, allowing close examination of the lining of your upper GI tract. The endoscope pumps air into your stomach and duodenum, making them easier to see.

During the upper GI endoscopy, the doctor may:

- Take small samples of tissue, cells, or fluid in your upper GI tract for testing.
- Stop any bleeding.
- Perform other procedures, such as opening up strictures.

The upper GI endoscopy most often takes between 15 and 30 minutes. The endoscope does not interfere with your breathing, and many people fall asleep during the procedure.

WHAT SHOULD YOU EXPECT AFTER AN UPPER GASTROINTESTINAL ENDOSCOPY?

After an upper GI endoscopy, you can expect the following:

- To stay at the hospital or outpatient center for 1 to 2 hours after the procedure so the sedative can wear off
- To rest at home for the rest of the day
- Bloating or nausea for a short time after the procedure
- A sore throat for 1 to 2 days
- To go back to your normal diet once your swallowing returns to normal

After the procedure, you – or a friend or family member who is with you if you are still groggy – will receive instructions on how to care for yourself when you are home. You should follow all instructions.

Some results from an upper GI endoscopy are available right away. Your doctor will share these results with you or, if you choose, with your friend or family member. A pathologist will examine the samples of tissue, cells, or fluid that were taken to help make a diagnosis. Biopsy results take a few days or longer to come back. The pathologist will send a report to your health-care professional to discuss with you.

WHAT ARE THE RISKS OF AN UPPER GASTROINTESTINAL ENDOSCOPY?

Upper GI endoscopy is considered a safe procedure. The risks of complications from an upper GI endoscopy are low, but may include:

- Bleeding from the site where the doctor took the tissue samples or removed a polyp
- Perforation in the lining of your upper GI tract
- An abnormal reaction to the sedative, including breathing or heart problems

Bleeding caused by the procedure often is minor and stops without treatment. Serious complications such as perforation are uncommon. Your doctor may need to perform surgery to treat some complications. Your doctor can also treat an abnormal reaction to a sedative with medicines or IV fluids during or after the procedure.

Seek Care Right Away

If you have any of the following symptoms after an upper GI endoscopy, seek medical care right away:

- Chest pain
- Problems breathing
- Problems swallowing or throat pain that gets worse
- Vomiting – particularly if your vomit is bloody or looks like coffee grounds
- Pain in your abdomen that gets worse
- Bloody or black, tar-colored stool
- Fever

Section 25.8 | **Laryngoscopy**

WHAT IS LARYNGOSCOPY?

A laryngoscopy is a close-up examination of your larynx, which is located at the top of your windpipe, and is also known as the "voice box." The vibration of your vocal cords, which are located in your larynx, produces sound and enables you to speak. An "ear, nose, and throat" (ENT) specialist will use an instrument called "laryngoscope" to view your throat. This process is called "laryngoscopy."

WHY IS A LARYNGOSCOPY DONE?

A laryngoscopy is performed if you have one of the following conditions:

- Voice problems, such as a hoarse or weak voice
- Throat or ear pain that does not go away
- A lump in the neck region

- Bad breath or a cough that does not go away
- Breathing or swallowing problems
- A laryngoscopy can also be used to:
- Remove a sample of tissue from the throat or vocal cords so that the tissue can be looked at under a microscope (This medical test is called a "biopsy.")
- Check the throat for redness, swelling, or blockage
- Remove something that is lodged in the throat

RISK FACTORS

Laryngoscopy is considered a safe procedure; however, risks associated with the procedure may include:

- Breathing and heart problems
- Spasm of the vocal cords
- Ulcers in the lining of the mouth or throat
- Injury to the tongue or lips
- Major bleeding

HOW DO YOU PREPARE FOR A LARYNGOSCOPY?

Your physician might want to take x-rays or other imaging tests before taking a laryngoscopy. In the case of a direct laryngoscopy, you will be advised not to eat or drink anything before you go to the medical center. You will also be asked to stop taking some or all of your medications for at least a week prior to the procedure or as directed by the physician.

THE PROCEDURE

Your physician will determine if you need an indirect or direct laryngoscopy.

- Indirect laryngoscopy is a simple procedure; a small mirror is held at the back of your throat and the physician shines a light on the mirror to view the throat. A medicine is applied to numb your throat as you are awake and lying down during the procedure. This procedure is not recommended for infants, young children, or those who have been diagnosed with acute epiglottitis.

- Direct laryngoscopy allows the physician to use a tube called a "laryngoscope" to examine your throat. General anesthesia given in the medical center will keep you in a state of sleep during the procedure. The physician may use a flexible or a stiff tube to remove any foreign object stuck in the throat.

RESULTS

The doctor might collect a tissue specimen or remove a growth or a foreign object during the laryngoscopy procedure. A biopsy performed on the tissue specimen or growth may take three to five days to complete. Your doctor will explain your results with you and, if needed, discuss treatment options with you or refer you to another doctor.

Normal Result

If your throat, larynx, and vocal cords look normal, then your test result is normal.

Abnormal Result

The following conditions may indicate an abnormal result:

- Redness or swelling of the vocal chords (usually caused by acid reflux)
- Thinning of the muscles and tissues in the voice box
- Inflammation in the throat
- Nodules or polyps on the vocal chords
- Cancer of the throat or voice box

FOLLOW-UP CARE

Gargling with salt water can ease a sore throat. Over-the-counter (OTC) pain relievers or throat lozenges are effective as well.

References

1. "A Close-Up Look at Laryngoscopy," Healthline Media, April 20, 2016.
2. "Laryngoscopy," Canadian Cancer Society (CCS), July 11, 2017.

Section 25.9 | **Flexible Sigmoidoscopy**

This section includes text excerpted from "Flexible Sigmoidoscopy," National Institute of Diabetes and Digestive and Kidney Diseases (NIDDK), July 2016. Reviewed October 2021.

WHAT IS FLEXIBLE SIGMOIDOSCOPY?

Flexible sigmoidoscopy is a procedure in which a trained medical professional uses a flexible, narrow tube with a light and tiny camera on one end, called a "sigmoidoscope" or "scope," to look inside your rectum and lower colon, also called the "sigmoid colon" and "descending colon." Flexible sigmoidoscopy can show irritated or swollen tissue, ulcers, polyps, and cancer.

WHY DO DOCTORS USE FLEXIBLE SIGMOIDOSCOPY?

A flexible sigmoidoscopy can help a doctor find the cause of unexplained symptoms, such as:

- Bleeding from your anus
- Changes in your bowel activity such as diarrhea
- Pain in your abdomen
- Unexplained weight loss

Doctors also use flexible sigmoidoscopy as a screening tool for colon polyps and colon and rectal cancer. Screening may find diseases at an early stage, when a doctor has a better chance of curing the disease.

Screening for Colon and Rectal Cancer

Your doctor will recommend screening for colon and rectal cancer at age 45 if you do not have health problems or other factors that make you more likely to develop colon cancer.

Factors that make you more likely to develop colorectal cancer include:

- Someone in your family has had polyps or cancer of the colon or rectum
- A personal history of inflammatory bowel disease, such as ulcerative colitis or Crohn disease

- Other factors, such as if you weigh too much or smoke cigarettes

If you are more likely to develop colorectal cancer, your doctor may recommend screening at a younger age, and you may need to be tested more often.

If you are older than age 75, talk with your doctor about whether you should be screened.

Most doctors recommend colonoscopy to screen for colon cancer because colonoscopy shows the entire colon and can remove colon polyps. However, preparing for and performing a flexible sigmoidoscopy may take less time and you may not need anesthesia. Health-care providers may combine flexible sigmoidoscopy with other tests.

If your doctor finds abnormal tissue or one or more polyps during a flexible sigmoidoscopy, you should have a colonoscopy to examine the rest of your colon.

Government health insurance plans, such as Medicare, and private health insurance plans sometimes change whether and how often they pay for cancer screening tests. Check with your insurance plan to find out how often your insurance will cover a screening flexible sigmoidoscopy.

HOW DO YOU PREPARE FOR A FLEXIBLE SIGMOIDOSCOPY?

To prepare for a flexible sigmoidoscopy, you will need to talk with your doctor, change your diet, and clean out your bowel.

Talk with Your Doctor

You should talk with your doctor about any medical conditions you have and all prescribed and over-the-counter medicines, vitamins, and supplements you take, including:

- Arthritis medicines
- Aspirin or medicines that contain aspirin
- Blood thinners
- Diabetes medicines

- Nonsteroidal anti-inflammatory drugs, such as ibuprofen or naproxen
- Vitamins that contain iron or iron supplements

Change Your Diet and Clean Out Your Bowel

A health-care professional will give you written bowel prep instructions to follow at home before the procedure. A health-care professional orders a bowel prep so that little or no stool is present in your intestine. A complete bowel prep lets you pass stool that is clear and liquid. Stool inside your colon can prevent your doctor from clearly seeing the lining of your intestine.

You may need to follow a clear liquid diet the day before the procedure. The instructions will provide specific direction about when to start and stop the clear liquid diet. In most cases, you may drink or eat the following:

- Fat-free bouillon or broth
- Gelatin in flavors such as lemon, lime, or orange
- Plain coffee or tea, without cream or milk
- Sports drinks in flavors such as lemon, lime, or orange
- Strained fruit juice, such as apple or white grape – doctors recommend avoiding orange juice and red or purple liquids.
- Water

Your doctor will tell you how long before the procedure you should have nothing by mouth.

A health-care professional will ask you to follow the directions for a bowel prep before the procedure. The bowel prep will cause diarrhea, so you should stay close to a bathroom.

Different bowel preps may contain different combinations of laxatives – pills that you swallow or powders that you dissolve in water and other clear liquids – and enemas. Some people will need to drink a large amount, often a gallon, of liquid laxative over a scheduled amount of time – most often the night before the procedure.

You may find this part of the bowel prep difficult; however, completing the prep is very important. Your doctor will not be able to see your sigmoid colon clearly if the prep is incomplete.

Call a health-care professional if you have side effects that prevent you from finishing the prep.

HOW DO DOCTORS PERFORM A FLEXIBLE SIGMOIDOSCOPY?

A trained medical professional performs a flexible sigmoidoscopy during an office visit or at a hospital or an outpatient center. You typically do not need sedatives or anesthesia, and the procedure takes about 20 minutes.

For the procedure, you will be asked to lie on a table while the doctor inserts a sigmoidoscope into your anus and slowly guides it through your rectum and into your sigmoid colon. The scope pumps air into your large intestine to give the doctor a better view. The camera sends a video image of your intestinal lining to a monitor, allowing the doctor to examine the tissues lining your sigmoid colon and rectum. The doctor may ask you to move several times on the table to adjust the scope for better viewing. Once the scope has reached your transverse colon, the doctor slowly withdraws it and examines the lining of your sigmoid colon again.

During the procedure, your doctor may remove polyps and send them to a lab for testing. Colon polyps are common in adults and are harmless in most cases. However, most colon cancer begins as a polyp, so removing polyps early is an effective way to prevent cancer.

If your doctor finds abnormal tissue, she or he may perform a biopsy. You would not feel the biopsy.

If your doctor found polyps or other abnormal tissue during a flexible sigmoidoscopy, your doctor may suggest you return for a colonoscopy.

WHAT SHOULD YOU EXPECT AFTER A FLEXIBLE SIGMOIDOSCOPY?

After a flexible sigmoidoscopy, you can expect the following:

- You may have cramping in your abdomen or bloating during the first hour after the procedure.

- You can resume regular activities right away after the procedure.
- You can return to a normal diet.

A health-care professional will give you written instructions on how to take care of yourself after the procedure and will review them with you. You should follow all instructions.

If the doctor removed polyps or performed a biopsy, you may have light bleeding from your anus. This bleeding is normal. Some results from a flexible sigmoidoscopy are available right after the procedure, and your doctor will share these results with you. A pathologist will examine the biopsy tissue. Biopsy results take a few days or longer to come back.

WHAT ARE THE RISKS OF A FLEXIBLE SIGMOIDOSCOPY?

The risks of a flexible sigmoidoscopy include:

- Bleeding
- Perforation of the colon
- Severe pain in your abdomen
- Death, although this risk is rare

Bleeding and perforation are the most common complications from flexible sigmoidoscopy. Most cases of bleeding occur in patients who have polyps removed. The doctor can treat bleeding that occurs during the flexible sigmoidoscopy right away. However, you may have delayed bleeding up to 2 weeks after the procedure. The doctor diagnoses and treats delayed bleeding with a colonoscopy or repeat flexible sigmoidoscopy. The doctor may need to treat perforation with surgery.

Seek Care Right Away

If you have any of the following symptoms after a flexible sigmoidoscopy, seek care right away:

- Severe pain in your abdomen
- Fever
- Continued bloody bowel movements or continued bleeding from your anus

- Dizziness
- Weakness

Section 25.10 | **Endoscopic Retrograde Cholangiopancreatography**

This section includes text excerpted from "Endoscopic Retrograde Cholangiopancreatography (ERCP)," National Institute of Diabetes and Digestive and Kidney Diseases (NIDDK), June 2016. Reviewed October 2021.

WHAT IS ENDOSCOPIC RETROGRADE CHOLANGIOPANCREATOGRAPHY?

Endoscopic retrograde cholangiopancreatography (ERCP) is a procedure that combines upper gastrointestinal (GI) endoscopy and x-rays to treat problems of the bile and pancreatic ducts.

WHAT ARE THE BILE AND PANCREATIC DUCTS?

Your bile ducts are tubes that carry bile from your liver to your gallbladder and duodenum. Your pancreatic ducts are tubes that carry pancreatic juice from your pancreas to your duodenum. Small pancreatic ducts empty into the main pancreatic duct. Your

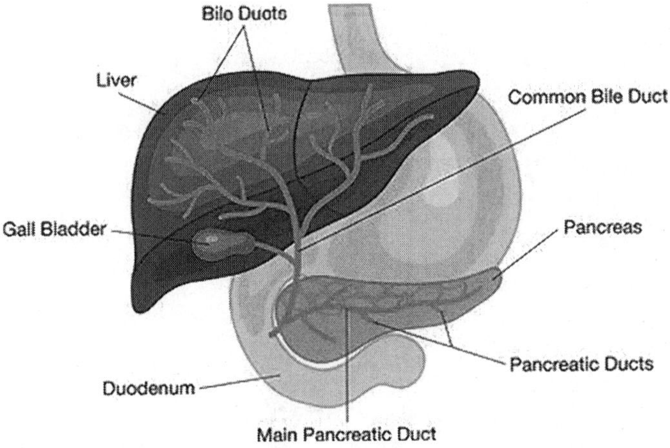

Figure 25.2. Bile and Pancreatic Ducts

common bile duct and main pancreatic duct join before emptying into your duodenum.

WHY DO DOCTORS USE ENDOSCOPIC RETROGRADE CHOLANGIOPANCREATOGRAPHY?

Doctors use ERCP to treat problems of the bile and pancreatic ducts. Doctors also use ERCP to diagnose problems of the bile and pancreatic ducts if they expect to treat problems during the procedure. For diagnosis alone, doctors may use noninvasive tests – tests that do not physically enter the body – instead of ERCP. Noninvasive tests such as magnetic resonance cholangiopancreatography (MRCP) – a type of magnetic resonance imaging (MRI) – are safer and can also diagnose many problems of the bile and pancreatic ducts.

Doctors perform ERCP when your bile or pancreatic ducts have become narrowed or blocked because of:

- Gallstones that form in your gallbladder and become stuck in your common bile duct
- Infection
- Acute pancreatitis
- Chronic pancreatitis
- Trauma or surgical complications in your bile or pancreatic ducts
- Pancreatic pseudocysts
- Tumors or cancers of the bile ducts
- Tumors or cancers of the pancreas

HOW DO YOU PREPARE FOR ENDOSCOPIC RETROGRADE CHOLANGIOPANCREATOGRAPHY?

To prepare for ERCP, talk with your doctor, arrange for a ride home, and follow your doctor's instructions.

Talk with Your Doctor

You should talk with your doctor about any allergies and medical conditions you have and all prescribed and over-the-counter medicines, vitamins, and supplements you take, including:

- Arthritis medicines
- Aspirin or medicines that contain aspirin
- Blood thinners
- Blood pressure medicines
- Diabetes medicines
- Nonsteroidal anti-inflammatory drugs (NSAIDs) such as ibuprofen and naproxen

Your doctor may ask you to temporarily stop taking medicines that affect blood clotting or interact with sedatives. You typically receive sedatives during ERCP to help you relax and stay comfortable.

Tell your doctor if you are, or may be, pregnant. If you are pregnant and need ERCP to treat a problem, the doctor performing the procedure may make changes to protect the fetus from x-rays. Research has found that ERCP is generally safe during pregnancy.

Arrange for a Ride Home

For safety reasons, you cannot drive for 24 hours after ERCP, as the sedatives or anesthesia used during the procedure needs time to wear off. You will need to make plans for getting a ride home after ERCP.

Do Not Eat, Drink, Smoke, or Chew Gum

To see your upper GI tract clearly, you doctor will most likely ask you not to eat, drink, smoke, or chew gum during the 8 hours before ERCP.

HOW DO DOCTORS PERFORM ENDOSCOPIC RETROGRADE CHOLANGIOPANCREATOGRAPHY?

Doctors who have specialized training in ERCP perform this procedure at a hospital or an outpatient center. An intravenous (IV) needle will be placed in your arm to provide a sedative. Sedatives help you stay relaxed and comfortable during the procedure. A health-care professional will give you a liquid anesthetic to gargle or will spray anesthetic on the back of your throat. The anesthetic numbs your throat and helps prevent gagging during the procedure. The health-care staff will monitor your vital signs and keep you as comfortable as possible. In some cases, you may receive general anesthesia.

You will be asked to lie on an examination table. The doctor will carefully feed the endoscope down your esophagus, through your stomach, and into your duodenum. A small camera mounted on the endoscope will send a video image to a monitor. The endoscope pumps air into your stomach and duodenum, making them easier to see.

During ERCP, the doctor:

- Locates the opening where the bile and pancreatic ducts empty into the duodenum
- Slides a thin, flexible tube called a "catheter" through the endoscope and into the ducts
- Injects a special dye, also called "contrast medium," into the ducts through the catheter to make the ducts more visible on x-rays
- Uses a type of x-ray imaging, called "fluoroscopy," to examine the ducts and look for narrowed areas or blockages

The doctor may pass tiny tools through the endoscope to:

- Open blocked or narrowed ducts
- Break up or remove stones
- Perform a biopsy or remove tumors in the ducts
- Insert stents – tiny tubes that a doctor leaves in narrowed ducts to hold them open. A doctor may also insert temporary stents to stop bile leaks that can occur after gallbladder surgery.

The procedure most often takes between 1 and 2 hours.

WHAT SHOULD YOU EXPECT AFTER ENDOSCOPIC RETROGRADE CHOLANGIOPANCREATOGRAPHY?

After ERCP, you can expect the following:

- You will most often stay at the hospital or outpatient center for 1 to 2 hours after the procedure so the sedation or anesthesia can wear off. In some cases, you may need to stay overnight in the hospital after ERCP.
- You may have bloating or nausea for a short time after the procedure.
- You may have a sore throat for 1 to 2 days.
- You can go back to a normal diet once your swallowing has returned to normal.
- You should rest at home for the remainder of the day.

Following the procedure, you – or a friend or family member who is with you if you are still groggy – will receive instructions on how to care for yourself after the procedure. You should follow all instructions.

Some results from ERCP are available right away after the procedure. After the sedative has worn off, the doctor will share results with you or, if you choose, with your friend or family member.

If the doctor performed a biopsy, a pathologist will examine the biopsy tissue. Biopsy results take a few days or longer to come back.

WHAT ARE THE RISKS OF ENDOSCOPIC RETROGRADE CHOLANGIOPANCREATOGRAPHY?

The risks of ERCP include complications such as the following:

- Pancreatitis
- Infection of the bile ducts or gallbladder
- Excessive bleeding, called "hemorrhage"
- An abnormal reaction to the sedative, including respiratory or cardiac problems
- Perforation in the bile or pancreatic ducts, or in the duodenum near the opening where the bile and pancreatic ducts empty into it
- Tissue damage from x-ray exposure
- Death, although this complication is rare

Research has found that these complications occur in about 5 to 10 percent of ERCP procedures. People with complications often need treatment at a hospital.

Seek Care Right Away

If you have any of the following symptoms after ERCP, seek medical attention right away:

- Bloody or black, tar-colored stool
- Chest pain
- Fever
- Pain in your abdomen that gets worse
- Problems breathing
- Problems swallowing or throat pain that gets worse
- Vomiting – particularly if your vomit is bloody or looks like coffee grounds

Section 25.11 | Diagnostic Laparoscopy

Diagnostic laparoscopy or laparoscopy is a minimally invasive procedure performed with an instrument called a "laparoscope." It is a long, thin tube with a high-resolution camera and high-intensity light at one end. The laparoscope allows the doctor to examine the organs in the abdomen or pelvis. The instrument is passed through a small incision in the abdomen, and the camera at the end of the tube sends images to a video monitor. In some cases, this procedure may also allow the doctor to obtain biopsy samples. With the help of a laparoscope, the doctor can get a real-time look inside the abdomen at the:

- Appendix
- Gallbladder
- Liver
- Pancreas
- Stomach
- Spleen
- Uterus
- Ovaries
- Fallopian tubes

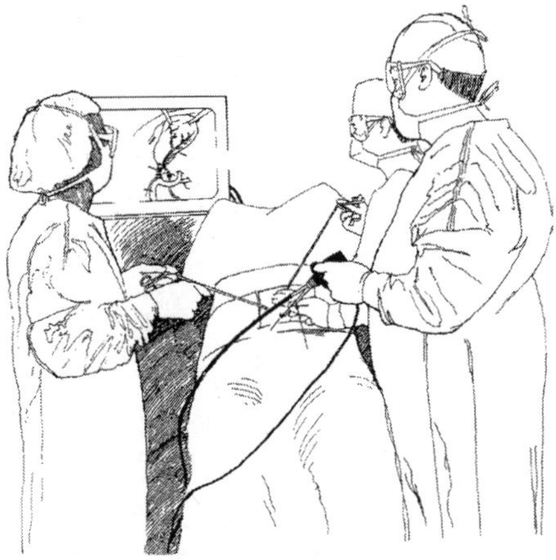

Figure 25.3. Laparoscopy Procedure *(Source: "Laparoscopic Cholecystectomy to Remove the Gallbladder," National Institute of Diabetes and Digestive and Kidney Diseases (NIDDK).)*

Imaging techniques such as ultrasound, computed tomography (CT) scan, and magnetic resonance imaging (MRI) scan are often used to diagnose problems in the abdomen. But if these tests are not able to provide enough information, a laparoscopy is performed.

RISKS OF LAPAROSCOPY

Laparoscopy is a very safe procedure that allows the doctor to make an accurate diagnosis of the condition. Possible risks can include:

- Bleeding
- Damage to organs in the abdomen
- Blood clot
- Inflammation in the abdominal wall
- Complications of general anesthesia such as dizziness
- Infection

TESTS DONE BEFORE A LAPAROSCOPIC SURGERY

Before the surgery, the health-care provider would require some medical information about the patient and order a few tests such as:

- Pathology report
- Lab work
- Tissue specimens
- Operative report
- Previous x-rays from a different facility

HOW IS A LAPAROSCOPY PERFORMED?

The procedure is performed under general anesthesia, and the patient needs to lie down in a slightly tilted position, with the head lower than the feet. General anesthesia is administered via an intravenous line (IV), and any special medication can be provided by it as well as fluids for hydration. An incision is made below the navel, and a small tube called a "cannula" is inserted. The cannula inflates the abdomen with carbon dioxide making it easier to view the organs. After the abdomen is inflated, the laparoscope is inserted. A secondary incision may be made near the pubic hairline if required. This incision helps to conduct minor surgical procedures. After the surgery, the patient is required to stay in the recovery room for an hour. In most cases, the patients are discharged four hours after the surgery. Follow-up appointments will be scheduled within 2–8 weeks of the surgery.

References

1. Giorgi, Anna. "Laparoscopy," Healthline, October 6, 2018.
2. "Laparoscopy," Cleveland Clinic, November 25, 2020.

Chapter 26 | Cardiac Catheterization

Cardiac catheterization is a medical procedure used to diagnose and treat some heart conditions. It lets doctors take a close look at the heart to identify problems and perform other tests or procedures on your heart.

Your doctor may recommend cardiac catheterization to find out the cause of symptoms such as chest pain or irregular heartbeat, or to find out whether you have ischemic heart disease due to blockages in the coronary arteries. Before the procedure, your doctor may need to do diagnostic tests, such as blood tests, heart imaging tests, or a stress test, to determine how well your heart is working and to help guide the procedure.

During cardiac catheterization, a long, thin, flexible tube called a "catheter" is put into a blood vessel in your arm, groin or upper thigh, or neck. The catheter is then threaded to your heart. Your doctor may use it to examine your heart valves or take samples of blood or heart muscle. Your doctor also may use ultrasound or inject a dye into your coronary arteries to see whether your arteries are narrowed or blocked. Cardiac catheterization may also be used instead of some heart surgeries to repair heart defects and replace heart valves.

Cardiac catheterization is safe for most people. Complications are rare, but can include bleeding and blood clots. Your doctor will monitor your condition and may recommend medicines to prevent blood clots.

This chapter includes text excerpted from "Cardiac Catheterization," National Heart, Lung, and Blood Institute (NHLBI), March 30, 2020.

WHO NEEDS IT

When Is Cardiac Catheterization Recommended?

Your doctor may recommend cardiac catheterization to help with diagnoses or plan treatment. It can be useful when your doctor wants to do any of the following:

- Better understand the results from other tests and procedures, such as echocardiography (echo), cardiac MRI, and cardiac CT scan, especially if other studies could not define the problem or if the results from other studies differ from what your doctor finds when examining you.
- Diagnose the cause of your chest pain, arrhythmia, or other signs and symptoms of a heart problem or evaluate you during an emergency such as a heart attack. The procedure may help your doctor diagnose heart conditions such as pulmonary hypertension, cardiomyopathy, ischemic heart disease, and heart valve diseases such as aortic stenosis and mitral regurgitation.
- Evaluate you before a possible heart transplant.
- Look at the pulmonary arteries for conditions, including pulmonary embolism, that can occur as a result of venous thromboembolism. The pulmonary arteries are the blood vessels that carry blood from your heart to your lungs, where the blood receives oxygen.
- Measure oxygen levels and pressures of the blood in your heart, such as in your ventricles, atria, and pulmonary arteries.

Your doctor may perform additional procedures to diagnose or treat your condition during cardiac catheterization. Some of these procedures include:

- Biopsies to take small samples of the heart tissue for further laboratory testing. Biopsies can be used for genetic testing or to check for myocarditis, a type of heart inflammation, or transplant rejection.

- Coronary angiography to look at the heart or blood vessels by injecting dye through the catheter.
- Minor heart surgery to treat congenital heart defects and replace or widen narrowed heart valves.
- Percutaneous coronary intervention (PCI) to open narrowed or blocked areas of the coronary arteries. PCI may include balloon dilation, or angioplasty, or stent placement. Most people who have heart attacks or underlying ischemic heart diseases have narrowed or blocked coronary arteries.

Who Should Not Have Cardiac Catheterization?

Your doctor may wait to do the procedure or recommend that you do not have cardiac catheterization if you have one of the following conditions:

- Abnormal electrolyte levels in your blood
- Acute gastrointestinal bleeding
- Acute kidney failure, or severe kidney disease that is not being treated with dialysis
- Acute stroke
- Blood that is too thin from medicines such as warfarin or other causes
- High blood levels of a heart medicine called "digoxin"
- Previous severe allergic reaction to the dye that is used during cardiac catheterization
- Severe anemia, which is a lower-than-normal red blood cell count or hemoglobin
- Unexplained fever
- Untreated infection

BEFORE CARDIAC CATHETERIZATION

Before cardiac catheterization, you will meet with your cardiologist, a doctor who specializes in the heart. The doctor will ask you about your medical history, including what medicines you are taking and any allergies you may have, and do a physical exam. Your doctor will also give you instructions on how to prepare for the procedure.

Diagnostic Tests and Procedures

You may have some of the following tests before your catheterization procedure:

- Electrocardiogram (ECG or EKG) to look at your heart's rhythm and other electrical activity of your heart. It can show arrhythmias, heart attacks, and other problems with the heart.
- Chest x-ray to look at your lungs, your heart, your major blood vessels, and other structures in the chest
- Echocardiogram (echo) to look at the structure and function of your heart.
- Stress test to look at how well your heart works during physical stress. The stress may be physical exercise such as walking on a treadmill, or it may be a medicine given to have the same effect.
- Cardiac CT scan to look for narrowing of your heart's blood vessels, and problems with the heart, larger blood vessels, and heart valves. These pictures also may help your doctor plan for procedures to open the coronary arteries.
- Cardiac MRI to provide information on the structure and function of your heart, as well as the type and severity of heart disease.
- Blood tests, including a complete blood count (CBC), to check your hemoglobin and platelet levels; blood chemistry tests to check how well your liver and kidneys are working; and tests to check your blood's ability to clot.

Preparing for the Procedure

Talk to your doctor about your medical history, including any medicines you take, other surgical procedures you have had, and any medical conditions you have, such as diabetes or kidney disease.

Your doctor will talk to you about how to prepare for the procedure, including:

- When to arrive at the hospital and where to go
- When you should stop eating or drinking

- If and when you should start or stop taking medicines
- How long you should expect to stay
- What happens during the procedure
- What to expect after the procedure, including potential complications, such as bleeding or soreness
- Instructions to follow after the procedure, including what medicines to take

DURING CARDIAC CATHETERIZATION

Cardiac catheterization takes place in a catheterization laboratory, or cath lab, which is similar to a small operating room. The procedure is often done in a hospital, but you may be able to have the procedure in a catheterization laboratory located in a medical clinic, depending on the reason you are having the procedure and the risk for complications.

How Is Cardiac Catheterization Done?

Before cardiac catheterization, an intravenous line (IV) will be placed in a vein in your arm. Through this IV you will get a medicine to either help you relax or make you sleep during the procedure.

You will get numbing medicine, or local anesthesia, at the site where the doctor will insert the catheter. This site is called the "access site" and may be in the upper thigh, arm, neck, or under the collarbone. The doctor places a needle into a blood vessel at the access site. A guidewire is inserted into the needle, and the needle is taken out. Then the doctor places a small tube called a "sheath" in the blood vessel around the guidewire. The guidewire is removed. The catheter is then inserted through the sheath. Your doctor watches x-ray images to see where to place the tip of the catheter.

Once the catheter is in place, your doctor may use it to perform tests or treatments on your heart. For example, she or he may inject a dye into the catheter to look at blood flow in the heart. The dye will enter your blood vessels and make your coronary arteries visible in x-ray pictures.

Possible Risks and Complications

Cardiac catheterization is a relatively safe procedure, and complications are rare. Possible complications include the following:

- Allergic reaction to the dye used. This reaction may be hives or a more serious reaction.
- Arrhythmias
- Bleeding at the access site or inside your abdomen
- Blood clot formation at the access site, inside your abdomen, in a blood vessel, or in your heart
- Collapsed lung, called "pneumothorax," resulting in air in the space between your lung and chest wall
- Damage to blood vessels, heart valves, or your heart
- Heart attack
- Hypothermia, especially in small children
- Infection
- Low blood pressure from bleeding or as a reaction to the procedure
- Need for blood transfusion
- Need for emergency surgery to repair a tear in the aorta or coronary artery and restore blood flow to the heart. This may be done using a coronary artery bypass graft (CABG).
- Side effects of general anesthesia, if used. These can include nausea, vomiting, confusion, or an allergic reaction.
- Stroke

Although not an immediate risk, repeated radiation exposure from x-rays used to place the catheter in the heart, especially with children, may increase the risk of cancer and leukemia, damage to skin, and cataracts later in life.

AFTER CARDIAC CATHETERIZATION

After the procedure, your doctor will remove the catheters, sheath, and guidewire. A dressing, accompanied by pressure, is applied to the site where the catheter was inserted to stop the bleeding. The pressure may be held by hand or with a sandbag or other device.

You will be moved to a recovery room, where you will lie in bed. Your heartbeat and blood pressure will be monitored.

Depending on your health before the cardiac catheterization and what additional procedures were done during the cardiac catheterization, you may have to spend the night in the hospital. You should follow your doctor's instructions on what medicines to take and when to resume activity.

LIFE AFTER CARDIAC CATHETERIZATION

If you have had cardiac catheterization, it is important that you receive follow-up care, know about the possible complications that may occur after the procedure, and follow the treatment plan that your doctor recommends for your condition.

Receive Follow-Up Care

It is important to get routine follow-up care after you have cardiac catheterization. Talk with your doctor about how often you should schedule office visits.

- Adopt a heart-healthy lifestyle, especially if your cardiac catheterization was needed because of ischemic heart disease or heart attack.
- Follow any instructions for when to resume physical activity and lifting and at what levels.
- Follow instructions on how to care for the site where the doctor accessed your blood vessel, including when you can take a bath or swim.
- Keep any follow-up appointments or tests.
- Take any medicines as directed by your doctor.
- Talk to your doctor about any blood tests you may need if you were placed on blood thinners after your procedure.

Learn the Warning Signs of Complications and Have a Plan

Complications from cardiac catheterization are rare, but can be serious. A small bruise and tenderness at the access site is normal.

Call your doctor immediately if you experience any of the following, as they may be signs of serious complications.

- Bleeding from the access site that cannot be stopped with firm pressure
- Chest pain or shortness of breath
- Dizziness
- Fever
- Increased pain, redness, or bruising at the access site
- Irregular, very slow, or fast heartbeat
- Swelling at the access site
- Yellow or green discharge draining from the access site
- Your leg or arm that was used for access becoming numb or weak or any part of it turning cold or blue

Other serious complications after catheterization, although rare, include heart attack and stroke. If you think that you are or someone else is having the following symptoms, call 911 immediately.

Heart attack signs and symptoms include:

- Chest pain or discomfort in the center of the chest or upper abdomen that lasts for more than a few minutes or goes away and comes back. It can feel like pressure, squeezing, fullness, heartburn, or indigestion.
- Nausea, vomiting, light-headedness or fainting, or breaking out in a cold sweat. These symptoms of a heart attack are more common in women.
- Shortness of breath, which may occur with or before chest discomfort.
- Upper body discomfort in one or both arms or the back, neck, jaw, or upper part of the stomach.

If you think someone may be having a stroke, act F.A.S.T. and perform the following simple test:

- **F – Face.** Ask the person to smile. Does one side of the face droop?
- **A – Arms**. Ask the person to raise both arms. Does one arm drift downward?

- **S – Speech.** Ask the person to repeat a simple phrase. Is their speech slurred or strange?
- **T – Time.** If you observe any of these signs, call for help immediately. Early treatment is essential.

Chapter 27 | Transesophageal Echocardiography

WHAT IS TRANSESOPHAGEAL ECHOCARDIOGRAPHY?

Transesophageal echocardiography, or TEE, is a test that uses sound waves to create high-quality moving pictures of the heart and its blood vessels.

The TEE is a type of echocardiography (echo). Echo shows the size and shape of the heart and how well the heart chambers and valves are working.

Echo can pinpoint areas of heart muscle that are not contracting well because of poor blood flow or injury from a previous heart attack.

Echo also can detect possible blood clots inside the heart, fluid buildup in the pericardium (the sac around the heart), and problems with the aorta. The aorta is the main artery that carries oxygen-rich blood from your heart to your body.

During echo, a device called a "transducer" is used to send sound waves (called "ultrasound") to the heart. As the ultrasound waves bounce off the structures of the heart, a computer in the echo machine converts them into pictures on a screen.

The TEE involves a flexible tube (probe) with a transducer at its tip. Your doctor will guide the probe down your throat and into your esophagus (the passage leading from your mouth to your stomach). This approach allows your doctor to get more detailed pictures of your heart because the esophagus is directly behind the heart.

This chapter includes text excerpted from "Transesophageal Echocardiography," National Heart, Lung, and Blood Institute (NHLBI), February 20, 2010. Reviewed October 2021.

The TEE can help doctors diagnose heart and blood vessel diseases and conditions in adults and children. Doctors also may use TEE to guide cardiac catheterization, help prepare for surgery, or assess a patient's status during or after surgery.

Doctors may use TEE in addition to transthoracic echo (TTE), the most common type of echo. If TTE pictures do not give doctors enough information, they may recommend TEE to get more detailed pictures.

The TEE has a low risk of complications in both adults and children. Even newborns can have TEE.

TYPES OF TRANSESOPHAGEAL ECHOCARDIOGRAPHY

Standard transesophageal echocardiography pictures are two-dimensional (2D). It is also possible to get three-dimensional (3D) pictures from TEE. These pictures provide even more details about the structure and function of the heart and its blood vessels.

Doctors can use 3D TEE to help diagnose heart problems, such as congenital heart disease and heart valve disease. Doctors also may use this technology to assist with heart surgery.

WHO NEEDS TRANSESOPHAGEAL ECHOCARDIOGRAPHY?

Doctors may recommend transesophageal echocardiography to help diagnose a heart or blood vessel disease or condition. TEE can be used for adults and children.

Doctors also may use TEE to guide cardiac catheterization, help prepare for surgery, or assess a patient's status during or after surgery.

Transesophageal Echocardiography as a Diagnostic Tool

The TEE helps doctors detect problems with the structure and function of the heart and its blood vessels.

In general, transthoracic echo (TTE) is the first echo test used to diagnose heart and blood vessel problems. However, you might have TEE if your doctor needs more information or more detailed pictures than TTE can provide.

For TTE, the transducer (the device that sends the sound waves) is placed on the chest, outside of the body. This means the sound waves may not always have a clear path to the heart and blood vessels. For example, obesity, scarring from previous heart surgery, or certain lung problems (such as a collapsed lung) may block the sound waves.

For TEE, the transducer is at the tip of a flexible tube (probe). Your doctor will guide the probe down your throat and into your esophagus (the passage leading from your mouth to your stomach).

This approach allows your doctor to get more detailed pictures of your heart because the esophagus is directly behind the heart.

Doctors may use TEE to help diagnose:

- Coronary heart disease
- Congenital heart disease
- Heart attack
- Aortic aneurysm
- Endocarditis
- Cardiomyopathy
- Heart valve disease
- Injury to the heart or aorta (the main artery that carries oxygen-rich blood from your heart to your body)

The TEE also can show blood clots that may have caused a stroke or that may affect treatment for atrial fibrillation, a type of arrhythmia.

Transesophageal Echocardiography and Cardiac Catheterization

Cardiac catheterization is a medical procedure used to diagnose and/or treat certain heart conditions. During this procedure, a long, thin, flexible tube called a "catheter" is put into a blood vessel in your arm, groin (upper thigh), or neck and threaded to your heart.

Doctors may use TEE to help guide the catheter while they are doing the procedure.

Through the catheter, doctors can do tests and treatments on your heart. For example, cardiac catheterization might be used to repair holes in the heart, heart valve disease, and abnormal heart rhythms.

Transesophageal Echocardiography and Surgery

Doctors may use TEE to prepare for a patient's surgery and identify possible risks. For example, they may use TEE to look for possible sources of blood clots in the heart or aorta. Blood clots can cause a stroke during surgery.

The TEE might be used in the operating room after a patient receives medicine to make her or him sleep during the surgery. The test can show the heart's structure and function and help guide the surgery.

The TEE also helps doctors assess a patient's status during surgery. For example, TEE can help check for blood flow and blood pressure problems.

At the end of surgery, TEE might be used again to check how well the surgery worked. For example, TEE can show whether heart valves are working well. TEE also can show how well the heart is pumping.

People having surgery that is not related to the heart also may have TEE to check their heart function if they have known heart disease or a critical illness.

WHAT TO EXPECT BEFORE TRANSESOPHAGEAL ECHOCARDIOGRAPHY

The TEE most often is done in a hospital. You usually will need to fast (not eat or drink) for several hours prior to the test. Your doctor will let you know exactly how long you should fast.

You should let your doctor know whether you are taking any blood-thinning medicines, have trouble swallowing, or are allergic to any medicines. If you have dentures or oral prostheses, you will need to remove them before the test.

You may be given medicine to help you relax during TEE. If so, you will have to arrange for a ride home after the test because the medicine can make you sleepy.

Talk with your doctor about whether you need to take any special steps before having TEE. Your doctor can tell you whether you need to change how you take your regular medicines on the day of the test or whether you need to make other changes.

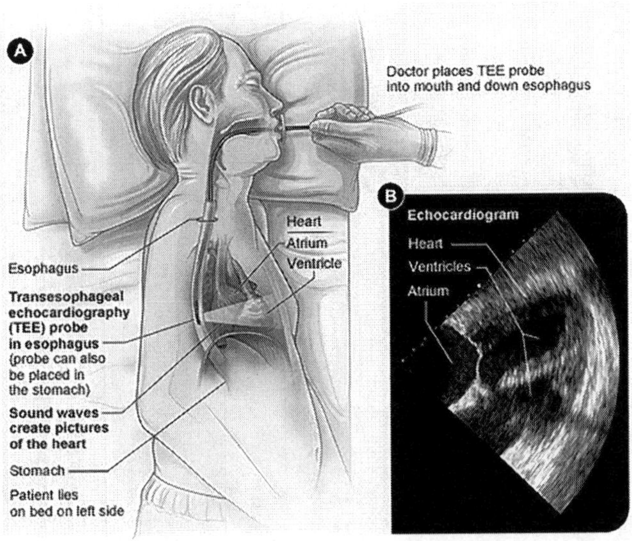

Figure 27.1. Transesophageal Echocardiography and Echocardiogram

Note: *Figure A shows a transesophageal echocardiography probe in the esophagus, which is located behind the heart. Sound waves from the probe create high-quality pictures of the heart. Figure B shows an echocardiogram of the heart's lower and upper chambers (ventricles and atrium, respectively).*

WHAT TO EXPECT DURING TRANSESOPHAGEAL ECHOCARDIOGRAPHY

During transesophageal echocardiography, your doctor or your child's doctor will use a probe with a transducer at its tip. The transducer sends sound waves (ultrasound) to the heart. Probes come in many sizes; smaller probes are used for children and newborns.

The back of your mouth will be numbed with gel or spray before the probe is put down your throat. You may feel some discomfort as the probe is guided into your esophagus (the passage leading from your mouth to your stomach).

Adults having TEE may get medicine to help them relax during the test. The medicine will be injected into a vein.

Children always receive medicine to help them relax or sleep if they are having TEE. This helps them remain still so the doctor can safely insert the probe and take good pictures of the heart and blood vessels.

Your doctor will insert the probe into your mouth or nose. She or he will then gently guide it down your throat into your esophagus. Your esophagus lies directly behind your heart. During this process, your doctor will take care to protect your teeth and mouth from injury.

Your blood pressure, blood oxygen level, and other vital signs will be checked during the test. You may be given oxygen through a tube in your nose.

The TEE takes less than an hour. However, if you received medicine to help you relax, you might be watched for a few hours after the test for side effects from the medicine.

WHAT TO EXPECT AFTER TRANSESOPHAGEAL ECHOCARDIOGRAPHY

After having transesophageal echocardiography, your or your child's blood pressure, blood oxygen level, and other vital signs will continue to be closely watched. You can likely go home a few hours after having the test.

After the TEE, you may have a sore throat for a few hours. You should not eat or drink for 30 to 60 minutes after having TEE. Most people can return to their normal activities within about 24 hours of the test.

Talk with your doctor or your child's doctor to learn more about what to expect after having TEE.

WHAT DOES TRANSESOPHAGEAL ECHOCARDIOGRAPHY SHOW?

The Transesophageal echocardiography provides high-quality moving pictures of your heart and blood vessels. These pictures help doctors detect and treat heart and blood vessel diseases and conditions.

The TEE creates pictures from inside the esophagus (the passage leading from the mouth to the stomach) or, sometimes, from inside the stomach. Because the esophagus lies directly behind the heart, TEE provides closeup pictures of the heart.

The TEE also offers different views and may provide more detailed pictures than transthoracic echocardiography (TTE), the most common type of echo. (For TTE, the transducer is placed on the chest, outside of the body.)

Your doctor may recommend TEE if she or he needs more information than TTE can provide. TEE can help diagnose and assess heart and blood vessel diseases and conditions in adults and children. Examples of these diseases and conditions include:

- Coronary heart disease
- Congenital heart disease
- Heart attack
- Aortic aneurysm
- Endocarditis
- Cardiomyopathy
- Heart valve disease
- Injury to the heart or aorta (the main artery that carries oxygen-rich blood from your heart to your body)

The TEE also can show blood clots that may have caused a stroke or that may affect treatment for atrial fibrillation, a type of arrhythmia.

Doctors also may use TEE during cardiac catheterization. TEE can help doctors guide the catheter (thin, flexible tube) through the blood vessels. TEE also can help doctors prepare for surgery or assess a patient's status during or after surgery.

WHAT ARE THE RISKS OF TRANSESOPHAGEAL ECHOCARDIOGRAPHY?

The transesophageal echocardiography has a very low risk of serious complications in both adults and children. To reduce your risk, your health-care team will carefully check your heart rate and other vital signs during and after the test.

Some risks are associated with the medicine that might be used to help you relax during TEE. You may have a bad reaction to the medicine, problems breathing, or nausea (feeling sick to your stomach). Usually, these problems go away without treatment.

Your throat also might be sore for a few hours after the test. Although rare, the probe used during TEE can damage the esophagus (the passage leading from your mouth to your stomach).

Chapter 28 | Electrocardiogram

WHAT IS AN ELECTROCARDIOGRAM TEST?

An electrocardiogram (EKG) test is a simple, painless procedure that measures electrical signals in your heart. Each time your heart beats, an electrical signal travels through the heart. An EKG can show if your heart is beating at a normal rate and strength. It also helps show the size and position of your heart's chambers. An abnormal EKG can be a sign of heart disease or damage.

WHAT IS IT USED FOR?

An EKG test is used to find and/or monitor various heart disorders. These include:

- Irregular heartbeat (known as "arrhythmia")
- Blocked arteries
- Heart damage
- Heart failure
- Heart attack. EKGs are often used in the ambulance, emergency room, or other hospital room to diagnose a suspected heart attack.

An EKG test is sometimes included in a routine exam for middle-aged and older adults, as they have a higher risk of heart disease than younger people.

This chapter includes text excerpted from "Electrocardiogram," MedlinePlus, National Institutes of Health (NIH), December 10, 2020.

WHY DO YOU NEED AN ELECTROCARDIOGRAM TEST?

You may need an EKG test if you have symptoms of a heart disorder. These include:

- Chest pain
- Rapid heartbeat
- Arrhythmia (it may feel like your heart has skipped a beat or is fluttering)
- Shortness of breath
- Dizziness
- Fatigue

You may also need this test if you:

- Have had a heart attack or other heart problems in the past
- Have a family history of heart disease
- Are scheduled for surgery. Your health-care provider may want to check your heart health before the procedure.
- Have a pacemaker. The EKG can show how well the device is working.
- Are taking medicine for heart disease. The EKG can show if your medicine is effective, or if you need to make changes in your treatment.

WHAT HAPPENS DURING AN ELECTROCARDIOGRAM TEST

An EKG test may be done in a provider's office, outpatient clinic, or a hospital. During the procedure:

- You will lie on an exam table.
- A health-care provider will place several electrodes (small sensors that stick to the skin) on your arms, legs, and chest. The provider may need to shave or trim excess hair before placing the electrodes.
- The electrodes are attached by wires to a computer that records your heart's electrical activity.
- The activity will be displayed on the computer's monitor and/or printed out on paper.
- The procedure only takes about three minutes.

WILL YOU NEED TO DO ANYTHING TO PREPARE FOR THE TEST?

You do not need any special preparations for an EKG test.

ARE THERE ANY RISKS TO THE TEST?

There is very little risk to having an EKG. You may feel a little discomfort or skin irritation after the electrodes are removed. There is no risk of electric shock. The EKG does not send any electricity to your body. It only records electricity.

WHAT DO THE RESULTS MEAN?

Your health-care provider will check your EKG results for a consistent heartbeat and rhythm. If your results were not normal, it may mean you have one of the following disorders:

- Arrhythmia
- A heartbeat that is too fast or too slow
- Inadequate blood supply to the heart
- A bulge in the heart's walls. This bulge is known as an "aneurysm."
- Thickening of the heart's walls
- A heart attack (Results can show if you have had a heart attack in the past or if you are having an attack during the EKG.)

If you have questions about your results, talk to your health-care provider.

Chapter 29 | Stress Testing

A stress test measures how healthy your heart is and how well it works during physical stress. Some heart problems are easier to identify when your heart is working hard to pump blood throughout your body, such as when you exercise.

A stress test is used to help diagnose and evaluate heart problems such as ischemic heart disease, heart valve disease, or heart failure. Your doctor may recommend this test if you have symptoms of a heart problem, such as shortness of breath, chest pain, dizziness, and a rapid or irregular heartbeat. If your doctor does find a problem, the stress test also can help your doctor choose the right treatment plan and determine what types of physical activity are safe for you.

A stress test usually involves physical exercise such as walking on a treadmill or riding a stationary bicycle. The test may be done in a hospital or doctor's office. As you exercise, your doctor will measure your heart rate and blood pressure and your heart's electrical activity. If you are not able to exercise, your doctor will give you medicine that will make your heart work hard and beat faster, as if you were exercising.

Your doctor will carefully monitor you throughout the test to minimize the risk of complications caused by the exercise or medicine used to raise your heart rate. Intense exercise during the test can cause some heart problems to get worse. If your doctor gives you medicine to make your heart beat harder instead of having you exercise, there is a small risk of developing certain heart problems after the test.

This chapter includes text excerpted from "Stress Test," National Heart, Lung, and Blood Institute (NHLBI), September 27, 2019.

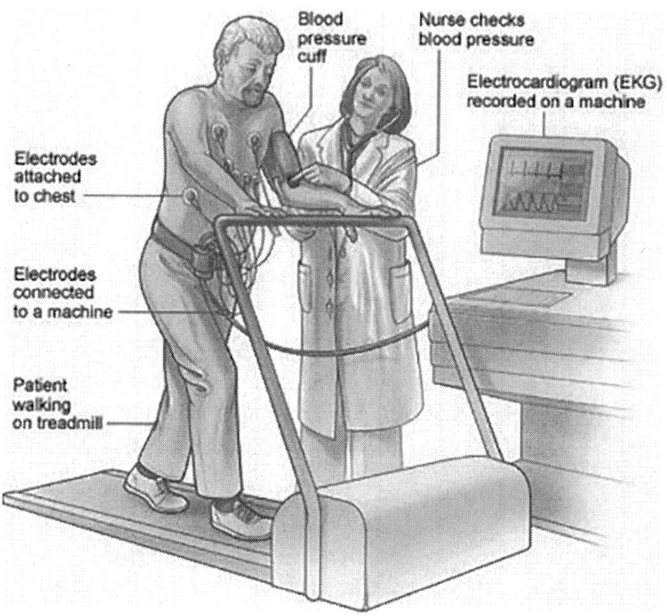

Figure 29.1. Stress Exercise Test

WHAT TO EXPECT

A stress test is usually done in a hospital or doctor's office. Your doctor will give you instructions to prepare for the test and tell you what to expect during and after the test.

Before the Stress Test

Your doctor may ask you not to take some of your prescription medicines or to avoid coffee, tea, or any drinks with caffeine on the day of your test, because these may affect your results. Your doctor will ask you to wear comfortable clothes and shoes for the test.

For the stress test, your doctor will put sticky patches called "electrodes" on your chest and attach a blood pressure cuff to your arm and a pulse monitor to your finger or other part of your body. Your doctor will measure your heart activity and blood pressure before you start the test.

During the Stress Test

You will slowly start to exercise on a treadmill or stationary bicycle, and then gradually increase the treadmill speed or bicycle resistance until your heart is working at the target heart rate for your age. Most often, a stress test includes an electrocardiogram to measure your heart's electrical activity as you exercise on a treadmill or on a stationary bicycle. Your doctor may also measure your blood oxygen level, blood pressure, and heart rate. During the test, you will exercise for 10 to 15 minutes. Your doctor will stop the test if you show any sign of a heart problem, or if you are too tired to continue the test.

If you are not able to exercise, your doctor will give you medicine over a 10- to 20-minute period through an intravenous (IV) line into one of your blood vessels.

Your doctor may also take images of your heart during or right after the stress test to see how well blood is flowing through your heart and how well your heart pumps blood when it beats. These pictures can be taken by echocardiography or by injecting a radioactive dye into one of your veins, called a "nuclear heart scan." The amount of radiation in the dye is considered safe for you and those around you. However, if you are pregnant, you should not have this test because of risks it might pose to your unborn child.

If your doctor also wants to see how well your lungs are working, you may be asked to wear a mask or mouthpiece to measure the gases that you breathe out during the stress test.

After the Stress Test

After the stress test, your doctor will measure your heart activity and blood pressure to make sure that both measurements are back within the normal range. You should be able to return to your normal activities right away. If you had a test that involved radioactive dye, your doctor may ask you to drink plenty of fluids to flush it out of your body.

If your stress test shows that your heart is healthy, you may not need further testing or treatment. Your doctor may order other diagnostic tests or imaging tests if the stress test results suggest that you may have a heart condition, if you are physically unable to exercise, or if you continue having symptoms, such as shortness of breath or chest pain.

Chapter 30 | **Holter and Event Monitors**

WHAT ARE HOLTER AND EVENT MONITORS?

Holter and event monitors are small, portable electrocardiogram devices that record your heart's electrical activity for long periods of time while you do your normal activities.

These monitors can record how fast your heart is beating, whether the rhythm of your heartbeats is steady or irregular, and the strength and timing of the electrical impulses passing through each part of your heart. Information from these recordings helps doctors diagnose an arrhythmia, or irregular heartbeat, and check whether treatments for the irregular heartbeat are working.

There are many types of monitors, such as episodic monitors, autodetect recorders, 30-day event recorders, and transtelephonic event monitors. Your doctor will decide which monitor is best for you. Most monitors have electrodes with sticky adhesive patches that attach to the skin on your chest. Some monitors and electrodes used for long-term recording may be implanted under your skin to make it easier for you to bathe and perform your daily activities. Your doctor will explain how to wear and use the monitor and tell you whether you need to adjust your activity during the testing period. You should avoid magnets, metal detectors, microwave ovens, electric blankets, electric toothbrushes, and electric razors while using your monitor. Usually, you will be instructed to keep electronic devices such as cell phones, MP3 players, and tablets away from the monitor. After you are finished using the monitor,

This chapter includes text excerpted from "Holter and Event Monitors," National Heart, Lung, and Blood Institute (NHLBI), December 6, 2007. Reviewed October 2021 you will return it to your doctor's office or the place where you picked it up. If you were using an implantable recorder, your doctor will remove it from your chest.

There is a small risk that the sticky patches that attach the electrodes to your chest can irritate your skin. You may have an allergic reaction to the electrode adhesive, but the reaction will go away once the electrodes are removed. If you are using an implantable recorder, you may get an infection or have pain where the device was placed under your skin. Your doctor can prescribe medicine to treat these problems.

How Holter and Event Monitors Work*

Holter and event monitors also are used to detect "silent" myocardial ischemia. In this condition, not enough oxygen-rich blood reaches the heart muscle. "Silent" means that no symptoms occur. Cardiac monitors also can check whether prescribed treatments for an arrhythmia or silent myocardial ischemia are working. Holter and event monitors are similar to an electrocardiogram (an "EKG"). An EKG is a simple test that detects and records the heart's electrical activity. It is a common test for diagnosing heart rhythm problems. However, a standard EKG only records the heartbeat for a few seconds. It does not detect heart rhythm problems unless they occur during the test. Holter and event monitors are small, portable devices that can be worn during normal daily activities thereby allowing the monitor to record a heart's electrical activity for a longer time than an EKG.

Although similar, Holter and event monitors are not the same. A Holter monitor records the heart's electrical activity the entire time a patient is wearing it. An event monitor records the heart's electrical activity only at certain times while being worn. Unlike Holter monitors, event monitors do not continuously record the heart's electrical activity, they only record during symptoms.

**Excerpted from "Report on Form 8-K/A filed with the SEC on November 26, 2014" U.S. Securities and Exchange Commission (SEC), September 30, 2014.*

Chapter 31 | Electroencephalogram

An electroencephalogram (EEG) is a noninvasive, medical-grade test that measures the electrical activity in the brain. The procedure of the test is called "electroencephalography" and is prescribed to detect any abnormalities in brain function. The test measures plural electrical impulses released by synaptic activities in the brain in specific regions, during certain activities such as sleeping or in response to various stimuli such as sight, sound, or touch. The impulses are recorded as waves with peaks and valleys. The test is conducted by placing electrodes on the scalp surface, and these electrodes are placed all over an elastic cap that resembles a shower cap. This is done to ensure uniformity in measurements.

WHY IS AN ELECTROENCEPHALOGRAM PERFORMED?

An EEG is performed to diagnose and determine brain activity alterations. The test is useful, especially in diagnosing brain disorders that can include epilepsy and seizure disorder. Other brain disorders that can be diagnosed with the help of an EEG include:

- Brain damage caused due to injury
- Brain dysfunction (encephalopathy)
- Brain inflammation (encephalitis)
- Stroke
- Brain tumor
- Sleep irregularities such as narcolepsy can be determined along with another sleep study called "polysomnogram"

- Memory problems
- Dementia
- Developmental delays
- Behavior problems
- Growth abnormalities in the nervous system
- Learning disorders
- Attention disorders such as attention deficit hyperactivity disorder (ADHD)

An EEG can also be performed to monitor brain activity in a comatose patient. In addition, a continuous EEG is used to determine anesthesia doses in patients under a medically induced coma. This test is also used to monitor brain activity during neurosurgery.

When using an EEG to diagnose epilepsies, the seizure activity will display as rapid, spiking waves, also known as an "epileptiform." Patients with lesions on the brain may record slow EEG waves. Alzheimer disease and other psychoses that influence brain activity can also be diagnosed with an EEG.

HOW TO PREPARE FOR AN ELECTROENCEPHALOGRAM

- Before attending a scheduled EEG, the health-care provider will describe the procedure to the patient, who can then ask any questions they might have before the procedure.
- The patient will then be required to sign a consent form that must be read carefully and clarified in case of any doubts.
- The patient must avoid using any form of hair products such as hairsprays, gels, and conditioners the previous night. Instead, the patient is required to wash their hair with shampoo the previous night.
- The patient must avoid wearing dangling earrings or pull-over clothes and can go for unbuttoned or zipped up clothes.
- The patient must not consume caffeine or undergo fasting for at least 8–12 hours before the EEG.

- The patient should inform the doctor and technician about any medications or herbal supplements they might be consuming.

HOW IS AN ELECTROENCEPHALOGRAM PERFORMED?

An EEG procedure can be administered on an outpatient basis or as part of an overnight stay at the hospital. The procedure is unlikely to cause significant discomfort. Before the procedure begins, the technician will mark areas on the scalp with a specialized pencil to indicate where electrodes are attached. A cream may be applied at these points to enhance the recordings.

The general procedure of an EEG follows the below steps:

- First, the patient is provided with a reclining bed or chair to lay on.
- Approximately, 16–25 electrodes will be placed on the scalp either individually or via a cap. These electrodes will be placed on marked points.
- The patient is then asked to close their eyes, relax, and lie still.
- As the recording begins, the patient is advised to remain motionless throughout the test as the technician monitors any disrupting movements such as swallowing or blinking from an adjacent room. The recording may be paused to allow the patient to reposition themselves.
- Once the initial recording at rest is completed, the technician will begin recording by testing the patient with different stimuli initiating brain activity that does not show up when at rest. For example, some stimuli may include bright flashing lights or being asked to breathe rapidly and deeply for 3 minutes.
- An EEG will take approximately 45 minutes to 2 hours to complete.
- EEGs done to evaluate sleep disorders will be done while the patient is asleep.
- Longer neural monitoring may require a 24-hour EEG.

AFTER THE ELECTROENCEPHALOGRAM

After completing the test, the electrodes are removed, and the applied paste is washed off from the skin surface either with warm water, acetone, or witch hazel. It may also require an additional hair wash at home. If any sedatives have been administered, the patient may need to rest for some time. It is advisable in such a case to make commute arrangements for safety. Patients may experience redness or soreness at the points where the electrodes were placed. These effects will lessen after a few hours. The health-care provider will instruct patients on further steps.

TYPES OF ELECTROENCEPHALOGRAMS

Two basic types of electroencephalograms are available:

- **Routine EEG.** It is mostly done within 24 hours after the first occurrence of a seizure in an individual. The test can be performed with or without video monitoring.
- **Ambulatory EEG.** This test uses wearable equipment that patients can use to monitor their brain activity while going about their normal day-to-day activities. If this type of EEG requires video, another individual must record videos of the patient.

WAVES RECORDED DURING AN ELECTROENCEPHALOGRAM

There are different types of waves that are recorded during an EEG depending on the measurement of activity in the brain, such as:

- **Delta.** These waves occur within 1–4 hertz and are used in sleep labs or tests to measure sleep depth.
- **Alpha.** These waves are noticed when the mind is in a calm state of wakefulness and show a frequency range of 7–12 hertz.
- **Beta.** The waves record frequencies between 12–30 hertz and are observed during body movements.
- **Gamma.** The waves record at frequencies higher than 30 hertz and are typically within 40 hertz. These waves are noticed during data exchange between brain regions, sensory processing, and attentive focusing.

- **Theta.** These waves occur between the frequency range of 4–7 hertz and are associated with cognitive processes, memory encoding, and retrieval.

RESULTS OF AN ELECTROENCEPHALOGRAM

A neurologist will interpret the EEG recordings, after which the results are sent to the referring doctor. During a later appointment, the doctor will discuss the results of the EEG with the patient.

While discussing normal results, the EEG will show electrical activity in the brain as waves. These waves will be recorded during different levels of consciousness. Each activity has specific ranges of frequencies that are considered normal.

Abnormal results on an EEG may be caused due to:

- Epilepsy
- Hemorrhage
- Dead tissue due to blocked blood flow
- Migraines
- Alcohol or drug abuse
- Head injury
- Encephalitis
- Tumor

RISKS OF AN ELECTROENCEPHALOGRAM

Electroencephalogram procedures do not pose significant risks or cause major medical complications. And yet, individuals having a seizure disorder may experience a seizure caused by exposure to stimuli such as flashing lights or deep breathing during an EEG procedure, which will be handled by the health-care team.

References

1. "EEG (Electroencephalogram)," Mayo Clinic, April 15, 2020.
2. "Electroencephalogram (EEG)," Johns Hopkins Medicine, n.d.
3. Blocka, Karla. "EEG (Electroencephalogram)," Healthline, September 29, 2018.

4. Peters, Brandon. "What Is an Electroencephalogram (EEG)?" Verywell Health, September 12, 2020.
5. Freedman, Megan. "EEG (Electroencephalogram)," Healthgrades, November 22, 2020.
6. Farnsworth, Bryn. "What Is EEG (Electroencephalography) and How Does It Work?" iMotions, July 13, 2021.

Chapter 32 | Electromyography

WHAT ARE ELECTROMYOGRAPHY AND NERVE CONDUCTION STUDIES?

Electromyography (EMG) and nerve conduction studies are tests that measure the electrical activity of muscles and nerves. Nerves send out electrical signals to make your muscles react in certain ways. As your muscles react, they give off these signals, which can then be measured.

- An EMG test looks at the electrical signals your muscles make when they are at rest and when they are being used.
- A nerve conduction study measures how fast and how well the body's electrical signals travel down your nerves.

Electromyography tests and nerve conduction studies can both help find out if you have a disorder of your muscles, nerves, or both. These tests can be done separately, but they are usually done at the same time.

WHAT ARE THEY USED FOR?

Electromyography and nerve conduction studies are used to help diagnose a variety of muscle and nerve disorders. An EMG test helps find out if muscles are responding the right way to nerve signals. Nerve conduction studies help diagnose nerve damage or disease. When EMG tests and nerve conduction studies are done

This chapter includes text excerpted from "Electromyography (EMG) and Nerve Conduction Studies," MedlinePlus, National Institutes of Health (NIH), March 3, 2021.

together, it helps providers tell if your symptoms are caused by a muscle disorder or a nerve problem.

WHY DO YOU NEED AN ELECTROMYOGRAPHY TEST AND A NERVE CONDUCTION STUDY?

You may need these tests if you have symptoms of a muscle or nerve disorder. These symptoms include:

- Muscle weakness
- Tingling or numbness in arms, legs, hands, feet, and/or face
- Muscle cramps, spasms, and/or twitching
- Paralysis of any muscles

WHAT HAPPENS DURING AN ELECTROMYOGRAPHY TEST AND NERVE CONDUCTION STUDY

For an EMG test:

- You will sit or lie down on a table or bed.
- Your provider will clean the skin over the muscle being tested.
- Your provider will place a needle electrode into the muscle. You may have slight pain or discomfort when the electrode is inserted.
- The machine will record the muscle activity while your muscle is at rest.
- Then you will be asked to tighten (contract) the muscle slowly and steadily.
- The electrode may be moved to record activity in different muscles.
- The electrical activity is recorded and shown on a video screen. The activity is displayed as wavy and spiky lines. The activity may also be recorded and sent to an audio speaker. You may hear popping sounds when you contract your muscle.

For a nerve conduction study:

- You will sit or lie down on a table or bed.

- Your provider will attach one or more electrodes to a certain nerve or nerves using tape or a paste. The electrodes, called "stimulating electrodes," deliver a mild electrical pulse.
- Your provider will attach different types of electrodes to the muscle or muscles controlled by those nerves. These electrodes will record the responses to the electrical stimulation from the nerve.
- Your provider will send a small pulse of electricity through the stimulating electrodes to stimulate the nerve to send a signal to the muscle.
- This may cause a mild tingling feeling.
- Your provider will record the time it takes for your muscle to respond to the nerve signal.
- The speed of the response is called the "conduction velocity."

If you are having both tests, the nerve conduction study will be done first.

DO YOU NEED TO DO ANYTHING TO PREPARE FOR THESE TESTS?

Tell your health-care provider if you have a pacemaker or cardiac defibrillator. Special steps will need to be taken before the test if you have one of these devices.

Wear loose, comfortable clothing that allows easy access to the test area or can be easily removed if you need to change into a hospital gown.

Make sure your skin is clean. Do not use lotions, creams, or perfumes for a day or two before the test.

ARE THERE ANY RISKS TO THE TESTS?

You may feel a little pain or cramping during an EMG test. You may have a tingly feeling, like a mild electric shock, during a nerve conduction study.

WHAT DO THE RESULTS MEAN?

If your results were not normal, it can indicate a variety of different conditions. Depending on which muscles or nerves are affected, it may mean one of the following:

- **Carpal tunnel syndrome.** A condition that affects nerves in the hand and arm. It is usually not serious, but can be painful.
- **Herniated disc.** A condition that happens when a part of your spine, called a "disc," is damaged. This puts pressure on the spine, causing pain and numbness.
- **Guillain-Barré syndrome (GBS).** An autoimmune disorder that affects the nerves. It can lead to numbness, tingling, and paralysis. Most people recover from the disorder after treatment.
- **Myasthenia gravis.** A rare disorder that causes muscle fatigue and weakness.
- **Muscular dystrophy.** An inherited disease that seriously affects muscle structure and function.
- **Charcot-Marie-Tooth (CMT) disease.** An inherited disorder that causes nerve damage, mostly in the arms and legs.
- **Amyotrophic lateral sclerosis (ALS).** Also known as "Lou Gehrig disease." This is a progressive, ultimately fatal, disorder that attacks nerve cells in your brain and spinal cord. It affects all the muscles you use to move, speak, eat, and breathe.

Chapter 33 | Electronystagmography

Vertigo is a disorder that causes a feeling of being thrown off balance. When a person experiences these dizzy episodes, she or he may feel as if they are spinning or as if the world around them is swirling.

Vertigo can be caused by any illness or injury to the auditory nerve. This might involve the following:

- Bleeding (hemorrhage), clots, or atherosclerosis of the ear's blood supply are all examples of blood vessel problems.
- Ear cancers such as cholesteatoma
- Congenital malformations
- Aminoglycoside antibiotics, certain antimalarial medications, loop diuretics, and salicylates are among the medicines that are toxic to the ear nerves.
- Multiple sclerosis (MS)
- Progressive supranuclear palsy
- Rubella

WHAT IS ELECTRONYSTAGMOGRAPHY?

Electronystagmography (ENG or electrooculography) is a test that is used to assess patients with vertigo and other hearing and visual problems. This test examines eye movements to determine the functionality of two brain nerves, which are:

- The eighth cranial nerve, which connects the brain to the ears, commonly known as the "vestibular nerve"

- The oculomotor nerve that connects the brain to the eyes

TYPES OF ELECTRONYSTAGMOGRAPHY

The ENG is a set of tests that includes one or more of the following parameters:

Test for Calibration

This includes using your eyes to follow a light that is roughly 6–10 feet away. The test is usually carried out to determine if you have ocular dysmetria – a condition in which movements of the pupil of the eye overshoot their target.

Test Using a Pendulum

This procedure, as the name implies, assesses one's ability to follow a light with their eyes as it travels like a clock's pendulum.

Test of Optokinetics

This test assesses your ability to follow a light as it travels swiftly across, out of, and back into your field of vision while keeping your head steady.

Positional Assessment

This entails moving your head and possibly your entire body, rather than simply your eyes. For example, you could be requested to tilt your head rapidly to one side or sit up fast after lying down. The quantity of eye movement caused by this activity is measured.

Caloric Test Using Water

With a syringe, warm or cool water is injected into the ear canal until it reaches the tympanic membrane. Your eyes will respond automatically to this stimulation if there is no issue. The stimulus for this test might be air rather than water, especially in people with a compromised tympanic membrane.

Test for Gaze Nystagmus

This includes sitting or lying down and looking at a fixed light in the middle or to the side. This test assesses your ability to maintain your attention on an item without your eyes shifting unintentionally.

HOW TO PREPARE FOR ELECTRONYSTAGMOGRAPHY

You will most likely be asked to follow the below steps, before taking the tests:

- Your doctor should be informed about any medication that you are taking. They may request that you avoid taking them 72 hours before the test.
- Caffeine and alcohol should be avoided at least 48 hours before an ENG.
- It is not recommended to eat immediately before the procedure.
- Earwax and ear obstructions might affect findings; therefore, if your ear canals are not clear, a medical assistant may flush them before the operation.
- It is better to plan for a ride home after the procedure.

HOW IS ELECTRONYSTAGMOGRAPHY PERFORMED?

Electrode patches are placed above, below, and on both sides of the person's eyes and can be affixed to a headband or adhesive patches. Another patch is then placed on the brow. At different times, the health-care practitioner will spray cold water or pump air into each ear canal. When the inner ear and surrounding nerves are activated by water or air, the patches capture eye movements. Nystagmus is a fast, side-to-side eye movement that occurs when cold water enters the ear. The ear is then filled with warm water or air. The eyes should now quickly travel toward the heated water and then gently move away.

The person may also be required to monitor items with their eyes, such as flashing lights or moving objects. The ENG test is generally a 90-minute procedure.

AFTER THE PROCEDURE

- The electrodes will be removed and the electrode paste will be wiped away once the test is over.
- You might be advised not to massage your eyes to avoid spreading the electrode paste.
- You may be asked to lay down or sit for a few minutes to recuperate if you show indications of weakness, dizziness, or nausea.
- Your doctor will tell you when you may resume taking any medications you discontinued before the test.
- Depending on your condition, your doctor may give you additional or different instructions following the surgery.

RESULTS OF ELECTRONYSTAGMOGRAPHY

Note that normal value ranges may differ between laboratories. Discuss the significance of your specific test findings with your health-care practitioner. Anomalies in the data might indicate injury to the inner ear nerve or other areas of the brain that govern eye movements.

References

1. "Electronystagmography (ENG)," Johns Hopkins Medicine, June 29, 2011.
2. "Electronystagmography," MedlinePlus, National Institutes of Health (NIH), September 1, 2021.
3. "What Is Electronystagmography?" WebMD, November 20, 2020.
4. "Electronystagmography (ENG)," Healthline, June 6, 2016.

Part 5 | **Screening and Assessments for Specific Conditions and Diseases**

Chapter 34 | Prenatal Tests

Every woman has certain tests during pregnancy. Some women, depending on their age, family history, or ethnicity, may undergo additional testing.

Some tests are screening tests, and others are diagnostic tests. If your health-care provider orders a screening test, keep in mind that such tests do not diagnose problems. They evaluate risk. So a screening test result that comes back abnormal does not mean there is a problem with your infant. It means that more information is needed. Your health-care provider can explain what the test results mean and possible next steps.

ROUTINE TESTS

Glucose challenge screening. Usually given between 24 and 28 weeks of pregnancy, this screening assesses your risk for gestational diabetes. You will consume a sugary drink and get a blood test 1 hour later to measure your blood sugar levels. If you are at high risk – for example, if you have a family history of diabetes, are obese, had a large baby in a previous pregnancy, or are having twins – you should discuss this with your health-care provider get a test for blood glucose earlier in your pregnancy.

Group B Streptococcus infection screening. This test is performed between 35 and 37 weeks of pregnancy to look for bacteria group B *Streptococcus* (GBS) that can cause pneumonia or other serious infections in your infant. Swabs will be used to take cells from your vagina and rectum. Women who test positive for GBS will need antibiotics when in labor.

This chapter includes text excerpted from "What Tests Might I Need during Pregnancy?" *Eunice Kennedy Shriver* National Institute of Child Health and Human Development (NICHD), January 31, 2017. Reviewed October 2021.

Ultrasound exam. You will likely have an ultrasound exam between 18 and 20 weeks of pregnancy to check for any problems with the developing fetus. During an ultrasound exam, gel is spread on your belly and a special tool is moved over it to create a "picture" of the fetus on a monitor.

Urine test. At each prenatal visit, you will give a urine sample, which will be tested for signs of diabetes, urinary tract infections, and preeclampsia.

SCREENING FOR CHROMOSOMAL AND NEURAL TUBE DEFECTS AND OTHER CONDITIONS

Nuchal translucency (NT) screening. This screening test uses ultrasonography to measure the thickness of the back of the fetus's neck between 11 and 14 weeks. This information, combined with the mother's age and the results of the serum screen, helps health-care providers determine the fetus's potential risk for chromosomal abnormalities and other problems.

First trimester screen. Blood is drawn to test for PAPP-A and free beta-human chorionic gonadotropin (beta-hCG) and may be combined with performing a nuchal translucency ultrasound. This test will provide the risk for Down syndrome as well as other chromosomal problems.

Maternal serum screen (also called "quad screen," "triple test," "triple screen," "multiple marker screen," or "alpha-fetoprotein" (AFP)). Blood is drawn to measure the levels of certain substances that determine the risk of the fetus having chromosomal abnormalities and neural tube defects (NTDs). This screening test is done between 15 and 20 weeks of pregnancy.

Chorionic villus sampling (CVS). If your fetus is at risk for a chromosomal defect or other genetic disorders, your doctor may recommend this test when you are between 10 and 13 weeks pregnant. In this test, a needle is inserted through the cervix or the abdomen to remove a small sample of cells from the placenta.

Amniocentesis. Given between 15 and 20 weeks of pregnancy, this test is used to diagnose chromosomal disorders, such as Down syndrome and your infant's risk for NTDs, such as spina bifida. After a local anesthetic is given, a thin needle is inserted into the abdomen to draw out a small amount of amniotic fluid and cells from the sac surrounding the fetus. The fluid is sent to a lab for testing.

Cell-free fetal deoxyribonucleic acid (DNA). A new, noninvasive test uses the mother's blood to look for increased amounts of material from chromosomes 21, 18, and 13. This test can be given as early as 10 weeks to women whose age, family history, or standard screening results put them at higher risk for having a child with a chromosome disorder. The test is not recommended for women who are at low risk or are carrying multiple fetuses.

Carrier screening for cystic fibrosis (CF). A blood or saliva test determines if you and your partner are carriers for this genetic disease that affects breathing and digestion. Both parents must be a carrier for their child to get CF.

ADDITIONAL TESTING THAT YOUR HEALTH-CARE PROVIDER MAY RECOMMEND

Glucose tolerance test. If the 1-hour glucose challenge screening is above a certain level, your health-care provider may order this test. You will fast for at least 8 hours before the test. Your blood is drawn to test your "fasting blood glucose level." You will consume a sugary drink, and your blood will be taken every hour for 3 hours to see how your body reacts to the sugar. You may then be diagnosed with gestational diabetes.

Nonstress test. This test is performed in the third trimester (28 weeks or later) to monitor the fetus's health. A belt placed around your belly measures the fetal heart rate while the fetus is at rest and while the fetus is moving or kicking. This test can determine if the fetus is getting enough oxygen.

Biophysical profile (BPP). This test, given in the third trimester of pregnancy, monitors the fetus's breathing, movement, muscle tone, and heart rate as well as the amount of amniotic fluid to determine fetal well-being. The BPP includes an ultrasound test and a nonstress test.

Chapter 35 | Infertility Tests

Health-care providers evaluate men and women differently to diagnose infertility. Health-care providers evaluate men and women differently to diagnose infertility.

EVALUATING FEMALE FERTILITY

In evaluating a woman's fertility, a health-care provider will ask specific questions about her health history. These include:

- Prior pregnancies
- Prior miscarriages
- The regularity of her menstrual period
- The presence of pelvic pain
- Whether she has abnormal vaginal bleeding or discharge
- Whether she has a history of pelvic infection or previous pelvic surgery

Initial screening may also involve a physical exam, including a pelvic exam or pelvic ultrasound, a Pap test, and blood tests to look at overall health. The health-care provider may look for signs of milk production in the breasts, which suggests a hormone imbalance, and other physical symptoms of polycystic ovary syndrome (PCOS) and other conditions that affect fertility.

A health-care provider may also conduct the following laboratory tests and evaluations:

This chapter includes text excerpted from "How Is Infertility Diagnosed?" *Eunice Kennedy Shriver* National Institute of Child Health and Human Development (NICHD), January 31, 2017. Reviewed October 2021.

- A blood test around day 23 of the woman's menstrual cycle can measure the amount of a hormone called "progesterone." This test can tell whether ovulation has occurred and whether the ovaries are producing a normal amount of this hormone.
- Tests may also measure levels of other hormones that are important for fertility. The levels of follicle-stimulating hormone (FSH) and anti-Müllerian hormone (AMH) in the blood can help determine the quantity of a woman's remaining egg supply. FSH stimulates egg production and a hormone called "estradiol." High FSH levels may mean that a woman has ovarian failure or is in perimenopause or menopause. Low levels of FSH may mean a woman has stopped producing eggs. AMH is produced only in ovarian follicles, so the levels of AMH in the blood indicate the presence of growing follicles.
- Other tests may include those to examine the fallopian tubes and determine whether there is blockage that prevents movement of the egg from the ovaries. These include the following:
    - **X-ray hysterosalpingogram.** A health-care provider injects a radiographic dye into the cervix to fill the uterus. If the fallopian tubes are clear of blockages, the dye will flow out the end of the fallopian tube into the peritoneal cavity. Movement of the dye is monitored by x-ray fluoroscopy.
    - Laparoscopy is a surgery in which a small viewing instrument, called a "laparoscope," is inserted through a small cut in the abdomen to examine the female reproductive organs. If the procedure identifies blockages in the fallopian tubes, the blockages can be surgically treated with instruments attached to the laparoscope.
- A health-care provider may examine the inside of the uterus to look for scarring, uterine fibroids, or polyps. The following procedures are used to examine the uterus:

    - **Transvaginal ultrasound.** An ultrasound looks at the internal organs using sound waves. A wand inserted into the vagina applies sound waves to the body. This provides a health-care provider a better view of the female reproductive organs, including the uterus and ovaries.
    - **Hysteroscopy.** A hysteroscope is a long, thin camera that is inserted through the vagina and into the uterus.
    - **Saline sonohysterogram.** In this procedure, a health-care provider injects sterile saline into the cervix to fill the uterus. Once the uterine cavity is full, it is easier to see its inner lining. The pelvic organs are visualized with transvaginal ultrasound. It is also possible to see fluid move into the peritoneal cavity at the same time, which indicates that at least one tube is open.
- Health-care providers may test a woman older than age 35 to get a snapshot of the number of remaining follicles or if her follicles mature to the stage of ovulation. This type of testing includes performing a transvaginal ultrasound to look at the ovaries and measuring hormones in the blood on certain days of the menstrual cycle.

EVALUATING MALE FERTILITY

The evaluation of a man's fertility includes looking for signs of hormone deficiency, such as increased body fat, decreased muscle mass, and decreased facial and body hair. The evaluation also includes questions about the man's health history, including:

- Past injury to the testicles or penis
- Recent high fevers
- Childhood diseases, such as mumps
- Low sexual desire (libido)

A physical examination of the testes and penis allows for identification of problems, such as:

- Infection, signaled by discharge or prostate swelling
- Hernia
- Malformed tubes that transport sperm
- Hormone deficiency as indicated by small testes or lack of facial and body hair
- Presence of a mass in the testicles
- Varicocele (abnormal veins in the scrotum)

A health-care provider may also ask a man to provide a sample of semen to assess the health and quality of his sperm. To give a semen sample, the man is requested to refrain from ejaculation for around 48 hours before the test. He then provides a sample by masturbating into a cup or by having intercourse using a special condom (without contraceptive) that collects semen without affecting the sperm. A man may need to provide a semen sample on more than one occasion, because sperm production can vary over time depending on the man's current health status, activities, and stress level.

Other tests may include:

- Measurement of hormones in the blood, including testosterone and follicle-stimulating hormone (FSH), thyroid hormones, and prolactin.
- **Biopsy of the testicle.** A health-care provider uses a needle to extract sperm from the testicle.
- **Genetic testing.** In cases where no or very few sperm are found in the semen, a health-care provider may do genetic testing before starting fertility treatments. Testing can identify chromosome abnormalities that may cause the lack of sperm or lead to developmental problems among offspring.

Chapter 36 | **Vision Tests**

Chapter Contents

Section 36.1 | **Common Vision Tests**

Experts recommend that people undergo regular, comprehensive eye examinations to check the clarity of their vision and the health of their eyes. A typical eye examination includes a number of tests designed to evaluate the structure and function of the eye and measure different aspects of eyesight. Some of the most common vision tests check the patient's ability to see details from a distance or close up, see colors, track moving objects, and see objects on the periphery of the field of vision. All of these tests help the ophthalmologist or optometrist determine whether corrective measures are needed to improve the quality of the patient's vision.

Some of the vision tests that are most likely to be performed during an eye examination include the following:

VISUAL ACUITY TEST

The visual acuity test measures the sharpness or clarity of the patient's near vision and distance vision. Both tests are usually conducted by asking the patient to read rows of letters on an eye chart. The test of distance vision, known as a "Snellen test" after the Dutch ophthalmologist who created it, uses a wall chart with rows of letters that gradually decrease in size from top to bottom. The patient typically stands about 20 feet (6 meters) away from the chart, covers one eye, and tries to read the letters on each line. The size of the letters on one of the lines corresponds to normal visual acuity, or what a person with normal eyesight can read from a distance of 20 feet.

Using the Snellen measurement system, a person with normal visual acuity is said to have 20/20 vision. The numerator (top number) of the Snellen fraction refers to the patient's distance from the eye chart, while the denominator (bottom number) refers to the distance at which a person with normal visual acuity can read that line. About 35 percent of adults have 20/20 vision without corrective lenses. A person with 20/40 vision would have visual acuity that is worse than normal, while a person with 20/10 vision would have visual acuity that is better than normal. The goal of corrective measures such as eyeglasses, contact lenses, and laser surgery is to bring a patient's vision to 20/20, and about 75 percent of adults can reach that goal with correction.

The test of close-up vision is conducted using a Jaeger chart, which is a small card containing a few lines of printed text that get smaller moving from top to bottom. The patient holds the card about 14 inches from their face to determine the smallest print they can read comfortably. In the test of near vision, both eyes are tested at the same time. Many people experience a deterioration of their near vision as part of the normal aging process, so they require reading glasses or bifocals in middle age.

REFRACTION

The most common problems affecting visual acuity – nearsightedness (myopia) and farsightedness (hyperopia) – occur when the lens and cornea in the eye do not focus light on the retina accurately. Instead, the light is bent or refracted so that it is focused in front of or behind the retina, causing blurry vision when the patient looks at objects far away (myopia) or up close (hyperopia). The refraction test is used to determine the exact amount of the refraction error in each eye so that it can be corrected with an eyeglass prescription.

To perform a refraction, an eye doctor uses an instrument called a "phoropter" to show the patient a series of lenses. The patient must decide which lens option provides greater clarity in their vision. The lens power is fine-tuned through this interactive process until the eye doctor determines the final prescription for corrective lenses.

RETINOSCOPY

Retinoscopy is a test that can be used to approximate the results of a refraction. The patient looks through a series of lenses in a phoropter while the eye doctor shines a light into their eyes. When the light reflects onto the correct spot on the retina in the back of the patient's eye, the doctor can determine the lens power needed to correct the refraction error. This test can be used to speed up the refraction process or to determine the corrective lens prescription for young children and other people who may have trouble providing accurate feedback during other vision tests.

Machines called "autorefractors" and "aberrometers" can also be used to estimate the results of a refraction test. The autorefractor works the same way as a manual retinoscopy. The machine shines a light into the patient's eyes and determines the corrective lens power needed to focus the light accurately on the retina. An aberrometer is a sophisticated machine that uses wavefront technology to detect abnormalities in the way light travels through a patient's eye. It is usually used to determine the precise corrections to be made during surgical vision correction procedures.

COLOR VISION TEST

Another test commonly performed in a comprehensive eye examination is designed to test the patient's ability to distinguish between colors. About 8 percent of men and 0.5 percent of women worldwide have a color vision deficiency or color blindness. Although most cases are hereditary, deficiencies in color vision can sometimes indicate problems with eye health. The typical color vision test asks patients to find colored numbers or symbols hidden within a pattern of different-colored dots. People with normal color vision are able to identify the numbers or symbols, while those with color vision deficiencies will have difficulty distinguishing one or more colors. Color vision tests are sometimes used to screen people for employment in jobs that require good color perception, such as electricians, pilots, and truck drivers.

COVER TEST

A comprehensive eye examination also includes a simple test designed to check the patient's binocular vision, or how well their eyes work together. The cover test is performed by asking the patient to stare at an object while the doctor alternately covers one eye, then the other. The doctor watches to make sure that each eye is able to maintain its focus on the fixed object while it is covered and then uncovered.

OCULAR MOTILITY TEST

Ocular motility is the eyes' ability to follow a moving object or shift focus quickly between two separate objects. To test ocular motility, an eye doctor will typically ask the patient to follow the movement of a small light with their eyes while keeping their head still. Ideally, the patient's eyes should move smoothly and in tandem. To test quick eye movements, an eye doctor may hold two objects some distance apart and ask the patient to move their eyes back and forth between them.

STEREOPSIS TEST

Stereopsis, also known as "depth perception," is the eyes' ability to discern the three-dimensional nature of objects. The two eyes must work together as a team to perceive depth. In the most common stereopsis test, the patient wears special 3D glasses while viewing a series of test patterns. For each pattern, the patient is asked to identify which letter or symbol appears closer.

SLIT LAMP EXAM

A slit lamp is a microscope that an eye doctor uses to examine the structures of the eye under magnification. This type of test can detect a variety of eye conditions and diseases, such as cataracts, macular degeneration, or corneal ulcers. It is often performed with the patient's pupils dilated in order to provide the best possible view of the internal structures of the eye. Pupil dilation is achieved by placing special drops in the patient's eyes. The effects can last for several hours, during which time the patient will likely be sensitive to light and have trouble focusing on close objects. If the patient will be exposed to bright light during this time, it is important for them to wear sunglasses to minimize glare and avoid damaging the eyes.

GLAUCOMA TEST

Glaucoma is a serious eye condition caused by a buildup of pressure inside the eye when the fluid does not circulate properly. This interocular pressure can cause progressive damage to the optic nerve that carries visual signals to the brain, resulting in permanent, total blindness. Since people with glaucoma rarely experience any early symptoms or warning signs, it is important to get tested regularly. The most common glaucoma test, known as "noncontact tonometry" (NCT), involves a small puff of air being blown into the patient's open eye. The tonometer measures the eye's resistance to the puff of air in order to calculate its internal pressure. NCT is quick and painless, and the machine never touches the patient's eye.

VISUAL FIELD TEST

A visual field test is used to detect gaps or blind spots in the patient's peripheral or side vision. Blind spots, known as "scotomas," in the normal field of vision can indicate the presence of certain eye diseases or brain damage from a stroke or tumor. There are several different methods of testing a patient's field of vision. In a confrontation test, the patient covers one eye and stares at the doctor's eye or nose. The doctor slowly moves their hand from the edge of the patient's visual field toward the center, and the patient indicates the point at which they are able to see the hand. In a perimetry test, the patient stares at a dot inside a machine called a "perimeter." The machine flashes lights at various points around the visual field, and the patient pushes a button each time they see a flash. At the end of the test, the machine prints a report showing any gaps or blind spots within the patient's field of vision.

If any of the above tests indicate problems with the patient's eye health or vision, the patient may be referred to a specialist for further testing.

References

1. Heiting, Gary; Palombi, Jennifer. "What to Expect during a Comprehensive Eye Exam," All About Vision, September 2016.
2. "Vision Tests," WebMD, 2017.

Section 36.2 | **Comprehensive Dilated Eye Exam**

This section includes text excerpted from "Get a Dilated Eye Exam," National Eye Institute (NEI), May 19, 2021.

WHAT IS A DILATED EYE EXAM?

A dilated eye exam is the best thing you can do for your eye health! It is the only way to check for eye diseases early on, when they are easier to treat – and before they cause vision loss.

The exam is simple and painless. Your eye doctor will check for vision problems that make it hard to see clearly, such as being nearsighted or farsighted. Then your doctor will give you some eye drops to dilate (widen) your pupil and check for eye diseases.

Since many eye diseases have no symptoms or warning signs, you could have a problem and not know it. Even if you think your eyes are healthy, getting a dilated eye exam is the only way to know for sure.

HOW OFTEN DO YOU NEED TO GET A DILATED EYE EXAM?

How often you need a dilated eye exam depends on your risk for eye disease. Talk to your doctor about what is right for you.

Get a dilated eye exam every 1 to 2 years if you:

- Are over age 60
- Are African American and over age 40
- Have a family history of glaucoma

If you have diabetes or high blood pressure, ask your doctor how often you need an exam. Most people with diabetes or high blood pressure need to get a dilated eye exam at least once a year.

WHAT HAPPENS DURING A DILATED EYE EXAM

The exam includes:

- A visual acuity test to check how clearly you see. Your doctor will ask you to read letters that are up close and far away.
- A visual field test to check your peripheral (side) vision. Your doctor will test how well you can see objects off to the sides of your vision without moving your eyes.

- An eye muscle function test to check for problems with the muscles around your eyeballs. Your doctor will move an object around and ask you to follow it with your eyes.
- A pupil response test to check how light enters your eyes. Your doctor will shine a small flashlight into your eyes and check how your pupils react to the light.
- A tonometry test to measure the pressure in your eyes. Your doctor will use a machine to blow a quick puff of air onto your eye, or gently touch your eye with a special tool. Do not worry – it does not hurt!
- Dilation to check for problems with the inner parts of your eye. Your doctor will give you some eye drops to dilate (widen) your pupil. This helps the doctor see inside your eye.

Depending on your needs, your doctor may include other tests too. Ask your doctor if you have questions.

HOW DOES DILATION WORK?

Dilating your pupil lets more light into your eye – just like opening a door lets light into a dark room. Dilation helps your eye doctor check for many common eye problems, including diabetic retinopathy, glaucoma, and age-related macular degeneration (AMD).

WHAT HAPPENS AFTER A DILATED EYE EXAM

For a few hours after a dilated eye exam, your vision may be blurry and you may be sensitive to light. Ask a friend or family member to drive you home from your appointment.

If your eye doctor finds refractive errors in your vision, you may get a prescription for eyeglasses or contact lenses to help you see more clearly.

If your eye doctor finds signs of an eye disease, you can talk about treatment options and decide what is right for you.

If you are seeing clearly and there are no signs of eye disease, you are all set until your next exam. Make an appointment for your

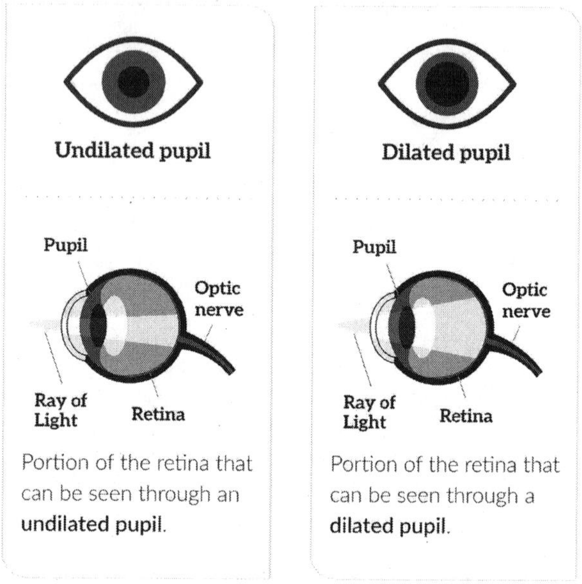

Figure 36.1. Eye Dilation

next dilated eye exam before you leave the office – that way, you would not forget!

Section 36.3 | Color Blindness Testing

This section includes text excerpted from "Color Blindness," National Eye Institute (NEI), July 3, 2019.

WHAT IS COLOR BLINDNESS?

If you have color blindness, it means you see colors differently than most people. Most of the time, color blindness makes it hard to tell the difference between certain colors.

Usually, color blindness runs in families. There is no cure, but special glasses and contact lenses can help. Most people who are color blind are able to adjust and do not have problems with everyday activities.

WHAT ARE THE TYPES OF COLOR BLINDNESS?

The most common type of color blindness makes it hard to tell the difference between red and green. Another type makes it hard to tell the difference between blue and yellow. People who are completely color blind do not see color at all, but that is not very common.

WHAT ARE THE SYMPTOMS OF COLOR BLINDNESS?

The main symptom of color blindness is not seeing colors the way most people do. If you are color blind, you may have trouble seeing:

- The difference between colors
- How bright colors are
- Different shades of colors

Symptoms of color blindness are often so mild that you may not notice them. And since we get used to the way we see colors, many people with color blindness do not know they have it.

People with very serious cases of color blindness might have other symptoms, too – such as quick side-to-side eye movements (nystagmus) or sensitivity to light.

ARE YOU AT RISK FOR COLOR BLINDNESS?

Men have a much higher risk than women for color blindness. You are also more likely to have color blindness if you:

- Have a family history of color blindness
- Have certain eye diseases, such as glaucoma or age-related macular degeneration (AMD)
- Have certain health problems, such as diabetes, Alzheimer disease (AD), or multiple sclerosis (MS)
- Take certain medicines
- Are white

If you think you may have color blindness, talk with your doctor about getting checked.

WHAT CAUSES COLOR BLINDNESS

The most common kinds of color blindness are genetic, meaning they are passed down from parents.

Color blindness can also happen because of damage to your eye or your brain. And color vision may get worse as you get older – often because of cataracts (cloudy areas in the lens of the eye).

HOW CAN YOU FIND OUT IF YOU HAVE COLOR BLINDNESS?

Your eye doctor can usually use a simple test to tell you if you are color blind.

During the test, your eye doctor will show you a circle made of many different colored dots. The circle has a shape inside it that is made out of dots – such as a number, a letter, or a squiggly line. This shape is easy to see if you do not have color blindness, but people who are color blind have a hard time seeing it.

WHAT IS THE TREATMENT FOR COLOR BLINDNESS?

There is no cure for color blindness that is passed down in families, but most people find ways to adjust to it. Children with color blindness may need help with some classroom activities, and adults with color blindness may not be able to do certain jobs, such as being a pilot or graphic designer. Keep in mind that most of the time, color blindness does not cause serious problems.

If your color blindness is happening because of another health problem, your doctor will treat the condition that is causing the problem. If you are taking a medicine that causes color blindness, your doctor may adjust how much you take or suggest you switch to a different medicine.

If color blindness is causing problems with everyday tasks, there are devices and technology that can help, including:

- **Glasses and contacts.** Special contact lenses and glasses may help people who are color blind tell the difference between colors.
- **Visual aids.** You can use visual aids, apps, and other technology to help you live with color blindness. For example, you can use an app to take a photo with your phone or tablet and then tap on part of the photo to find out the color of that area.

Talk over your options with your eye doctor. Remember these tips:

- Ask your doctor about visual aids and technology that can help you with everyday tasks.
- Encourage family members to get checked for color blindness, since it can run in families.

Chapter 37 | Balance Tests

WHAT ARE BALANCE TESTS?

Balance tests are a group of tests that check for balance disorders. A balance disorder is a condition that makes you feel unsteady on your feet and dizzy. Dizziness is a general term for different symptoms of imbalance. Dizziness can include vertigo, a feeling that you or your surroundings are spinning, and lightheadedness, a feeling like you are going to faint. Balance disorders can be mild, or so severe that you may have trouble walking, climbing stairs, or doing other normal activities.

Different systems in your body need to work together for you to have good balance. The most important system is called the "vestibular system." This system is located in your inner ear and includes special nerves and structures that help you keep your balance. Your vision and sense of touch are also essential for good balance. Problems with any of these systems can lead to a balance disorder.

Balance disorders can happen at any age, but are more common in older people. It is one of the main reasons that older adults tend to fall more often than younger people.

WHAT ARE THEY USED FOR?

Balance tests are used to find out if you have a problem with your balance, and if so, what is causing it. There are many causes of balance disorders. They include:

- **Benign paroxysmal positional vertigo (BPPV).** Your inner ear contains calcium crystals, which help control balance. BPPV happens when these crystals get shifted out of position. It can make you feel like the room is

This chapter includes text excerpted from "Balance Tests," MedlinePlus, National Institutes of Health (NIH), September 9, 2021.

spinning or your surroundings are moving. BPPV is the most common cause of vertigo in adults.
- **Meniere disease.** This disorder causes dizziness, bouts of hearing loss, and tinnitus (ringing in the ears).
- **Vestibular neuritis.** This refers to an inflammation inside the inner ear. It is usually caused by a virus. Symptoms include nausea and vertigo.
- **Migraines.** A migraine is a type of throbbing, severe headache. It is different than other types of headaches. It can cause nausea and dizziness.
- **Head injury.** You may get vertigo or other balance symptoms after a head injury.
- **Medicine side effect.** Dizziness can be a side effect of certain medicines.

Once you learn the cause of your balance disorder, you can take steps to help manage or treat your condition.

WHY DO YOU NEED A BALANCE TEST?

You may need a balance test if you have symptoms of a balance disorder. Symptoms include:
- Dizziness
- Feeling like you are in motion or spinning, even when standing still (vertigo)
- Loss of balance while walking
- Staggering while walking
- Ringing in the ears (tinnitus)
- Feeling like you are going to faint (lightheadedness) and/or a floating sensation
- Blurred vision or double vision
- Confusion

WHAT HAPPENS DURING A BALANCE TEST

Balance testing may be done by a primary health-care provider or a specialist in disorders of the ear. These include:
- An audiologist, a health-care provider who specializes in diagnosing, treating, and managing hearing loss.

- An otolaryngologist (ENT), a doctor specializing in treating diseases and conditions of the ears, nose, and throat.

Diagnosing balance disorders usually requires several tests. You may get one or more of the following tests:

Electronystagmography (ENG) and videonystagmography (VNG) tests. These tests record and measure your eye movements. Your vision system needs to work right for you to have good balance. For an ENG test, electrodes (small sensors that stick to the skin) will be placed over the skin around your eyes. For a VNG test, special goggles will be placed on your eyes. Both tests include the following steps:

- You will sit in an exam chair in a dark room.
- You will be asked to look at and follow patterns of light on a screen.
- You will be asked to move into different positions as you watch this light pattern.
- Then warm and cool water or air will be put in each ear. This should cause the eyes to move in specific ways. If the eyes do not respond in these ways, it may mean there is damage to the nerves of the inner ear.

Rotary test, also known as a "rotary chair test." This test also measures your eye movements. During this test:

- You will sit in a computer-controlled, motorized chair.
- You will put on special goggles that will record your eye movements as the chair slowly moves back and forth and in a circle.

Posturography, also known as "computerized dynamic posturography" (CDP). This test measures your ability to maintain balance while standing. During this test:

- You will stand barefoot on a platform, wearing a safety harness.
- There will be a landscape screen around you.
- The platform will move around to test your ability to remain standing on a moving surface.

Vestibular evoked myogenic potentials (VEMPs) test. This test measures how certain muscles respond in reaction to sound. It can show if there is a problem in your inner ear. During this test:

- You will recline in a chair.
- You will put on earphones.
- Sensor pads will be attached to your neck, forehead, and under your eyes. These pads will record your muscle movements.
- Clicks and/or bursts of tones will be sent to your earphones.
- While the sound is playing, you will be asked to lift your head or eyes for short periods of time.

Dix-Hallpike maneuver. This test measures how your eye reacts to abrupt movements. During this test:

- Your provider will move you quickly from sitting to lying down position and/or move your head in different positions.
- Your provider will check your eye movements to see if you have a false sense of motion or spinning.

A newer version of this test is called a "video head impulse test" (vHIT). During a vHIT test, you will wear goggles that record your eye movements while a provider gently turns your head in different positions.

You may also get one or more hearing tests, since many balance disorders are related to hearing problems.

WILL YOU NEED TO DO ANYTHING TO PREPARE FOR A BALANCE TEST?

You should wear loose, comfortable clothes. Depending on the test, you may need to make changes in your diet or avoid certain medicines for a day or two before your test. Your health-care provider will let you know if there are any special instructions to follow.

ARE THERE ANY RISKS TO BALANCE TESTS?

Certain tests may make you feel dizzy or nauseous. But, these feelings usually go away within a few minutes. You may want to make arrangements for someone to drive you home, in case the dizziness lasts for a longer period of time.

WHAT DO THE RESULTS MEAN?

If your results were not normal, your provider may order more tests and/or put you on a treatment plan. Depending on the cause of your balance disorder, your treatment may include:

- Medicine to treat an infection
- Medicine to help control dizziness and nausea
- **Positioning procedure.** If you were diagnosed with BPPV, your provider may perform a series of specialized movements of your head and chest. This can help reposition particles in your inner ear that have gotten out of place. The procedure is also known as the "Epley maneuver," or "canalith repositioning."
- **Balance retraining therapy, also known as "vestibular rehabilitation."** A provider specializing in balance rehabilitation may design a program of exercises and other steps to improve your balance and prevent falls. This may include learning to use a cane or a walker.
- **Diet and lifestyle changes.** If you were diagnosed with Meniere disease or migraine headaches, certain lifestyle changes may ease your symptoms. These can include increasing physical activity, avoiding certain foods, and quitting smoking. Ask your health-care provider about which changes may be best for you.
- **Surgery.** If medicines or other treatments are not working, you may need surgery to correct a problem in your inner ear. The type of surgery will depend on the specific cause of your balance disorder.

If you have questions about your results, talk to your health-care provider.

Chapter 38 | Eating Disorders: Suggested Medical Tests

Many people with eating disorders either deny that a problem exists or try to hide it from friends, family members, and medical professionals. As a result, diagnosing an eating disorder can be a difficult process, and such conditions as anorexia nervosa, bulimia nervosa, and binge-eating disorder often go undetected for long periods of time. However, doctors have a variety of assessment tools and medical tests available to aid in the diagnosis of eating disorders. If an eating disorder is suspected, the diagnostic process is likely to include the following:

- A full medical history, including information about both physical and emotional health
- A mental-health screening to look for underlying psychological problems, evaluate eating habits, and assess attitudes about food and body image
- A complete physical examination to check for signs of eating disorders as well as health problems related to malnutrition
- Additional medical tests – including x-rays and chemical analysis of blood and urine – to look for evidence of damage to the heart, kidneys, gastrointestinal tract, and other organs

In the process of diagnosing eating disorders, doctors must rule out other health conditions that may present similar symptoms, such as hyperthyroidism, inflammatory bowel syndrome, immunodeficiency, chronic infection, diabetes, and cancer. In addition, doctors must look for evidence of diseases that often co-exist with eating disorders, such as depression, anxiety, obsessive-compulsive disorder, schizophrenia, and substance abuse.

COMMONLY USED MEDICAL TESTS

The initial step in diagnosing eating disorders usually involves administering questionnaires and conducting interviews to gather information about the patient's eating history, body image, and attitudes about food. Interviews are often conducted by a psychologist or psychiatrist in the presence of a supportive friend or family member of the patient. Medical professionals may also administer psychometric tests that are specifically designed to elicit information about eating disorders, such as the Eating Disorders Examination (EDE), the Eating Disorders Examination-Questionnaire (EDE-Q), and the SCOFF questionnaire. The results of these screening assessments help doctors determine whether further testing and evaluation is appropriate.

The next step in diagnosing eating disorders may involve administering a number of different medical tests to detect and rule out physical symptoms and health complications related to eating disorders. Some of the most commonly used tests include:

- A complete blood count, including levels of cholesterol, protein, and electrolytes
- A urinalysis to evaluate kidney function
- An oral glucose tolerance test (OGTT) to assess the body's ability to metabolize sugar
- An enzyme-linked immunosorbent assay (ELISA) to check for antibodies to various viruses and bacteria
- A secretin-CCK test to evaluate pancreas and gall bladder function
- A blood urea nitrogen (BUN) test to evaluate protein metabolism and kidney function
- A BUN-to-creatinine ratio to check for evidence of severe dehydration, kidney failure, congestive

heart failure, cirrhosis of the liver, and other serious conditions
- A serum cholinesterase test to assess liver function and check for signs of malnutrition
- A luteinizing hormone (LH) response to gonadotropin-releasing hormone (GnRH) to evaluate pituitary gland function
- Thyroid-stimulating hormone (TSH) and parathyroid hormone (PTH) tests to assess thyroid function
- A creatine kinase test to evaluate enzyme levels in the heart, brain, and muscles
- An echocardiogram or electrocardiogram (EKG) to assess heart function
- An electroencephalogram (EEG) to measure electrical activity in the brain
- An upper GI series to look for problems in the upper gastrointestinal tract
- X-rays or a barium enema to assess issues in the lower gastrointestinal tract

MAKING A DIAGNOSIS

The results of these various medical tests can help medical professionals diagnose an eating disorder as well as pinpoint the specific type of disorder in order to provide effective treatment. To receive a diagnosis of anorexia nervosa, a patient typically has a distorted self-image and an intense fear of gaining weight, which translates into an inability or refusal to maintain a healthy weight for their age, height, and body type. Severely restricting food intake, abusing laxatives or diuretics in an effort to eliminate calories, and exercising excessively are common symptoms of anorexia. In females, the loss of menstrual function for at least three months is another key indicator.

The criteria for diagnosing bulimia nervosa include patterns of purging food from the body through self-induced vomiting or other methods at least twice a week for three months. Bulimia can be difficult to diagnose because patients usually binge and purge secretly and deny that they have a problem. In addition, most people with bulimia fall within their normal weight range. Dental and gum problems, stomach and digestive issues, dehydration, fatigue, and other symptoms related to repeated vomiting are key factors in the diagnosis of bulimia.

The diagnosis of binge-eating disorder often occurs when a patient seeks medical help with losing weight or dealing with an obesity-related health problem. Medical tests aid in the diagnosis by ruling out physical illnesses and detecting health consequences of the eating disorder. With all types of eating disorders, early diagnosis is important to reduce the patient's risk of long-term health problems and improve the chances of successful treatment and recovery.

References

1. "Anorexia Nervosa – Exams and Tests," WebMD, November 14, 2014.
2. "Bulimia Nervosa – Exams and Tests," WebMD, November 14, 2014.
3. "Diagnosing Binge Eating Disorder," WebMD, 2016.
4. Mandal, Ananya. "Eating Disorders Diagnosis," News Medical, 2016.

Chapter 39 | **Allergy Testing**

Chapter Contents

Section 39.1 | **Allergy Blood Test**

This section includes text excerpted from "Allergy Blood Test," MedlinePlus, National Institutes of Health (NIH), July 30, 2020.

WHAT IS AN ALLERGY BLOOD TEST?

Allergies are a common and chronic condition that involves the body's immune system. Normally, your immune system works to fight off viruses, bacteria, and other infectious agents. When you have an allergy, your immune system treats a harmless substance, like dust or pollen, as a threat. To fight this perceived threat, your immune system makes antibodies called "immunoglobulin E" (IgE).

Substances that cause an allergic reaction are called "allergens." Besides dust and pollen, other common allergens include animal dander, foods, including nuts and shellfish, and certain medicines, such as penicillin. Allergy symptoms can range from sneezing and a stuffy nose to a life-threatening complication called "anaphylactic shock." Allergy blood tests measure the amount of IgE antibodies in the blood. A small amount of IgE antibodies is normal. A larger amount of IgE may mean you have an allergy.

WHAT IS IT USED FOR?

Allergy blood tests are used to find out if you have an allergy. One type of test called a "total IgE test" measures the overall number of IgE antibodies in your blood. Another type of allergy blood test called a "specific IgE test" measures the level of IgE antibodies in response to individual allergens.

WHY DO YOU NEED AN ALLERGY BLOOD TEST?

Your health-care provider may order allergy testing if you have symptoms of an allergy. These include:

- Stuffy or runny nose
- Sneezing
- Itchy, watery eyes
- Hives (a rash with raised red patches)

- Diarrhea
- Vomiting
- Shortness of breath
- Coughing
- Wheezing

WHAT HAPPENS DURING AN ALLERGY BLOOD TEST

A health-care professional will take a blood sample from a vein in your arm, using a small needle. After the needle is inserted, a small amount of blood will be collected into a test tube or vial. You may feel a little sting when the needle goes in or out. This usually takes less than five minutes.

WILL YOU NEED TO DO ANYTHING TO PREPARE FOR THE TEST?

You do not need any special preparations for an allergy blood test.

ARE THERE ANY RISKS TO THE TEST?

There is very little risk to having an allergy blood test. You may have slight pain or bruising at the spot where the needle was put in, but most symptoms go away quickly.

WHAT DO THE RESULTS MEAN?

If your total IgE levels are higher than normal, it likely means you have some kind of allergy. But, it does not reveal what you are allergic to. A specific IgE test will help identify your particular allergy. If your results indicate an allergy, your health-care provider may refer you to an allergy specialist or recommend a treatment plan.

Your treatment plan will depend on the type and severity of your allergy. People at risk for anaphylactic shock, a severe allergic reaction that can cause death, need to take extra care to avoid the allergy-causing substance. They may need to carry an emergency epinephrine treatment with them at all times.

Be sure to talk to your health-care provider if you have questions about your test results and/or your allergy treatment plan.

IS THERE ANYTHING ELSE YOU NEED TO KNOW ABOUT AN ALLERGY BLOOD TEST?

An IgE skin test is another way to detect allergies, by measuring IgE levels and looking for a reaction directly on the skin. Your healthcare provider may order an IgE skin test instead of, or in addition to, an IgE allergy blood test.

Section 39.2 | **Patch Tests for Allergies**

An allergy is the sensitivity of the immune system, often known as an "overreaction." The immune system's job is to defend the body against external pathogens such as viruses and bacteria. When a person has an allergy, their immune system perceives a harmless material such as dust or pollen as a danger. The immune system then responds by causing an allergic response to combat this threat.

Type I–IV hypersensitivities are the four basic forms of overreactions. Some of the most common allergies are caused by type I hypersensitivity allergens, such as dust mite, pollen, food, and animal dander. Different immune system overreactions are caused by different forms of hypersensitivities and might range from minor rashes to life-threatening autoimmune diseases.

WHAT IS PATCH TESTING?

A patch test is a type of skin test that is performed to determine the source of an allergic response on the skin and is also known as "allergic contact dermatitis." A reaction to anything that encounters the skin is known as "contact dermatitis." Inflammation (redness, itching) is common with this type of allergic response.

A dermatological clinic is a place that usually does patch testing. Different chemicals are applied to the skin and taped in place during patch testing. The patches are usually applied to the back of the body by using hypoallergenic tapes and are kept on for 2 days

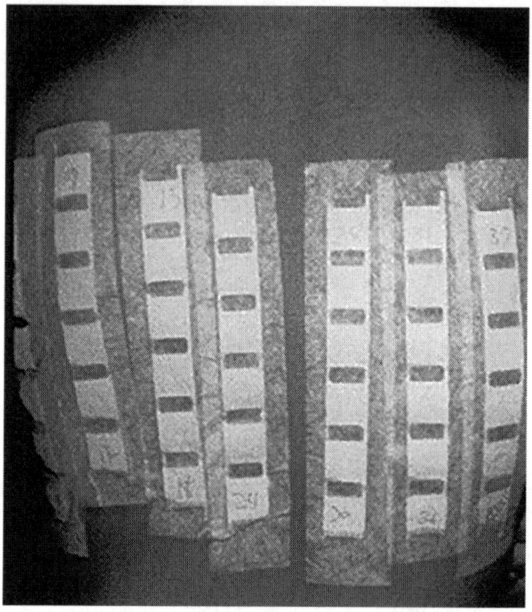

Figure 39.1. Patch Testing *(Source: "Occupational Dermatoses Slides 96 to 100," Centers for Disease Control and Prevention (CDC).)*

before being removed. The dermatologist will examine the skin region that was tested 2–4 days after the patches are removed. The patch test does not involve the usage of needles or needle pricks.

WHY ARE PATCH TESTS DONE?

Patch tests are commonly used to identify allergies, such as:

- Allergic rhinitis (hay fever)
- Asthma caused by allergies
- Eczema (dermatitis)
- Allergies to foods
- Allergy to penicillin
- Allergy to insect bite or venom

Adults and children of all ages, including babies, are typically safe with patch testing. If you have ever experienced a severe allergic reaction, such as the ones listed below, your health-care practitioner may advise against skin testing.

- A person might be allergic to some chemicals that even the tiniest quantity used in skin testing might cause a life-threatening reaction (anaphylaxis).
- **Any medicines that could affect your test findings.** Several antidepressants, and certain heartburn medicines are among them. Your doctor may determine that continuing to take these medications is better than stopping them briefly in preparation for a skin test.
- **Having particular skin problems.** There may not be enough clean, unaffected skin to do an effective test if severe eczema or psoriasis covers significant regions of skin on your arms and back – the standard testing sites. Other skin disorders, including dermatographism, might cause test findings to be inaccurate.

PREPARING FOR THE PATCH TEST

It is crucial to prepare your skin for your patch test. The below-mentioned points will assist you in obtaining more accurate and dependable results.

BEFORE PATCH TESTING

- Reduce exposure to the sun for 1–2 weeks.
- For at least 1 week before patch testing, avoid using topical medications (creams and ointments) on the back and any other region where patches may be applied. These medications can be used on other parts of the body where patches will not be applied.
- Moisturizers should not be used on the skin on the day of the patch test.
- Before and throughout the testing, you can continue to take any antihistamines as prescribed by your health-care provider.

DURING THE PATCH TEST

- Throughout the test, the patches and ink-marked test area must be maintained dry.
- Soaps, creams, ointments, and moisturizers should not be applied to the test area.
- Scratching, rubbing, loosening, or removing the patches is not recommended.
- Physical activities that loosen the tape should be avoided.
- Avoid exposing the test area to direct sunlight.
- Avoid hot places and activities that cause you to sweat excessively.

RESULTS OF A PATCH TEST

At the second and third sessions, the dermatologist will fill out a record form (usually 48- and 96-hour readings). Each test site's outcome is kept track of. The following is the system that is commonly used to understand results.

- (-) Negative
- (IR) Irritant response – sweat rash, follicular pustules, and burn-like responses are examples.
- (+/-) Unclear – a pink region under the test chamber that denotes unclear results.
- (+) Positive – slightly increased pink or red plaques are examples.
- (++) Strongly positive – papulovesicles are an example.
- (+++) Excessive reactivity – while blisters or ulcers are examples.

The significance varies depending on the location and kind of dermatitis, as well as the allergen in question. The interpretation of the results necessitates a great deal of knowledge and practice.

References

1. Chow, Elizabeth. "Allergy Patch Testing," The Australasian College of Dermatologists (ACD), April 20, 2017.
2. "Allergy Skin Tests," Mayo Clinic, April 4, 2020.

3. "Patch Tests," DermNet NZ, December 22, 2005.
4. "Patch Testing for Skin Allergies," Nationwide Children's Hospital, October 25, 2016.

Chapter 40 | **Infectious Disease Testing**

Chapter Contents

Section 40.1 | **Chlamydia Test**

This section includes text excerpted from "Chlamydia Test," MedlinePlus, National Institutes of Health (NIH), July 30, 2020.

Chlamydia is one of the most common sexually transmitted diseases (STDs). It is a bacterial infection spread through vaginal, oral, or anal sex with an infected person. Many people with chlamydia have no symptoms, so someone may spread the disease without even knowing they are infected. A chlamydia test looks for the presence of chlamydia bacteria in your body. The disease is easily treated with antibiotics. But, if it is not treated, chlamydia can cause serious complications, including infertility in women and swelling of the urethra in men.

WHAT IS CHLAMYDIA TEST USED FOR?

A chlamydia test is used to determine whether or not you have a chlamydia infection.

WHY DO YOU NEED A CHLAMYDIA TEST?

The Centers for Disease Control and Prevention (CDC) estimates that more than two and a half million Americans are infected with chlamydia every year. Chlamydia is especially common in sexually active people aged 15 to 24. Many individuals with chlamydia do not have symptoms, so the CDC and other health organizations recommend regular screening for groups at higher risk.

These recommendations include yearly chlamydia tests for:

- Sexually active women under the age of 25
- Women over the age of 25 with certain risk factors, which include:
  - Having new or multiple sex partners
  - Previous chlamydia infections
  - Having a sex partner with an STD
  - Using condoms inconsistently or incorrectly
- Men who have sex with men

In addition, chlamydia testing is recommended for:

- Pregnant women under the age of 25
- People who are human immunodeficiency virus (HIV)-positive

Some people with chlamydia will have symptoms. Your health-care provider may order a test if you experience symptoms such as:

For women:

- Stomach pain
- Abnormal vaginal bleeding or discharge
- Pain during sex
- Pain when urinating
- Frequent urination

For men:

- Pain or tenderness in the testicles
- Swollen scrotum
- Pus or other discharge from the penis
- Pain when urinating
- Frequent urination

WHAT HAPPENS DURING A CHLAMYDIA TEST

If you are a woman, your health-care provider will use a small brush or swab to take a sample of cells from your vagina for testing. You may also be offered the option of testing yourself at home using a test kit. Ask your provider for recommendations on which kit to use. If you do the test at home, be sure to follow all the directions carefully.

If you are a man, your health-care provider may use a swab to take a sample from your urethra, but it is more likely that a urine test for chlamydia will be recommended. Urine tests can also be used for women. During a urine test, you will be instructed to provide a clean catch sample.

The clean-catch method generally includes the following steps:

- Wash your hands.
- Clean your genital area with a cleansing pad given to you by your provider. Men should wipe the tip of their

penis. Women should open their labia and clean from front to back.

- Start to urinate into the toilet.
- Move the collection container under your urine stream.
- Collect at least an ounce or two of urine into the container, which should have markings to indicate the amounts.
- Finish urinating into the toilet.
- Return the sample container as instructed by your health-care provider.

WILL YOU NEED TO DO ANYTHING TO PREPARE FOR THE TEST?

If you are a woman, you may need to avoid using douches or vaginal creams for 24 hours before your test. Both men and women may be asked to avoid taking antibiotics for 24 hours before testing. Ask your health-care provider if there are any special instructions.

ARE THERE ANY RISKS TO THE TEST?

There are no known risks to having a chlamydia test.

WHAT DO THE RESULTS MEAN?

A positive result means you have been infected with chlamydia. The infection requires treatment with antibiotics. Your health-care provider will give you instructions on how to take your medicine. Be sure to take all the required doses. In addition, let your sexual partner know you tested positive for chlamydia, so she or he can be tested and treated promptly.

IS THERE ANYTHING ELSE YOU NEED TO KNOW ABOUT A CHLAMYDIA TEST?

Chlamydia testing enables diagnosis and treatment of the infection before it can cause serious health problems. If you are at risk for chlamydia due to your age and/or lifestyle, talk to your health-care provider about getting tested.

You can also take steps to prevent getting infected with chlamydia The best way to prevent chlamydia or any STD is to not have vaginal, anal, or oral sex. If you are sexually active, you can reduce your risk of infection by:

- Being in a long-term relationship with one partner who has tested negative for STDs
- Using condoms correctly every time you have sex

Section 40.2 | **Hepatitis Diagnostic Tests**

This section includes text excerpted from "Hepatitis Panel," MedlinePlus, National Institutes of Health (NIH), July 31, 2020.

Hepatitis is a type of liver disease. Viruses called "hepatitis A," "hepatitis B," and "hepatitis C" are the most common causes of hepatitis. A hepatitis panel is a blood test that checks to see if you have a hepatitis infection caused by one of these viruses.

The viruses are spread in different ways and cause different symptoms:

- Hepatitis A is most often spread by contact with contaminated feces (stool) or by eating tainted food. Though uncommon, it can also be spread through sexual contact with an infected person. Most people recover from hepatitis A without any lasting liver damage.
- Hepatitis B is spread through contact with infected blood, semen, or other bodily fluids. Some people recover quickly from a hepatitis B infection. For others, the virus can cause long-term, chronic liver disease (CLD).
- Hepatitis C is most often spread by contact with infected blood, usually through sharing of hypodermic needles. Though uncommon, it can also be spread through sexual contact with an infected person. Many people with hepatitis C develop chronic liver disease and cirrhosis.

A hepatitis panel includes tests for hepatitis antibodies and antigens. Antibodies are proteins that the immune system produces to help fight infections. Antigens are substances that cause an immune response. Antibodies and antigens can be detected before symptoms appear.

Other names include acute hepatitis panel, viral hepatitis panel, and hepatitis screening panel.

WHAT IS HEPATITIS PANEL USED FOR?

A hepatitis panel is used to find out if you have a hepatitis virus infection.

WHY DO YOU NEED A HEPATITIS PANEL?

You may need a hepatitis panel if you have symptoms of liver damage. These symptoms include:

- Jaundice, a condition that causes your skin and eyes to turn yellow
- Fever
- Fatigue
- Loss of appetite
- Dark-colored urine
- Pale-colored stool
- Nausea and vomiting

You may also need a hepatitis panel if you have certain risk factors. You may be at a higher risk for a hepatitis infection if you:

- Use illegal, injectable drugs
- Have a sexually transmitted disease (STD)
- Are in close contact with someone infected with hepatitis
- Are on long-term dialysis
- Were born between 1945 and 1965, often referred to as the "baby boom years." Though the reasons are not entirely understood, baby boomers are 5 times more likely to have hepatitis C than other adults.

WHAT HAPPENS DURING A HEPATITIS PANEL

A health-care professional will take a blood sample from a vein in your arm, using a small needle. After the needle is inserted, a small amount of blood will be collected into a test tube or vial. You may feel a little sting when the needle goes in or out. This usually takes less than five minutes.

You may also be able to use an at-home kit to test for hepatitis. While instructions may vary between brands, your kit will include a device to prick your finger (lancet). You will use this device to collect a drop of blood for testing.

WILL YOU NEED TO DO ANYTHING TO PREPARE FOR THE TEST?

You do not need any special preparations for a hepatitis panel.

ARE THERE ANY RISKS TO THE TEST?

There is very little risk to having a blood test. You may have slight pain or bruising at the spot where the needle was put in, but most symptoms go away quickly.

WHAT DO THE RESULTS MEAN?

A negative result means you probably do not have a hepatitis infection. A positive result may mean you have or previously had an infection from hepatitis A, hepatitis B, or hepatitis C. You may need more tests to confirm a diagnosis. If you have questions about your results, talk to your health-care provider.

IS THERE ANYTHING ELSE YOU NEED TO KNOW ABOUT A HEPATITIS PANEL?

There are vaccines for hepatitis A and hepatitis B. Talk to your health-care provider to see if you or your children should get vaccinated.

Section 40.3 | Human Immunodeficiency Virus and Sexually Transmitted Disease Testing

This section includes text excerpted from "Rapid Oral HIV Test: Patient Fact Sheet," U.S. Department of Veterans Affairs (VA), March 2017. Reviewed October 2021.

WHAT IS A RAPID ORAL HIV TEST?

This is a test for human immunodeficiency virus (HIV), the virus that causes acquired immunodeficiency virus (AIDS). With a rapid oral test, results take about 20 minutes. There are also rapid tests that use a blood sample. Rapid tests are usually used when results need to be delivered within a few minutes, such as in an outreach center or homeless clinic; otherwise, a traditional blood test is used. The rapid oral test is quite good at detecting chronic (long-standing) HIV infection, but not so good at detecting very recent HIV infection.

HOW DOES THE RAPID ORAL HIV TEST WORK?

When HIV enters the body, antibodies are produced. The test looks for HIV antibodies in your oral fluids. The test uses a swab to collect a sample from the inside of your mouth.

WHAT HAPPENS WHEN YOU AGREE TO BE TESTED

- The test is explained to you by a health provider.
- A health provider will ask you to swab your gums with a special swab.
- Results are ready in about 20 minutes.
- You will learn your HIV result and discuss what it means.
- Your provider will give you information about how to protect yourself and others from HIV.
- If your test result is positive, you will do a second, different, test using a blood sample that is sent to the lab.
- Your test result will be confidential (results will only be discussed with you).

WHAT DOES A NEGATIVE RAPID ORAL HIV TEST RESULT MEAN?

This means that HIV antibodies have not been found in your system. This could mean one of two things:

- You do not have HIV
- You have HIV, but it was not detected by the rapid oral test (this is a false-negative result).

It can take up to three months for your system to produce enough antibodies to be detected by the rapid oral test. If you have engaged in activities that might put you at risk of HIV infection in the past three months, you should repeat the test in a few weeks, or talk with your health-care provider about doing a standard blood test for HIV right away.

WHAT DOES A POSITIVE RAPID ORAL HIV TEST RESULT MEAN?

This means that HIV antibodies may be in your system. Positive results on the rapid test must always be confirmed by doing a second HIV test. This is because sometimes (rarely) the rapid oral test gives a false-positive result. A person is considered to be HIV positive only if two different test results are positive. The second HIV test is a blood test that is sent to the lab; the results may take up to 1 to 2 weeks to return.

IF YOUR POSITIVE RESULT IS CONFIRMED BY A SECOND TEST, THAT MEANS

- You have HIV and should be evaluated right away for treatment
- Your testing site will refer you to a clinic that has expertise in caring for people with HIV
- They may also refer you for counseling and other support services. The HIV treatment (medication) greatly improves health and can prevent transmission (infection) to others.

WHY SHOULD YOU GET TESTED?

- Many HIV-positive people do not know they are infected with HIV, because they have never been tested.

- Knowing your HIV status helps you protect yourself and others.
- Getting diagnosed early can greatly improve your health.
- Although there is no cure for HIV, there are many effective medicines that can control it.
- Most people with HIV who take their medication every day can live long, healthy lives.
- If you test negative, you may feel less anxious after testing, and you may be more committed to preventing yourself from becoming infected.
- An HIV test is part of routine medical care.

Section 40.4 | **Tuberculosis Test**

This section includes text excerpted from "Testing for Tuberculosis (TB)," Centers for Disease Control and Prevention (CDC), September 1, 2016. Reviewed October 2021.

Tuberculosis (TB) is a disease that is spread through the air from one person to another. When someone who is sick with TB coughs, speaks, laughs, sings, or sneezes, people nearby may breathe TB bacteria into their lungs. TB usually attacks the lungs, but can also attack other parts of the body, such as the brain, spine, or kidneys.

TB bacteria can live in the body without making a person sick. This is called "latent TB infection." People with latent TB infection do not feel sick, do not have TB symptoms, and cannot spread TB bacteria to others. Some people with latent TB infection go on to develop TB disease. People with TB disease can spread the bacteria to others, feel sick, and can have symptoms including fever, night sweats, cough, and weight loss.

There are two kinds of tests that are used to determine if a person has been infected with TB bacteria: the tuberculin skin test and TB blood tests.

TUBERCULIN SKIN TEST

What Is a Tuberculin Skin Test?

The Mantoux tuberculin skin test (TST) is a test to check if a person has been infected with TB bacteria.

How Does the Tuberculin Skin Test Work?

Using a small needle, a health-care provider injects a liquid (called "tuberculin") into the skin of the lower part of the arm. When injected, a small, pale bump will appear. This is different from a bacille Calmette-Guérin (BCG) shot (a TB vaccine that many people living outside of the United States receive).

The person given the TST must return within two or three days to have a trained health-care worker look for a reaction on the arm where the liquid was injected. The health-care worker will look for a raised, hard area or swelling, and if present, measure its size using a ruler. Redness by itself is not considered part of the reaction.

What Does a Positive Tuberculin Skin Test Result Mean?

The TST result depends on the size of the raised, hard area, or swelling. It also depends on the person's risk of being infected with TB bacteria and the progression to TB disease if infected.

- **Positive TST.** This means the person's body was infected with TB bacteria. Additional tests are needed to determine if the person has latent TB infection or TB disease. A health-care worker will then provide treatment as needed.
- **Negative TST.** This means the person's body did not react to the test, and that latent TB infection or TB disease is not likely.

Who Can Receive a Tuberculin Skin Test?

Almost everyone can receive a TST, including infants, children, pregnant women, people living with HIV, and people who have had a BCG shot. People who had a severe reaction to a previous TST should not receive another TST.

How Often Can a Tuberculin Skin Test Be Given?

Usually, there is no problem with repeated TSTs unless a person has had a severe reaction to a previous TST.

TESTING FOR TUBERCULOSIS IN PEOPLE WITH A BACILLE CALMETTE-GUERIN

People who have had a previous BCG shot may receive a TST. In some people, the BCG shot may cause a positive TST when they are not infected with TB bacteria. If a TST is positive, additional tests are needed.

TUBERCULOSIS BLOOD TESTS

What Is an Interferon Gamma Release Assay?

An interferon gamma release assay (IGRA) is a blood test that can determine if a person has been infected with TB bacteria. An IGRA measures how strong a person's immune system reacts to TB bacteria by testing the person's blood in a laboratory. Two IGRAs are approved by the U.S. Food and Drug Administration (FDA) and are available in the United States:

- QuantiFERON®–TB Gold In-Tube test (QFT–GIT)
- T–SPOT®.TB test (T–Spot)

How Does the Interferon Gamma Release Assay Work?

Blood is collected into special tubes using a needle. The blood is delivered to a laboratory as directed by the IGRA test instructions. The laboratory runs the test and reports the results to the health-care provider.

What Does a Positive Interferon Gamma Release Assay Result Mean?

- **Positive IGRA.** This means that the person has been infected with TB bacteria. Additional tests are needed to determine if the person has latent TB infection or TB disease. A health-care worker will then provide treatment as needed.

- **Negative IGRA.** This means that the person's blood did not react to the test and that latent TB infection or TB disease is not likely.

Who Can Receive an Interferon Gamma Release Assay?

Anyone can have an IGRA in place of a TST. This can be for any situation where a TST is recommended. In general, a person should have either a TST or an IGRA, but not both. There are rare exceptions when results from both tests may be useful in deciding whether a person has been infected with TB. IGRAs are the preferred method of TB infection testing for the following:

- People who have received the BCG shot
- People who have a difficult time returning for a second appointment to look at the TST after the test was given

How Often Can an Interferon Gamma Release Assay be Given?

There is no problem with repeated IGRAs.

Who Should Get Tested for Tuberculosis?

The Centers for Disease Control and Prevention (CDC) and the United States Preventive Services Task Force (USPSTF) recommend testing populations that are at increased risk for TB infection. Certain people should be tested for TB bacteria because they are more likely to get TB disease, including:

- People who have spent time with someone who has TB disease
- People with HIV infection or another medical problem that weakens the immune system
- People who have symptoms of TB disease (fever, night sweats, cough, and weight loss)
- People from a country where TB disease is common (most countries in Latin America, the Caribbean, Africa, Asia, Eastern Europe, and Russia)
- People who live or work somewhere in the United States where TB disease is more common (homeless shelters, prison or jails, or some nursing homes)
- People who use illegal drugs

CHOOSING A TUBERCULOSIS TEST

Choosing which TB test to use should be done by the person's health-care provider. Factors in selecting which test to use include the reason for testing, test availability, and cost. Generally, it is not recommended to test a person with both a TST and an IGRA.

DIAGNOSIS OF LATENT TUBERCULOSIS INFECTION OR DISEASE

If a person is found to be infected with TB bacteria, other tests are needed to see if the person has TB disease. TB disease can be diagnosed by medical history, physical examination, chest x-ray, and other laboratory tests. TB disease is treated by taking several drugs as recommended by a health-care provider.

If a person does not have TB disease, but has TB bacteria in the body, then latent TB infection is diagnosed. The decision about taking treatment for latent TB infection will be based on a person's chances of developing TB disease.

Chapter 41 | Celiac Disease Tests

WHAT IS CELIAC DISEASE?

Celiac disease is a chronic digestive and immune disorder that damages the small intestine. The disease is triggered by eating foods containing gluten. Gluten is a protein found naturally in wheat, barley, and rye, and is common in foods such as bread, pasta, cookies, and cakes. Many products contain gluten, such as prepackaged foods, lip balms and lipsticks, toothpastes, vitamin and nutrient supplements, and, rarely, medicines.

Celiac disease can be serious. The disease can cause long-lasting digestive problems and keep your body from getting all the nutrients it needs. Celiac disease can also affect the body outside the small intestine.

Celiac disease is different from gluten sensitivity or wheat intolerance. If you have gluten sensitivity, you may have symptoms like those of celiac disease, such as abdominal pain and tiredness. Unlike celiac disease, gluten sensitivity does not damage the small intestine.

Celiac disease is also different from a wheat allergy, a type of food allergy. In both cases, your body's immune system reacts to wheat. However, some symptoms of wheat allergies, such as having itchy eyes or a hard time breathing, are different from celiac disease. Wheat allergies also do not cause long-term damage to the small intestine.

This chapter includes text excerpted from "Celiac Disease," National Institute of Diabetes and Digestive and Kidney Diseases (NIDDK), October 2020.

WHAT CAUSES CELIAC DISEASE

Research suggests that celiac disease only occurs in people who have certain genes and eat food that contains gluten. Experts are studying other factors that may play a role in causing the disease.

Genes

Celiac disease almost always occurs in people who have one of two groups of normal gene variants, called "*DQ2*" and "*DQ8*". People who do not have these gene variants are very unlikely to develop celiac disease. About 30 percent of people have *DQ2* or *DQ8*. However, only about 3 percent of people with *DQ2* or *DQ8* develop celiac disease.

Researchers are studying other genes that may increase the chance of developing celiac disease in people who have *DQ2* or *DQ8*.

Gluten

Consuming gluten triggers the abnormal immune system response that causes celiac disease. However, not all people who have the gene variants *DQ2* or *DQ8* and eat gluten develop the disease. Research suggests that among children with a genetic predisposition for celiac disease, those who eat more gluten in early childhood may have a greater risk for celiac disease.

Other Factors

Researchers are studying other factors that may increase a person's chances of developing celiac disease. For example, research suggests that a higher number of infections in early life and certain digestive tract infections may increase the risk. Experts also think changes in the microbiome – the bacteria in the digestive tract that help with digestion – could play a role in the development of celiac disease.

WHAT ARE THE SYMPTOMS OF CELIAC DISEASE?

Symptoms of celiac disease vary widely, and a person may have multiple symptoms that come and go. If you have celiac disease, you may have digestive problems or other symptoms. Digestive symptoms are more common in children than in adults. Digestive symptoms of celiac disease may include:

- Bloating
- Chronic diarrhea
- Constipation
- Gas
- Lactose intolerance due to damage to the small intestine
- Loose, greasy, bulky, and bad-smelling stools
- Nausea or vomiting
- Pain in the abdomen

For children with celiac disease, being unable to absorb nutrients at a time when they are so important to normal growth and development can lead to:

- Damage to the permanent teeth's enamel
- Delayed puberty
- Failure to thrive, meaning that an infant or a child weighs less or is gaining less weight than expected for her or his age
- Mood changes or feeling annoyed or impatient
- Slowed growth and short height
- Weight loss

Some people with celiac disease have symptoms that affect other parts of the body. These symptoms may include:

- Dermatitis herpetiformis
- Fatigue, or feeling tired
- Joint or bone pain
- Mental-health problems, such as depression or anxiety
- Nervous system symptoms, such as headaches, balance problems, seizures, or peripheral neuropathy
- Reproductive problems in women and girls – which may include infertility, delayed start of menstrual periods, missed menstrual periods, or repeated miscarriages – and male infertility

- Symptoms involving the mouth, such as canker sores; a dry mouth; or a red, smooth, shiny tongue

Most people with celiac disease have one or more symptoms before they are diagnosed and begin treatment. Symptoms typically improve and may go away after a person begins eating a gluten-free diet. Symptoms may return if a person consumes small amounts of gluten.

Depending on how old you are when a doctor diagnoses your celiac disease, some symptoms, such as short height and tooth defects, may not improve. People with celiac disease who have no symptoms can still develop complications over time if they do not get treatment.

Dermatitis Herpetiformis

Dermatitis herpetiformis is an itchy, blistering skin rash that usually appears on the elbows, knees, buttocks, back, or scalp. Among people with untreated celiac disease, about 2 to 3 percent of children and 10 to 20 percent of adults have dermatitis herpetiformis. Some people with celiac disease may have the rash and no other symptoms. After a person starts a gluten-free diet, the rash may take some time to heal and may return if a person consumes small amounts of gluten.

HOW DO DOCTORS DIAGNOSE CELIAC DISEASE?

Doctors use information from your medical and family history, a physical exam, a dental exam, and medical test results to look for signs that you might have celiac disease and should be tested. Doctors typically diagnose celiac disease with blood tests and biopsies of the small intestine.

Medical and Family History

Your doctor will ask about your symptoms. Celiac disease is not diagnosed based on symptoms alone because some of the symptoms are like the symptoms of other digestive disorders, such as irritable bowel syndrome (IBS) or lactose intolerance. Some people with celiac disease have symptoms that affect parts of the body outside the digestive tract.

The doctor will review your medical history, including your history of conditions that are more common in people who have celiac disease. Your doctor will also ask about your family's medical history and whether anyone in your family has been diagnosed with celiac disease.

Physical Exam

During a physical exam, a doctor may:

- Check for signs of weight loss or growth problems
- Examine your skin for rashes, such as dermatitis herpetiformis
- Listen to sounds in the abdomen using a stethoscope
- Tap on the abdomen to check for pain or swelling

In some cases, a dentist may notice signs of celiac disease during an exam. Celiac disease may cause problems with the teeth and mouth, such as defects in tooth enamel or canker sores.

WHAT TESTS DO DOCTORS USE TO DIAGNOSE CELIAC DISEASE?

Doctors most often use blood tests and biopsies of the small intestine to diagnose or rule out celiac disease. Doctors do not recommend starting a gluten-free diet before diagnostic testing because a gluten-free diet can affect test results.

In some cases, doctors may order additional tests, such as skin biopsies and genetic tests, to help diagnose or rule out celiac disease.

Blood Tests

A health-care professional will take a blood sample from you and send the sample to a lab. Blood tests can show levels of certain antibodies that are often higher than normal in people who have untreated celiac disease. Blood tests may also show signs of health problems that could be related to celiac disease, such as anemia.

Biopsies of the Small Intestine

A doctor obtains biopsies of the small intestine during an upper GI endoscopy. For an upper GI endoscopy, a doctor uses an endoscope – a flexible tube with a camera – to see the lining of your upper GI tract, including the first part of your small intestine. The doctor passes an instrument through the endoscope to take small pieces of tissue from your small intestine. A pathologist will examine the tissue under a microscope to look for signs of celiac disease.

Skin Biopsies

A doctor may order skin biopsies if you have a rash that could be dermatitis herpetiformis. For skin biopsies, a doctor removes small pieces of skin tissue on and next to the rash. A pathologist will examine the tissue under a microscope to look for signs of dermatitis herpetiformis.

Genetic Testing

In some cases, a health-care professional may take a blood sample or use a swab to collect cells from the inside of your cheek. The sample will be tested for groups of gene variants called "*DQ2*" and "*DQ8*." If you do not have these gene variants, you are very unlikely to have celiac disease.

Having *DQ2* or *DQ8* alone does not mean you have celiac disease. Most people with these gene variants do not develop celiac disease. If you do have *DQ2* or *DQ8*, your doctor may recommend additional tests to check for or rule out celiac disease.

DO DOCTORS SCREEN FOR CELIAC DISEASE?

Screening is testing for diseases when you have no symptoms. Doctors in the United States do not routinely screen people for celiac disease. However, blood relatives of people with celiac disease and those with type 1 diabetes should talk with their doctor about their chances of getting the disease to see if they should be tested.

Chapter 42 | **Diabetes Tests**

Chapter Contents

Section 42.1 | Screening Tests for Diabetes

This section includes text excerpted from "Diabetes Tests and Diagnosis," National Institute of Diabetes and Digestive and Kidney Diseases (NIDDK), December 2016. Reviewed October 2021.

Your health-care professional can diagnose diabetes, prediabetes, and gestational diabetes through blood tests. The blood tests show if your blood glucose, also called "blood sugar," is too high.

Do not try to diagnose yourself if you think you might have diabetes. Testing equipment that you can buy over the counter, such as a blood glucose meter, cannot diagnose diabetes.

WHO SHOULD BE TESTED FOR DIABETES?

Anyone who has symptoms of diabetes should be tested for the disease. Some people will not have any symptoms but may have risk factors for diabetes and need to be tested. Testing allows health-care professionals to find diabetes sooner and work with their patients to manage diabetes and prevent complications.

Testing also allows health-care professionals to find prediabetes. Making lifestyle changes to lose a modest amount of weight if you are overweight may help you delay or prevent type 2 diabetes.

TYPE 1 DIABETES

Most often, testing for type 1 diabetes occurs in people with diabetes symptoms. Doctors usually diagnose type 1 diabetes in children and young adults. Because type 1 diabetes can run in families, a study called "TrialNet" offers free testing to family members of people with the disease, even if they do not have symptoms.

TYPE 2 DIABETES

Experts recommend routine testing for type 2 diabetes if you:

- Are age 45 or older
- Are between the ages of 19 and 44, are overweight or obese, and have one or more other diabetes risk factors
- Are a woman who had gestational diabetes

Medicare covers the cost of diabetes tests for people with certain risk factors for diabetes. If you have Medicare, find out if you qualify for coverage. If you have different insurance, ask your insurance company if it covers diabetes tests.

Though type 2 diabetes most often develops in adults, children also can develop type 2 diabetes. Experts recommend testing children between the ages of 10 and 18 who are overweight or obese and have at least two other risk factors for developing diabetes.

- Low birth weight
- A mother who had diabetes while pregnant with them
- Any risk factor mentioned in Risk Factors for Type 2 Diabetes (www.niddk.nih.gov/health-information/diabetes/overview/risk-factors-type-2-diabetes)

GESTATIONAL DIABETES

All pregnant women who do not have a prior diabetes diagnosis should be tested for gestational diabetes. If you are pregnant, you will take a glucose challenge test between 24 and 28 weeks of pregnancy.

WHAT TESTS ARE USED TO DIAGNOSE DIABETES AND PREDIABETES?

Health-care professionals most often use the fasting plasma glucose (FPG) test or the A1c test to diagnose diabetes. In some cases, they may use a random plasma glucose (RPG) test.

Fasting Plasma Glucose Test

The FPG blood test measures your blood glucose level at a single point in time. For the most reliable results, it is best to have this test in the morning, after you fast for at least 8 hours. Fasting means having nothing to eat or drink except sips of water.

A1c Test

The A1c test is a blood test that provides your average levels of blood glucose over the past 3 months. Other names for the A1c test are hemoglobin A1c, HbA1c, glycated hemoglobin, and glycosylated hemoglobin test. You can eat and drink before this test. When it comes to using the A1c to diagnose diabetes, your doctor will consider factors such as your age and whether you have anemia or another problem with your blood. The A1c test is not accurate in people with anemia.

If you are of African, Mediterranean, or Southeast Asian descent, your A1c test results may be falsely high or low. Your health-care professional may need to order a different type of A1c test.

Your health-care professional will report your A1c test result as a percentage, such as an A1c of 7 percent. The higher the percentage, the higher your average blood glucose levels.

People with diabetes also use information from the A1c test to help manage their diabetes.

Random Plasma Glucose Test

Sometimes health-care professionals use the RPG test to diagnose diabetes when diabetes symptoms are present and they do not want to wait until you have fasted. You do not need to fast overnight for the RPG test. You may have this blood test at any time.

WHAT TESTS ARE USED TO DIAGNOSE GESTATIONAL DIABETES?

Pregnant women may have the glucose challenge test, the oral glucose tolerance test, or both. These tests show how well your body handles glucose.

Glucose Challenge Test

If you are pregnant and a health-care professional is checking you for gestational diabetes, you may first receive the glucose challenge test. Another name for this test is the glucose screening test. In this test, a health-care professional will draw your blood 1 hour after you drink a sweet liquid containing glucose. You do not need to fast for this test. If your blood glucose is too high – 135 to 140 or more – you may need to return for an oral glucose tolerance test while fasting.

Oral Glucose Tolerance Test

The oral glucose tolerance test (OGTT) measures blood glucose after you fast for at least 8 hours. First, a health-care professional will draw your blood. Then you will drink the liquid containing glucose. For diagnosing gestational diabetes, you will need your blood drawn every hour for 2 to 3 hours.

High blood glucose levels at any two or more blood test times during the OGTT – fasting, 1 hour, 2 hours, or 3 hours – mean you have gestational diabetes. Your health-care team will explain what your OGTT results mean.

Health-care professionals also can use the OGTT to diagnose type 2 diabetes and prediabetes in people who are not pregnant. The OGTT helps health-care professionals detect type 2 diabetes and prediabetes better than the FPG test. However, the OGTT is a more expensive test and is not as easy to give. To diagnose type 2 diabetes and prediabetes, a health-care professional will need to draw your blood 1 hour after you drink the liquid containing glucose and again after 2 hours.

WHAT TEST NUMBERS TELL YOU IF YOU HAVE DIABETES OR PREDIABETES

Each test to detect diabetes and prediabetes uses a different measurement. Usually, the same test method needs to be repeated on a second day to diagnose diabetes. Your doctor may also use a second test method to confirm that you have diabetes.

Table 42.1 helps you understand what your test numbers mean if you are not pregnant.

WHICH TESTS HELP YOUR HEALTH-CARE PROFESSIONAL KNOW WHAT KIND OF DIABETES YOU HAVE?

Even though the tests described here can confirm that you have diabetes, they cannot identify what type you have. Sometimes health-care professionals are unsure if diabetes is type 1 or type 2. A rare type of diabetes that can occur in babies, called "monogenic diabetes," can also be mistaken for type 1 diabetes. Treatment depends on the type of diabetes, so knowing which type you have is important.

Table 42.1. Understand What Your Test Numbers Mean

Diagnosis	A1c (%)	Fasting Plasma Glucose (FPG)[a]	Oral Glucose Tolerance Test (OGTT)[ab]	Random Plasma Glucose Test (RPG)[a]
Normal	below 5.7	99 or below	139 or below	
Prediabetes	5.7 to 6.4	100 to 125	140 to 199	
Diabetes	6.5 or above	126 or above	200 or above	200 or above

[a]Glucose values are in milligrams per deciliter, or mg/dL.
[b]At 2 hours after drinking 75 grams of glucose. To diagnose gestational diabetes, health-care professionals give more glucose to drink and use different numbers as cutoffs.

To find out if your diabetes is type 1, your health-care professional may look for certain autoantibodies. Autoantibodies are antibodies that mistakenly attack your healthy tissues and cells. The presence of one or more of several types of autoantibodies specific to diabetes is common in type 1 diabetes, but not in type 2 or monogenic diabetes. A health-care professional will have to draw your blood for this test.

If you had diabetes while you were pregnant, you should get tested no later than 12 weeks after your baby is born to see if you have type 2 diabetes.

Section 42.2 | **A1c Test**

This section includes text excerpted from "The A1c Test and Diabetes," National Institute of Diabetes and Digestive and Kidney Diseases (NIDDK), April 2018. Reviewed October 2021.

WHAT IS THE A1c TEST?

The A1c test is a blood test that provides information about your average levels of blood glucose, also called "blood sugar," over the past 3 months. The A1c test can be used to diagnose type 2 diabetes and prediabetes. The A1c test is also the primary test used for diabetes management.

The A1c test is sometimes called the "hemoglobin A1c," "HbA1c," "glycated hemoglobin," or "glycohemoglobin" test. Hemoglobin is the part of a red blood cell that carries oxygen to the cells. Glucose attaches to or binds with hemoglobin in your blood cells, and the A1c test is based on this attachment of glucose to hemoglobin.

The higher the glucose level in your bloodstream, the more glucose will attach to the hemoglobin. The A1c test measures the amount of hemoglobin with attached glucose and reflects your average blood glucose levels over the past 3 months.

The A1c test result is reported as a percentage. The higher the percentage, the higher your blood glucose levels have been. A normal A1c level is below 5.7 percent.

WHY SHOULD A PERSON GET THE A1c TEST?

Testing can help health-care professionals:

- Find prediabetes and counsel you about lifestyle changes to help you delay or prevent type 2 diabetes
- Find type 2 diabetes
- Work with you to monitor the disease and help make treatment decisions to prevent complications

If you have risk factors for prediabetes or diabetes, talk with your doctor about whether you should be tested.

HOW IS THE A1c TEST USED TO DIAGNOSE TYPE 2 DIABETES AND PREDIABETES?

Health-care professionals can use the A1c test alone or in combination with other diabetes tests to diagnose type 2 diabetes and prediabetes. You do not have to fast before having your blood drawn for an A1c test, which means that blood can be drawn for the test at any time of the day.

If you do not have symptoms but the A1c test shows you have diabetes or prediabetes, you should have a repeat test on a different day using the A1c test or one of the other diabetes tests to confirm the diagnosis.

Table 42.2. A1c Results and What the Numbers Mean

Diagnosis*	A1c Level
Normal	below 5.7%
Prediabetes	5.7% to 6.4%
Diabetes	6.5% or above

**Any test used to diagnose diabetes requires confirmation with a second measurement, unless there are clear symptoms of diabetes.*

When using the A1c test for diagnosis, your doctor will send your blood sample taken from a vein to a lab that uses an NGSP-certified method. The NGSP, formerly called the "National Glycohemoglobin Standardization Program," certifies that makers of A1c tests provide results that are consistent and comparable with those used in the Diabetes Control and Complications Trial.

Blood samples analyzed in a doctor's office or clinic, known as "point-of-care tests," should not be used for diagnosis.

The A1c test should not be used to diagnose type 1 diabetes, gestational diabetes, or cystic fibrosis-related diabetes. The A1c test may give false results in people with certain conditions.

Having prediabetes is a risk factor for developing type 2 diabetes. Within the prediabetes A1c range of 5.7 to 6.4 percent, the higher the A1c, the greater the risk of diabetes.

IS THE A1c TEST USED DURING PREGNANCY?

Health-care professionals may use the A1c test early in pregnancy to see if a woman with risk factors had undiagnosed diabetes before becoming pregnant. Since the A1c test reflects your average blood glucose levels over the past 3 months, testing early in pregnancy may include values reflecting time before you were pregnant. The glucose challenge test or the oral glucose tolerance test (OGTT) are used to check for gestational diabetes, usually between 24 and 28 weeks of pregnancy. If you had gestational diabetes, you should be tested for diabetes no later than 12 weeks after your baby is born.

If your blood glucose is still high, you may have type 2 diabetes. Even if your blood glucose is normal, you still have a greater chance of developing type 2 diabetes in the future and should get tested every 3 years.

CAN OTHER BLOOD GLUCOSE TESTS BE USED TO DIAGNOSE TYPE 2 DIABETES AND PREDIABETES?

Yes. Health-care professionals also use the fasting plasma glucose (FPG) test and the OGTT to diagnose type 2 diabetes and prediabetes. For these blood glucose tests used to diagnose diabetes, you must fast at least 8 hours before you have your blood drawn. If you have symptoms of diabetes, your doctor may use the random plasma glucose test, which does not require fasting. In some cases, health-care professionals use the A1c test to help confirm the results of another blood glucose test.

CAN THE A1c TEST RESULT IN A DIFFERENT DIAGNOSIS THAN THE BLOOD GLUCOSE TESTS?

Yes. In some people, a blood glucose test may show diabetes when an A1c test does not. The reverse can also occur – an A1c test may indicate diabetes even though a blood glucose test does not. Because of these differences in test results, health-care professionals repeat tests before making a diagnosis.

People with differing test results may be in an early stage of the disease, when blood glucose levels have not risen high enough to show up on every test. In this case, health-care professionals may choose to follow the person closely and repeat the test in several months.

WHY DO DIABETES BLOOD TEST RESULTS VARY?

Lab test results can vary from day to day and from test to test. This can be a result of the following factors:

Blood Glucose Levels Move Up and Down

Your results can vary because of natural changes in your blood glucose level. For example, your blood glucose level moves up and

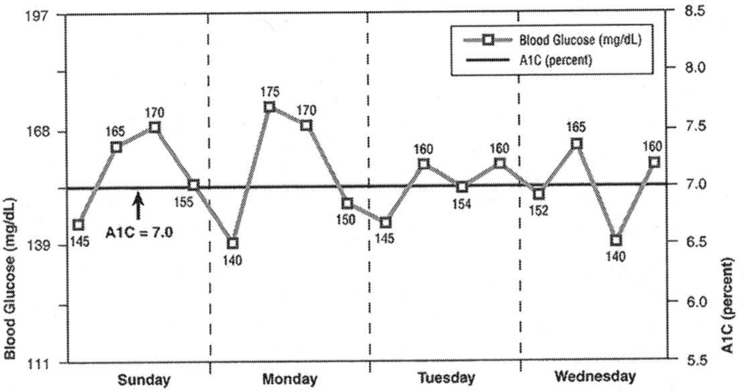

Figure 42.1. Blood Glucose Measurements Compared with A1c Measurements over 4 Days

Blood glucose (mg/dL) measurements were taken four times per day (fasting or prebreakfast, prelunch, predinner, and bedtime).

down when you eat or exercise. Sickness and stress also can affect your blood glucose test results. A1c tests are less likely to be affected by short-term changes than FPG or OGTT tests.

The following chart shows how multiple blood glucose measurements over 4 days compare with an A1c measurement.

The straight black line shows an A1c measurement of 7.0 percent. The blue line shows an example of how blood glucose test results might look from self-monitoring four times a day over a 4-day period.

A1c Tests Can Be Affected by Changes in Red Blood Cells or Hemoglobin

Conditions that change the life span of red blood cells, such as recent blood loss, sickle cell disease, erythropoietin treatment, hemodialysis, or transfusion, can change A1c levels.

A falsely high A1c result can occur in people who are very low in iron; for example, those with iron-deficiency anemia. Other causes of false A1c results include kidney failure or liver disease.

If you are of African, Mediterranean, or Southeast Asian descent or have family members with sickle cell anemia or a thalassemia, an A1c test can be unreliable for diagnosing or monitoring diabetes and prediabetes. People in these groups may have a different type of hemoglobin, known as a "hemoglobin variant," which can interfere with some A1c tests. Most people with a hemoglobin variant have no symptoms and may not know that they carry this type of hemoglobin. Health-care professionals may suspect interference – a falsely high or low result – when your A1c and blood glucose test results do not match.

Not all A1c tests are unreliable for people with a hemoglobin variant. People with false results from one type of A1c test may need a different type of A1c test to measure their average blood glucose level. The NGSP provides information for health-care professionals about which A1c tests are appropriate to use for specific hemoglobin variants.

Small Changes in Temperature, Equipment, or Sample Handling

Even when the same blood sample is repeatedly measured in the same lab, the results may vary because of small changes in temperature, equipment, or sample handling. These factors tend to affect glucose measurements – fasting and OGTT – more than the A1c test.

Health-care professionals understand these variations and repeat lab tests for confirmation. Diabetes develops over time, so even with variations in test results, health-care professionals can tell when overall blood glucose levels are becoming too high.

HOW PRECISE IS THE A1c TEST?

When repeated, the A1c test result can be slightly higher or lower than the first measurement. This means, for example, an A1c reported as 6.8 percent on one test could be reported in a range from 6.4 to 7.2 percent on a repeat test from the same blood sample. In the past, this range was larger but new, stricter quality-control standards mean more precise A1c test results.

Health-care professionals can visit www.ngsp.org to find information about the precision of the A1c test used by their lab.

HOW IS THE A1c TEST USED AFTER DIAGNOSIS OF DIABETES?

Your health-care professional may use the A1c test to set your treatment goals, modify therapy, and monitor your diabetes management.

Experts recommend that people with diabetes have an A1c test at least twice a year. Health-care professionals may check your A1c more often if you are not meeting your treatment goals.

WHAT A1c GOAL SHOULD YOU HAVE

People will have different A1c targets, depending on their diabetes history and their general health. You should discuss your A1c target with your health-care professional. Studies have shown that some people with diabetes can reduce the risk of diabetes complications by keeping A1c levels below 7 percent.

Managing blood glucose early in the course of diabetes may provide benefits for many years to come. However, an A1c level that is safe for one person may not be safe for another. For example, keeping an A1c level below 7 percent may not be safe if it leads to problems with hypoglycemia, also called "low blood glucose."

Less strict blood glucose control, or an A1c between 7 and 8 percent – or even higher in some circumstances – may be appropriate in people who have:

- Limited life expectancy
- Long-standing diabetes and trouble reaching a lower goal
- Severe hypoglycemia or inability to sense hypoglycemia (also called "hypoglycemia unawareness")
- Advanced diabetes complications such as chronic kidney disease, nerve problems, or cardiovascular disease

HOW DOES A1c RELATE TO ESTIMATED AVERAGE GLUCOSE?

Estimated average glucose (eAG) is calculated from your A1c. Some laboratories report eAG with A1c test results. The eAG number helps you relate your A1c to daily glucose monitoring levels. The eAG calculation converts the A1c percentage to the same units used by home glucose meters – milligrams per deciliter (mg/dL).

The eAG number will not match daily glucose readings because it is a long-term average – rather than your blood glucose level at a single time, as is measured with a home glucose meter.

WILL THE A1c TEST SHOW SHORT-TERM CHANGES IN BLOOD GLUCOSE LEVELS?

Large changes in your blood glucose levels over the past month will show up in your A1c test result, but the A1c test does not show sudden, temporary increases or decreases in blood glucose levels. Even though A1c results represent a long-term average, blood glucose levels within the past 30 days have a greater effect on the A1c reading than those in previous months.

Chapter 43 | Thyroid Tests

NEED FOR THE TEST

Health-care professionals use thyroid tests to check how well your thyroid is working and to find the cause of problems such as hyperthyroidism or hypothyroidism. The thyroid is a small, butterfly-shaped gland in the front of your neck that makes two thyroid hormones: thyroxine (T_4) and tri-iodothyronine (T_3). Thyroid hormones control how the body uses energy, so they affect nearly every organ in your body, even your heart.

Thyroid tests help health-care professionals diagnose thyroid diseases such as:

- Hyperthyroidism – when thyroid hormone levels are too high
- Graves disease, the most common cause of hyperthyroidism
- Hypothyroidism – when thyroid hormones levels are too low
- Hashimoto disease, of the most common cause of hypothyroidism
- Thyroid nodules and thyroid cancer

Your doctor will start with blood tests and may also order imaging tests.

This chapter contains text excerpted from the following sources: Text beginning with the heading "Need for the Test" is excerpted from "Thyroid Tests," National Institute of Diabetes and Digestive and Kidney Diseases (NIDDK), May 2017. Reviewed October 2021; Text under the heading "Diagnosis of Graves Disease" is excerpted from "Graves' Disease," National Institute of Diabetes and Digestive and Kidney Diseases (NIDDK), September 2017. Reviewed October 2021; Text under the heading "Diagnosis of Hashimoto Disease" is excerpted from "Hashimoto's Disease," Office on Women's Health (OWH), U.S. Department of Health and Human Services (HHS), October 18, 2018. Reviewed October 2021.

WHAT BLOOD TESTS DO DOCTORS USE TO CHECK THYROID FUNCTION?

Doctors may order one or more blood tests to check your thyroid function. Tests may include thyroid stimulating hormone (TSH), thyroxine (T_4), triiodothyronine (T_3), and thyroid antibody tests.

For these tests, a health-care professional will draw blood from your arm and send it to a lab for testing. Your doctor will talk to you about your test results.

Thyroid-Stimulating Hormone Test

Health-care professionals usually check the amount of TSH in your blood first. TSH is a hormone made in the pituitary gland that tells the thyroid how much T_4 and T_3 to make.

A high TSH level most often means you have hypothyroidism, or an underactive thyroid. This means that your thyroid is not making enough hormone. As a result, the pituitary keeps making and releasing TSH into your blood.

A low TSH level usually means you have hyperthyroidism, or an overactive thyroid. This means that your thyroid is making too much hormone, so the pituitary stops making and releasing TSH into your blood.

If the TSH test results are not normal, you will need at least one other test to help find the cause of the problem.

Thyroxine Tests

A high blood level of T_4 may mean you have hyperthyroidism. A low level of T_4 may mean you have hypothyroidism.

In some cases, high or low T_4 levels may not mean you have thyroid problems. If you are pregnant or are taking oral contraceptives, your thyroid hormone levels will be higher. Severe illness or using corticosteroids – medicines to treat asthma, arthritis, skin conditions, and other health problems – can lower T_4 levels. These conditions and medicines change the amount of proteins in your blood that "bind," or attach to T_4. Bound T_4 is kept in reserve in the blood until it is needed. "Free" T_4 is not bound to these proteins and is available to enter body tissues. Because changes in binding protein levels do not affect free T_4 levels, many health-care professionals prefer to measure free T_4.

Triiodothyronine Test

If your health-care professional thinks you may have hyperthyroidism even though your T_4 level is normal, you may have a T_3 test to confirm the diagnosis. Sometimes T_4 is normal yet T_3 is high, so measuring both T_4 and T_3 levels can be useful in diagnosing hyperthyroidism.

Thyroid Antibody Tests

Measuring levels of thyroid antibodies may help diagnose an autoimmune thyroid disorder such as Graves disease – the most common cause of hyperthyroidism – and Hashimoto disease – the most common cause of hypothyroidism. Thyroid antibodies are made when your immune system attacks the thyroid gland by mistake. Your health-care professional may order thyroid antibody tests if the results of other blood tests suggest thyroid disease.

WHAT IMAGING TESTS DO DOCTORS USE TO DIAGNOSE AND FIND THE CAUSE OF THYROID DISEASE?

Your health-care professional may order one or more imaging tests to diagnose and find the cause of thyroid disease. A trained technician usually does these tests in your doctor's office, outpatient center, or hospital. A radiologist, a doctor who specializes in medical imaging, reviews the images and sends a report for your health-care professional to discuss with you.

Ultrasound

Ultrasound of the thyroid is most often used to look for, or more closely at, thyroid nodules. Thyroid nodules are lumps in your neck. Ultrasound can help your doctor tell if the nodules are more likely to be cancerous.

For an ultrasound, you will lie on an exam table and a technician will run a device called a "transducer" over your neck. The transducer bounces safe, painless sound waves off your neck to make pictures of your thyroid. The ultrasound usually takes around 30 minutes.

Thyroid Scan

Health-care professionals use a thyroid scan to look at the size, shape, and position of the thyroid gland. This test uses a small amount of radioactive iodine to help find the cause of hyperthyroidism and check for thyroid nodules. Your health-care professional may ask you to avoid foods high in iodine, such as kelp, or medicines containing iodine for a week before the test.

For the scan, a technician injects a small amount of radioactive iodine or a similar substance into your vein. You also may swallow the substance in liquid or capsule form. The scan takes place 30 minutes after an injection, or up to 24 hours after you swallow the substance, so your thyroid has enough time to absorb it.

During the scan, you will lie on an exam table while a special camera takes pictures of your thyroid. The scan usually takes 30 minutes or less.

Thyroid nodules that make too much thyroid hormone show up clearly in the pictures. Radioactive iodine that shows up over the whole thyroid could mean you have Graves disease.

Even though only a small amount of radiation is needed for a thyroid scan and it is thought to be safe, you should not have this test if you are pregnant or breastfeeding.

Radioactive Iodine Uptake Test

A radioactive iodine uptake test, also called a "thyroid uptake test," can help check thyroid function and find the cause of hyperthyroidism. The thyroid "takes up" iodine from the blood to make thyroid hormones, which is why this is called an "uptake test." Your health-care professional may ask you to avoid foods high in iodine, such as kelp, or medicines containing iodine for a week before the test.

For this test, you will swallow a small amount of radioactive iodine in liquid or capsule form. During the test, you will sit in a chair while a technician places a device called a "gamma probe" in front of your neck, near your thyroid gland. The probe measures how much radioactive iodine your thyroid takes up from your blood. Measurements are often taken 4 to 6 hours after you swallow the radioactive iodine and again at 24 hours. The test takes only a few minutes.

If your thyroid collects a large amount of radioactive iodine, you may have Graves disease, or one or more nodules that make too much thyroid hormone. You may have this test at the same time as a thyroid scan.

Even though the test uses a small amount of radiation and is thought to be safe, you should not have this test if you are pregnant or breastfeeding.

WHAT TESTS DO DOCTORS USE IF YOU HAVE A THYROID NODULE?

If your health-care professional finds a nodule or lump in your neck during a physical exam or on thyroid imaging tests, you may have a fine needle aspiration biopsy to see if the lump is cancerous or noncancerous.

For this test, you will lie on an exam table and slightly bend your neck backward. A technician will clean your neck with an antiseptic and may use medicine to numb the area. An endocrinologist who treats people with endocrine gland problems such as thyroid disease, or a specially trained radiologist, will place a needle through the skin and use ultrasound to guide the needle to the nodule. Small samples of tissue from the nodule will be sent to a lab for testing. This procedure usually takes less than 30 minutes. Your health-care professional will talk with you about the test result when it is available.

DIAGNOSIS OF GRAVES DISEASE

Your health-care provider may suspect Graves disease based on your symptoms and findings during a physical exam. One or more blood tests can confirm that you have hyperthyroidism and may point to Graves disease as the cause.

Other clues that hyperthyroidism is caused by Graves disease are:

- An enlarged thyroid
- Signs of Graves eye disease, present in about one out of three people with Graves disease
- A history of other family members with thyroid or autoimmune problems

If the diagnosis is uncertain, your doctor may order further blood or imaging tests to confirm Graves disease as the cause.

A blood test can detect TSI. However, in mild cases of Graves disease, TSI may not show up in your blood. The next step may be one of two imaging tests that use small, safe doses of radioactive iodine. Your thyroid collects iodine from your bloodstream and uses it to make thyroid hormones; it will collect radioactive iodine in the same way.

- **Radioactive iodine uptake test.** This test measures the amount of iodine the thyroid collects from the bloodstream. If your thyroid collects large amounts of iodine, you may have Graves disease.
- **Thyroid scan.** This scan shows how and where iodine is distributed in the thyroid. With Graves disease, the entire thyroid is involved, so the iodine shows up throughout the gland. With other causes of hyperthyroidism such as nodules – small lumps in the gland – the iodine shows up in a different pattern.

DIAGNOSIS OF HASHIMOTO DISEASE

If you have symptoms of hypothyroidism, your doctor or nurse will do an exam and order one or more tests. Tests used to find out whether you have hypothyroidism and Hashimoto disease include:

- **Thyroid function test.** This blood test tells whether your body has the right amounts of TSH and thyroid hormone. A high level of TSH is a sign of an underactive thyroid. When the thyroid begins to fail, the pituitary gland makes more TSH to trigger the thyroid to make more thyroid hormone. When the damaged thyroid can no longer keep up, your thyroid hormone levels drop below normal.

- **Antibody test.** This blood test tells whether you have the antibodies that suggest Hashimoto disease. More than one in 10 people have the antibodies, but have normal thyroid function. Having only the antibodies does not cause hypothyroidism.

Chapter 44 | Heart and Vascular Disease Screening and Diagnostic Tests

Coronary heart disease (CHD) also known as "coronary artery disease" (CAD), "coronary microvascular disease" (MVD), "coronary syndrome X" (CSX), "ischemic heart disease," "nonobstructive CAD," "obstructive CAD."

Heart disease is a catch-all phrase for a variety of conditions that affect the heart's structure and function. CHD is a type of heart disease that develops when the arteries of the heart cannot deliver enough oxygen-rich blood to the heart. It is the leading cause of death in the United States.

The CHD is often caused by the buildup of plaque, a waxy substance, inside the lining of larger coronary arteries. This buildup can partially or totally block blood flow in the large arteries of the heart. Some types of this condition may be caused by disease or injury affecting how the arteries work in the heart. The MVD is another type of CHD. It occurs when the heart's tiny blood vessels do not work normally.

Symptoms of CHD may be different from person to person even if they have the same type of CHD. However, because many people

This chapter includes text excerpted from "Coronary Heart Disease," National Heart, Lung, and Blood Institute (NHLBI), August 9, 2021.

have no symptoms, they do not know they have CHD until they have chest pain, a heart attack, or sudden cardiac arrest.

If you have CHD, your doctor will recommend heart-healthy lifestyle changes, medicines, surgery, or a combination of these approaches to treat your condition and prevent complications.

CAUSES OF CORONARY HEART DISEASE

There are three main types of CHD: obstructive CAD, nonobstructive CAD, and MVD. CAD affects the large arteries on the surface of the heart. Many people have both obstructive and nonobstructive forms of this disease. The MVD affects the tiny arteries in the heart muscle.

The cause depends on the type of CHD. This condition may also have more than one cause, including plaque buildup or problems that affect how the heart's blood vessels work.

Plaque Buildup

Plaque buildup in the arteries is called "atherosclerosis." When this buildup happens in the heart's arteries over many years, the arteries become narrower and harden, reducing oxygen-rich blood flow to the heart. The result is CAD.

Problems Affecting the Blood Vessels

Problems with how the heart's blood vessels work can cause CHD. For example, the blood vessels may not respond to signals that the heart needs more oxygen-rich blood. Normally, the blood vessels widen to allow more blood flow when a person is physically active or under stress. But, if you have CHD, the size of these blood vessels may not change, or the blood vessels may even narrow.

The cause of these problems is not fully clear. But, it may involve:

- Damage or injury to the walls of the arteries or tiny blood vessels from chronic inflammation, high blood pressure, or diabetes
- Molecular changes are part of the normal aging process. Molecular changes affect the way genes and proteins are controlled inside cells.

In nonobstructive CAD, damage to the inner walls of the coronary arteries can cause them to spasm (suddenly tighten). This is called "vasospasm." The spasm causes the arteries to narrow temporarily and blocks blood flow to the heart.

These problems can also happen in the tiny blood vessels in the heart, causing MVD, sometimes called "coronary syndrome X" (CSX). MVD can happen with or without obstructive or nonobstructive CAD.

Plaque can attract platelets and white blood cells (WBCs) to the area of buildup in the large coronary arteries, causing inflammation. Inflammation can also prevent the small arteries of the heart from responding to the physical, electrical, and chemical signals that tell the arteries when the heart needs more oxygen-rich blood. This can lead to MVD. Research suggests that inflammation may also reduce levels of HDL cholesterol (sometimes called "good cholesterol").

SIGNS, SYMPTOMS, AND COMPLICATIONS OF CORONARY HEART DISEASE

Some people have severe symptoms of CHD. Others have no symptoms at all. If you have "silent" CHD, you may not have any symptoms until you have a heart attack or other complications.

Signs and Symptoms

An acute coronary event, such as a heart attack, may cause the following symptoms:

- Angina, which can feel like pressure, squeezing, burning, or tightness during physical activity. The pain or discomfort usually starts behind the breastbone, but it can also occur in the arms, shoulders, jaw, throat, or back. The pain may feel like indigestion.
- Cold sweats
- Dizziness
- Light-headedness
- Nausea or a feeling of indigestion
- Neck pain

- Shortness of breath, especially with activity
- Sleep disturbances
- Weakness

Women are somewhat less likely than men to experience chest pain. Instead, they are more likely to experience:

- Dizziness
- Fatigue
- Nausea
- Pressure or tightness in the chest
- Stomach pain

Women are also more likely than men to have no symptoms of CHD.

Chronic (long-term) CHD can cause symptoms such as the following:

- Angina
- Shortness of breath with physical activity
- Fatigue
- Neck pain

The symptoms may get worse as the buildup of plaque continues to narrow the coronary arteries. Chest pain or discomfort that does not go away or happens more often or while you are resting might be a sign of a heart attack. If you do not know whether your chest pain is angina or a heart attack, call 911 right away. All chest pain should be checked by a doctor.

Complications

The CHD can cause serious complications, including the following:

- Acute coronary syndrome, including angina or heart attack
- Arrhythmia
- Heart failure
- Cardiogenic shock
- Sudden cardiac arrest

Complications of CHD can be life-threatening and may lead to disability.

SCREENING AND PREVENTION OF CORONARY HEART DISEASE

You should start getting screening tests and risk assessments for coronary heart disease around age 20 if you do not have any risk factors for CHD. Children may need screening if they have risk factors, such as obesity, low levels of physical activity, or a family history of heart problems.

Afterward, your doctor may recommend preventive treatments such as heart-healthy lifestyle changes to help you lower your risk of CHD.

Screening Tests and Results

To screen for CHD, your doctor will:

- Assess risk factors to help evaluate your risk of developing CHD
- Check blood pressure readings to see whether you have high blood pressure
- Calculate your body mass index and waist circumference to see whether you have an unhealthy weight
- Order blood tests to see whether you have high blood cholesterol, high blood triglycerides, or diabetes

Screening usually occurs in a doctor's office, but sometimes screenings are done at health fairs, drugstores, or other places. Blood samples might be collected at your doctor's office, a hospital, or a laboratory.

Ask your doctor or nurse whether you need to fast (not eat or drink anything besides water) before the blood tests.

Risk Calculators

Your doctor may use a risk calculator to estimate your risk of having a heart attack, having a stroke, or dying from a heart or blood vessel disease in the next 10 years or throughout your lifetime.

For example, the atherosclerotic cardiovascular disease (ASCVD) estimator (tools.acc.org/ASCVD-Risk-Estimator-Plus/#!/calculate/estimate), considers your cholesterol levels, age, sex, race, and blood pressure. It also factors in whether you smoke or take medicines to manage your high blood pressure or cholesterol.

Ask about your risk during your annual checkup. Knowing your risk will help you and your doctor decide on healthy lifestyle changes and possibly medicines to lower your risk.

Risk assessments should be repeated every 4 to 6 years in adults 20 to 79 years of age who do not have heart or blood vessel disease.

No single risk calculator is appropriate for all people. Calculators can give you and your doctor a good idea about your risk, but your doctor might have to consider other factors to estimate your risk more accurately.

Commonly used risk calculators might not accurately estimate risk in certain situations, such as if you:

- Are an ethnic minority, such as South Asian
- Are a woman who has had complications during pregnancy or had early menopause. Your risk might be higher than predicted by the ASCVD risk estimator.
- Have metabolic syndrome or an inflammatory or autoimmune condition
- Have a family history of heart or blood vessel disease at a young age
- Take a statin to manage your cholesterol levels

In these cases, your doctor may suggest other tests for CHD even if the ASCVD risk estimator says you are not at high risk.

How to Prevent Coronary Heart Disease

Studies show that heart-healthy living – never smoking, eating healthy, and being physically active – throughout life can prevent CHD and its complications.

Work with your doctor to set up a plan that works for you based on your lifestyle, your home and neighborhood environments, and your culture. Working with a team of health-care providers may help with making changes in your diet, being physically active, managing other medical conditions, and helping you quit smoking.

DIAGNOSIS OF CORONARY HEART DISEASE

Your doctor will diagnose CHD based on your symptoms, your medical and family history, your risk factors, and the results from tests and procedures.

Because women and their doctors may not recognize CHD symptoms that are different from men's, women may not be diagnosed and treated as quickly as men. It is important to seek care right away if you have symptoms of CHD.

Medical History

Your doctor will ask about your eating and physical activity habits, your medical history, your family history, and risk factors for CHD. Your doctor may ask whether you have any other signs or symptoms. This information can help your doctor determine whether you have complications or other conditions that may cause CHD.

Diagnostic Tests and Procedures

To diagnose CHD, your doctor may order some of the following tests.

- Blood tests to check the levels of cholesterol, triglycerides, sugar, lipoproteins, or proteins, such as C-reactive protein, are a sign of inflammation.
- Electrocardiogram (EKG or ECG) to determine whether the heart's rhythm is steady or irregular. An EKG also records the strength and timing of electrical signals as they pass through the heart.
- Coronary calcium scan to measure the amount of calcium in the walls of your coronary arteries. Buildup of calcium can be a sign of atherosclerosis, CAD, or MVD. This test is a type of cardiac CT scan. Coronary calcium scans can also help assess CHD risk for people who smoke or for people who do not have heart symptoms.
- Stress tests to check how your heart works during physical stress. During stress testing, you walk or run on a treadmill or pedal a stationary bike to make your

heart work hard and beat fast. If you have a medical problem that prevents you from exercising, your doctor may give you medicine to make your heart work hard, as it would during exercise. To detect reduced blood flow to your heart muscle, while you exercise you will be monitored by ECG and possibly echocardiogram or a CT scan.

- Cardiac magnetic resonance imaging (MRI) to detect tissue damage or problems with blood flow in the heart or coronary arteries. It can help your doctor diagnose MVD or nonobstructive or obstructive CAD. Cardiac MRI can help explain results from other imaging tests such as chest x-rays and CT scans.
- Cardiac positron emission tomography (PET) scanning to assess blood flow through the small coronary blood vessels and into the heart tissues. This is a type of nuclear heart scan that can diagnose coronary MVD.
- Coronary angiography to show the insides of your coronary arteries. To get the dye into your coronary arteries, your doctor will use a procedure called "cardiac catheterization." This procedure is often used if other tests show that you are likely to have CAD. To diagnose MVD, your doctor will use coronary angiography with guidewire technology. A guidewire with sensors is inserted into the heart's arteries. The sensors measure how easily blood flows through the small vessels. Usually, measurements are done before and after giving you medicine to enhance blood flow in your heart.
- Coronary computed tomographic angiography (CCTA) to show the insides of your coronary arteries rather than an invasive cardiac catheterization. It is a noninvasive imaging test using CT scanning.

If you have CHD risk factors, your doctor may recommend diagnostic tests even if you do not have symptoms.

Nonobstructive CAD and MVD can be missed because patients or doctors may not recognize the warning signs. Diagnosing these types often requires more invasive tests or specialized tests, such as cardiac PET scans, that are not widely available.

TREATMENT OF CORONARY HEART DISEASE

Your treatment plan depends on how severe your disease is, the severity of your symptoms, and any other health conditions you may have. Possible treatments for CHD include heart-healthy lifestyle changes, medicines, or procedures such as coronary artery bypass grafting or percutaneous coronary intervention.

Your doctor will consider your 10-year risk calculation when deciding how best to treat your CHD.

Chapter 45 | **Bladder and Kidney Function Tests**

Chapter Contents

Section 45.1 | **Albumin Blood Test**

This section includes text excerpted from "Albumin Blood Test," MedlinePlus, National Institutes of Health (NIH), July 30, 2020.

WHAT IS AN ALBUMIN BLOOD TEST?

An albumin blood test measures the amount of albumin in your blood. Albumin is a protein made by your liver. Albumin helps keep fluid in your bloodstream so it does not leak into other tissues. It also carries various substances throughout your body, including hormones, vitamins, and enzymes. Low albumin levels can indicate a problem with your liver or kidneys.

WHAT IS IT USED FOR?

An albumin blood test is a type of liver function test. Liver function tests are blood tests that measure different enzymes and proteins in the liver, including albumin. An albumin test may also be part of a comprehensive metabolic panel, a test that measures several substances in your blood. These substances include electrolytes, glucose, and proteins such as albumin.

WHY DO YOU NEED AN ALBUMIN BLOOD TEST?

Your health-care provider may have ordered liver function tests or a comprehensive metabolic panel, which include tests for albumin, as part your regular checkup. You may also need this test if you have symptoms of liver or kidney disease.

Symptoms of liver disease include:

- Jaundice, a condition that causes your skin and eyes to turn yellow
- Fatigue
- Weight loss
- Loss of appetite
- Dark-colored urine
- Pale-colored stool

Symptoms of kidney disease include:

- Swelling around the abdomen, thighs, or face

- More frequent urination, especially at night
- Foamy, bloody, or coffee-colored urine
- Nausea
- Itchy skin

WHAT HAPPENS DURING AN ALBUMIN BLOOD TEST?

A health-care professional will take a blood sample from a vein in your arm, using a small needle. After the needle is inserted, a small amount of blood will be collected into a test tube or vial. You may feel a little sting when the needle goes in or out. This usually takes less than five minutes.

WILL YOU NEED TO DO ANYTHING TO PREPARE FOR THE TEST?

You do not need any special preparations to test for albumin in blood. If your health-care provider has ordered other blood tests, you may need to fast (not eat or drink) for several hours before the test. Your health-care provider will let you know if there are any special instructions to follow.

ARE THERE ANY RISKS TO THE TEST?

There is very little risk to having a blood test. You may have slight pain or bruising at the spot where the needle was put in, but most symptoms go away quickly.

WHAT DO THE RESULTS MEAN?

If your albumin levels are lower than normal, it may indicate one of the following conditions:

- Liver disease, including cirrhosis
- Kidney disease
- Malnutrition
- Infection
- Inflammatory bowel disease (IBD)
- Thyroid disease

Higher than normal levels of albumin may indicate dehydration or severe diarrhea.

If your albumin levels are not in the normal range, it does not necessarily mean you have a medical condition needing treatment. Certain drugs, including steroids, insulin, and hormones, can raise albumin levels. Other drugs, including birth control pills, can lower your albumin levels.

Section 45.2 | **Blood Urea Nitrogen Test**

This section includes text excerpted from "BUN (Blood Urea Nitrogen)," MedlinePlus, National Institutes of Health (NIH), July 30, 2020.

WHAT IS A BLOOD UREA NITROGEN TEST?

A blood urea nitrogen (BUN), or blood urea nitrogen test, can provide important information about your kidney function. The main job of your kidneys is to remove waste and extra fluid from your body. If you have kidney disease, this waste material can build up in your blood and may lead to serious health problems, including high blood pressure (HBP), anemia, and heart disease.

The test measures the amount of urea nitrogen in your blood. Urea nitrogen is one of the waste products removed from your blood by your kidneys. Higher than normal BUN levels may be a sign that your kidneys are not working efficiently.

People with early kidney disease may not have any symptoms. A BUN test can help uncover kidney problems at an early stage when treatment can be more effective.

WHAT IS IT USED FOR?

A BUN test is often part of a series of tests called a "comprehensive metabolic panel," and can be used to help diagnose or monitor a kidney disease or disorder.

WHY DO YOU NEED A BLOOD UREA NITROGEN TEST?

Your health-care provider may order a BUN test as part of a routine checkup or if you have or are at risk for a kidney problem. Although early kidney disease usually does not have any signs or symptoms, certain factors can put you at a higher risk. These include:

- Family history of kidney problems
- Diabetes
- HBP
- Heart disease

In addition, your BUN levels may be checked if you are experiencing symptoms of later stage kidney disease, such as:

- Needing to go the bathroom (urinate) frequently or infrequently
- Itching
- Recurring fatigue
- Swelling in your arms, legs, or feet
- Muscle cramps
- Trouble sleeping

WHAT HAPPENS DURING A BLOOD UREA NITROGEN TEST

A health-care professional will take a blood sample from a vein in your arm, using a small needle. After the needle is inserted, a small amount of blood will be collected into a test tube or vial. You may feel a little sting when the needle goes in or out. This usually takes less than five minutes.

WILL YOU NEED TO DO ANYTHING TO PREPARE FOR THE TEST?

You do not need any special preparations for a BUN test. If your health-care provider has also ordered other blood tests, you may need to fast (not eat or drink) for several hours before the test. Your health-care provider will let you know if there are any special instructions to follow.

ARE THERE ANY RISKS TO THE TEST?

There is very little risk to having a blood test. You may have slight pain or bruising at the spot where the needle was put in, but most symptoms go away quickly.

WHAT DO THE RESULTS MEAN?

Normal BUN levels can vary, but generally a high level of blood urea nitrogen is a sign that your kidneys are not working correctly. However, abnormal results do not always indicate that you have a medical condition needing treatment. Higher than normal BUN levels can also be caused by dehydration, burns, certain medicines, a high protein diet, or other factors, including your age. BUN levels normally increase as you get older. To learn what your results mean, talk to your health-care provider.

IS THERE ANYTHING ELSE YOU NEED TO KNOW ABOUT A BLOOD UREA NITROGEN TEST?

A BUN test is only one type of measurement of kidney function. If your health-care provider suspects you have kidney disease, additional tests may be recommended. These may include a measurement of creatinine, which is another waste product filtered by your kidneys, and a test called a "glomerular filtration rate" (GFR), which estimates how well your kidneys are filtering blood.

Section 45.3 | **Calcium Blood Test**

This section includes text excerpted from "Calcium Blood Test," MedlinePlus, National Institutes of Health (NIH), July 30, 2020.

WHAT IS A CALCIUM BLOOD TEST?

A calcium blood test measures the amount of calcium in your blood. Calcium is one of the most important minerals in your body. You need calcium for healthy bones and teeth. Calcium is also essential for proper functioning of your nerves, muscles, and heart. About 99 percent of your body's calcium is stored in your bones. The remaining 1 percent circulates in the blood. If there is too much or too little calcium in the blood, it may be a sign of bone disease, thyroid disease, kidney disease, or other medical conditions.

WHAT IS IT USED FOR?

There are two types of calcium blood tests:

- Total calcium, which measures the calcium attached to specific proteins in your blood.
- Ionized calcium, which measures the calcium that is unattached or "free" from these proteins.

Total calcium is often part of a routine screening test called a "basic metabolic panel." A basic metabolic panel is a test that measures different minerals and other substances in the blood, including calcium.

WHY DO YOU NEED A CALCIUM BLOOD TEST?

Your health-care provider may have ordered a basic metabolic panel, which includes a calcium blood test, as part of your regular checkup, or if you have symptoms of abnormal calcium levels.

Symptoms of high calcium levels include:

- Nausea and vomiting
- More frequent urination
- Increased thirst
- Constipation
- Abdominal pain
- Loss of appetite

Symptoms of low calcium levels include:

- Tingling in the lips, tongue, fingers, and feet
- Muscle cramps
- Muscle spasms
- Irregular heartbeat

Many people with high or low calcium levels do not have any symptoms. Your health-care provider may order a calcium test if you have a preexisting condition that may affect your calcium levels. These include:

- Kidney disease
- Thyroid disease
- Malnutrition
- Certain types of cancer

WHAT HAPPENS DURING A CALCIUM BLOOD TEST

A health-care professional will take a blood sample from a vein in your arm, using a small needle. After the needle is inserted, a small amount of blood will be collected into a test tube or vial. You may feel a little sting when the needle goes in or out. This usually takes less than five minutes.

WILL YOU NEED TO DO ANYTHING TO PREPARE FOR THE TEST?

You do not need any special preparations for a calcium blood test or a basic metabolic panel. If your health-care provider has ordered more tests on your blood sample, you may need to fast (not eat or drink) for several hours before the test. Your health-care provider will let you know if there are any special instructions to follow.

ARE THERE ANY RISKS TO THE TEST?

There is very little risk to having a blood test. You may have slight pain or bruising at the spot where the needle was put in, but most symptoms go away quickly.

WHAT DO THE RESULTS MEAN?

If your results show higher than normal calcium levels, it may indicate:

- Hyperparathyroidism, a condition in which your parathyroid glands produce too much parathyroid hormone
- Paget disease of the bone, a condition that causes your bones to become too big, weak, and prone to fractures
- Overuse of antacids that contain calcium
- Excessive intake of calcium from vitamin D supplements or milk
- Certain types of cancer

If your results show lower than normal calcium levels, it may indicate:

- Hypoparathyroidism, a condition in which your parathyroid glands produce too little parathyroid hormone
- Vitamin D deficiency
- Magnesium deficiency
- Inflammation of the pancreas (pancreatitis)
- Kidney disease

If your calcium test results are not in the normal range, it does not necessarily mean that you have a medical condition needing treatment. Other factors, such as diet and certain medicines, can affect your calcium levels. If you have questions about your results, talk to your health-care provider.

IS THERE ANYTHING ELSE YOU NEED TO KNOW ABOUT A CALCIUM BLOOD TEST?

A calcium blood test does not tell you how much calcium is in your bones. Bone health can be measured with a type of x-ray called a "bone density scan," or "dexa scan." A dexa scan measures the mineral content, including calcium, and other aspects of your bones.

Section 45.4 | **Calcium in Urine Test**

This section includes text excerpted from "Calcium in Urine Test," MedlinePlus, National Institutes of Health (NIH), July 30, 2020.

WHAT IS A CALCIUM IN URINE TEST?

A calcium in urine test measures the amount of calcium in your urine. Calcium is one of the most important minerals in your body. You need calcium for healthy bones and teeth. Calcium is also essential for proper functioning of your nerves, muscles, and heart. Almost all of your body's calcium is stored in your bones. A small amount circulates in the blood, and the remainder is filtered by the kidneys and passed into your urine. If urine calcium levels are too high or too low, it may mean you have a medical condition, such as kidney disease or kidney stones. Kidney stones are hard, pebble-like substances that can form in one or both kidneys when calcium or other minerals build up in the urine. Most kidney stones are formed from calcium.

Too much or too little calcium in the blood can also indicate a kidney disorder, as well as certain bone diseases, and other medical problems. So if you have symptoms of one of these disorders, your health-care provider may order a calcium blood test, along with a calcium in urine test. In addition, a calcium blood test is often included as part of a regular checkup.

WHAT IS IT USED FOR?

A calcium in urine test may be used to diagnose or monitor kidney function or kidney stones. It may also be used to diagnose disorders of the parathyroid, a gland near the thyroid that helps regulate the amount of calcium in your body.

WHY DO YOU NEED A CALCIUM IN URINE TEST?

You may need a calcium in urine test if you have symptoms of a kidney stone. These symptoms include:

- Severe back pain
- Abdominal pain
- Nausea and vomiting
- Blood in the urine
- Frequent urination

You may also need a calcium in urine test if you have symptoms of a parathyroid disorder.

Symptoms of too much parathyroid hormone include:

- Nausea and vomiting
- Loss of appetite
- Abdominal pain
- Fatigue
- Frequent urination
- Bone and joint pain

Symptoms of too little parathyroid hormone include:

- Abdominal pain
- Muscle cramps
- Tingling fingers
- Dry skin
- Brittle nails

WHAT HAPPENS DURING A CALCIUM IN URINE TEST

You will need to collect all your urine during a 24-hour period. This is called a "24-hour urine sample test." Your health-care provider or a laboratory professional will give you a container to collect your urine in and instructions on how to collect and store your samples. A 24-hour urine sample test generally includes the following steps:

- Empty your bladder in the morning and flush that urine down. Do not collect this urine. Record the time.
- For the next 24 hours, save all your urine in the container provided.
- Store your urine container in a refrigerator or a cooler with ice.
- Return the sample container to your health provider's office or the laboratory as instructed.

WILL YOU NEED TO DO ANYTHING TO PREPARE FOR THE TEST?

You may be asked to avoid certain foods and medicines for several days before the test. Your health-care provider will let you know if there are any special instructions to follow.

ARE THERE ANY RISKS TO THE TEST?

There is no known risk of having calcium in a urine test.

WHAT DO THE RESULTS MEAN?

If your results show higher than normal calcium levels in your urine, it may indicate:

- Risk for or the presence of a kidney stone

- Hyperparathyroidism, a condition in which your parathyroid gland produces too much parathyroid hormone
- Sarcoidosis, a disease that causes inflammation in the lungs, lymph nodes, or other organs
- Too much calcium in your diet from vitamin D supplements or milk

If your results show lower than normal calcium levels in your urine, it may indicate:

- Hypoparathyroidism, a condition in which your parathyroid gland produces too little parathyroid hormone
- Vitamin D deficiency
- A kidney disorder

If your calcium levels are not normal, it does not necessarily mean you have a medical condition needing treatment. Other factors, such as diet, supplements, and certain medicines, including antacids, can affect your urine calcium levels. If you have questions about your results, talk to your health-care provider.

IS THERE ANYTHING ELSE YOU NEED TO KNOW ABOUT A CALCIUM IN URINE TEST?

A calcium in urine test does not tell you how much calcium is in your bones. Bone health can be measured with a type of x-ray called a "bone density scan," or "dexa scan." A dexa scan measures the mineral content, including calcium, and other aspects of your bones.

Section 45.5 | **Chloride Blood Test**

This section includes text excerpted from "Chloride Blood Test," MedlinePlus, National Institutes of Health (NIH), July 30, 2020.

WHAT IS A CHLORIDE BLOOD TEST?

A chloride blood test measures the amount of chloride in your blood. Chloride is a type of electrolyte. Electrolytes are electrically charged minerals that help control the amount of fluids and the balance of acids and bases in your body. Chloride is often measured along with other electrolytes to diagnose or monitor conditions such as kidney disease, heart failure, liver disease, and high blood pressure (HBP).

WHAT IS IT USED FOR?

A chloride test is not normally given as an individual test. You usually get a chloride test as part of a routine blood screening or to help diagnose a condition related to an imbalance of acids or fluids in your body.

WHY DO YOU NEED A CHLORIDE BLOOD TEST?

Your health-care provider may have ordered a chloride blood test as part of an electrolyte panel, which is a routine blood test. An electrolyte panel is a test that measures chloride and other electrolytes, such as potassium, sodium, and bicarbonate. You may also need a chloride blood test if you have symptoms of an acid or fluid imbalance, including:

- Vomiting over a long period of time
- Diarrhea
- Fatigue
- Weakness
- Dehydration
- Trouble breathing

WHAT HAPPENS DURING A CHLORIDE BLOOD TEST

A health-care professional will take a blood sample from a vein in your arm, using a small needle. After the needle is inserted, a small amount of blood will be collected into a test tube or vial. You may feel a little sting when the needle goes in or out. This usually takes less than five minutes.

WILL YOU NEED TO DO ANYTHING TO PREPARE FOR THE TEST?

You do not need any special preparations for a chloride blood test or an electrolyte panel. If your health-care provider has ordered other blood tests, you may need to fast (not eat or drink) for several hours before the test. Your health-care provider will let you know if there are any special instructions to follow.

ARE THERE ANY RISKS TO THE TEST?

There is very little risk to having a blood test. You may have slight pain or bruising at the spot where the needle was put in, but most symptoms go away quickly.

WHAT DO THE RESULTS MEAN?

There are many reasons why your chloride levels may not be in the normal range. High levels of chloride may indicate:

- Dehydration
- Kidney disease
- Acidosis, a condition in which you have too much acid in your blood. It can cause nausea, vomiting, and fatigue.
- Alkalosis, a condition in which you have too much base in your blood. It can cause irritability, muscle twitching, and tingling in the fingers and toes.

Low levels of chloride may indicate:

- Heart failure
- Lung diseases
- Addison disease, a condition in which your body's adrenal glands do not produce enough of certain types of hormones. It can cause a variety of symptoms, including weakness, dizziness, weight loss, and dehydration.

If your chloride levels are not the normal range, it does not necessarily mean you have a medical problem needing treatment. Many factors can affect your chloride levels. If you have taken in too much fluid or have lost fluid because of vomiting or diarrhea, it can affect your chloride levels. Also, certain medicines such as antacids can cause abnormal results. To learn what your results mean, talk to your health-care provider.

IS THERE ANYTHING ELSE YOU NEED TO KNOW ABOUT A CHLORIDE BLOOD TEST?

Urine also contains some chloride. Your health-care provider may recommend a urine chloride test in addition to the blood test to get more information about your chloride levels.

Section 45.6 | **Urodynamic Testing**

This section includes text excerpted from "Urodynamic Testing," National Institute of Diabetes and Digestive and Kidney Diseases (NIDDK), February 2014. Reviewed October 2021.

WHAT IS THE URINARY TRACT?

The urinary tract is the body's drainage system for removing wastes and extra water. The urinary tract includes two kidneys, two ureters, a bladder, and a urethra. Blood flows through the kidneys, and the kidneys filter out wastes and extra water, making urine. The urine travels down two narrow tubes called the "ureters." The urine is then stored in a muscular, balloon-like organ called the "bladder." The bladder swells into a round shape when it is full and gets smaller as it empties. When the bladder empties, urine flows out of the body through the urethra.

WHAT IS THE LOWER URINARY TRACT AND HOW DOES IT WORK?

The lower urinary tract includes the bladder and urethra. The bladder sits in the pelvis and is attached to other organs, muscles, and the pelvic bones, which hold it in place. The urethra is a tube at

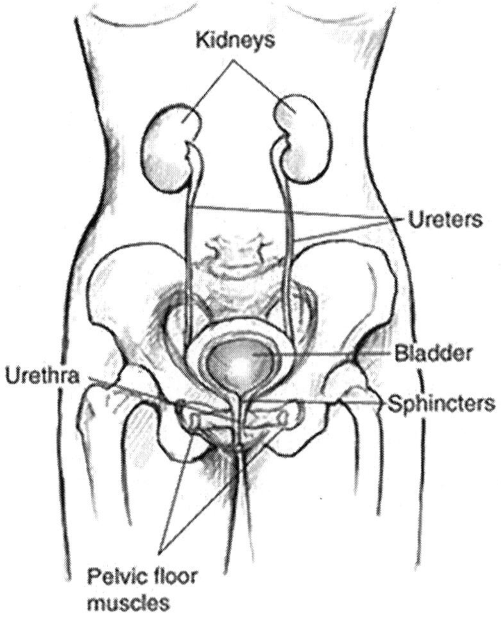

Figure 45.1. Front View of the Urinary Tract

the bottom of the bladder that carries urine from the bladder to the outside of the body.

The lower urinary tract works by coordinating the muscles of the bladder wall with the sphincters, which are circular muscles that surround the area of the bladder that opens into the urethra. The muscles of the bladder wall relax as the bladder fills with urine. If the urinary tract is healthy, the bladder can hold up to 2 cups, or 16 ounces, of urine comfortably for 2 to 5 hours. The sphincters close tightly like rubber bands around the bladder to help keep urine from leaking. As the bladder fills, the need to urinate becomes stronger and stronger, until the bladder reaches its limit. Urination is the process of emptying the bladder. To urinate, the brain signals the bladder muscles to tighten, squeezing urine out of the bladder. At the same time, the brain signals the sphincters to relax. As the sphincters relax, urine exits the bladder through the urethra. When all the signals occur in the correct order, normal urination occurs.

WHAT IS URODYNAMIC TESTING?

Urodynamic testing is any procedure that looks at how well the bladder, sphincters, and urethra are storing and releasing urine. Most urodynamic tests focus on the bladder's ability to hold urine and empty steadily and completely. Urodynamic tests can also show whether the bladder is having involuntary contractions that cause urine leakage. A health-care provider may recommend urodynamic tests if symptoms suggest problems with the lower urinary tract.

Lower urinary tract symptoms (LUTS) include:

- Urine leakage
- Frequent urination
- Painful urination
- Sudden, strong urges to urinate
- Problems starting a urine stream
- Problems emptying the bladder completely
- Recurrent urinary tract infections

Urodynamic tests range from simple observation to precise measurements using sophisticated instruments. For simple observation, a health-care provider may record:

- The length of time it takes a person to produce a urinary stream
- The volume of urine produced
- Ability or inability to stop the urine flow in midstream

For precise measurements, imaging equipment takes pictures of the bladder filling and emptying, pressure monitors record the pressures inside the bladder, and sensors record muscle and nerve activity. The health-care provider will decide the type of urodynamic test based on the person's health information, physical exam, and LUTS. The urodynamic test results help diagnose the cause and nature of a lower urinary tract problem.

Most urodynamic tests do not involve special preparations, though some tests may require a person to make a change in fluid intake or to stop taking certain medications. Depending on the test, a person may be instructed to arrive for testing with a full bladder.

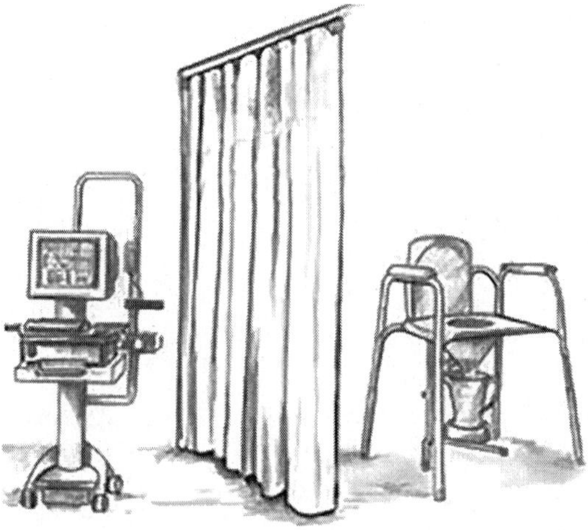

Figure 45.2. Uroflowmetry Equipment

WHAT ARE THE URODYNAMIC TESTS?

Urodynamic tests include:

- Uroflowmetry
- Postvoid residual measurement
- Cystometric test
- Leak point pressure measurement
- Pressure flow study
- Electromyography
- Video urodynamic tests

Uroflowmetry

Uroflowmetry is the measurement of urine speed and volume. Special equipment automatically measures the amount of urine and the flow rate – how fast the urine comes out. Uroflowmetry equipment includes a device for catching and measuring urine and a computer to record the data. During a uroflowmetry test, the person urinates privately into a special toilet or funnel that has a container for collecting the urine and a scale. The equipment creates a graph that shows changes in flow rate from second to second so the health-care provider can see when the flow rate is the highest and how many seconds it takes to get there. Results of this test will be abnormal if the bladder muscles are weak or urine flow is blocked. Another approach to measuring flow rate is to record the time it takes to urinate into a special container that accurately measures the volume of urine. Uroflowmetry measurements are performed in a health-care provider's office; no anesthesia is needed.

Postvoid Residual Measurement

This urodynamic test measures the amount of urine left in the bladder after urination. The remaining urine is called the "postvoid residual." Postvoid residual can be measured with ultrasound equipment that uses harmless sound waves to create a picture of the bladder. Bladder ultrasounds are performed in a health-care provider's office, radiology center, or hospital by a specially trained technician and interpreted by a doctor, usually a radiologist. Anesthesia is not needed. Postvoid residual can also be measured using a catheter – a thin flexible tube. A health-care provider inserts the catheter through the urethra up into the bladder to remove and measure the amount of remaining urine. A postvoid residual of 100 milliliters or more is a sign that the bladder is not emptying completely. Catheter measurements are performed in a health-care provider's office, clinic, or hospital with local anesthesia.

Cystometric Test

A cystometric test measures how much urine the bladder can hold, how much pressure builds up inside the bladder as it stores urine, and how full it is when the urge to urinate begins. A catheter is used to empty the bladder completely. Then a special, smaller catheter is placed in the bladder. This catheter has a pressure-measuring device called a "manometer." Another catheter may be placed in the rectum to record pressure there.

Once the bladder is emptied completely, the bladder is filled slowly with warm water. During this time, the person is asked to describe how the bladder feels and indicate when the need to urinate arises. When the urge to urinate occurs, the volume of water and the bladder pressure are recorded. The person may be asked to cough or strain during this procedure to see if the bladder pressure

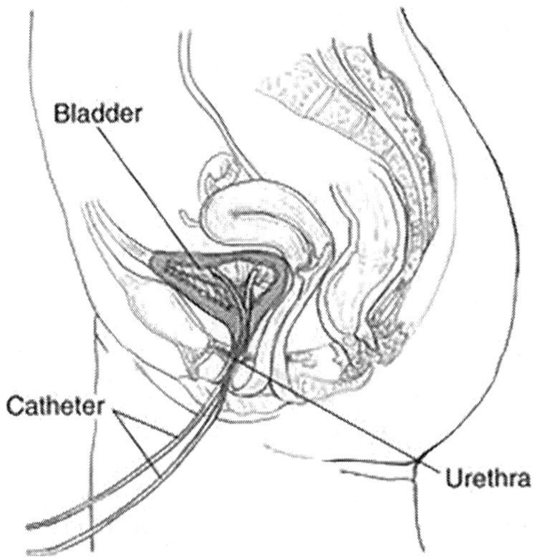

Figure 45.3. Cystometric Test

changes. A cystometric test can also identify involuntary bladder contractions. Cystometric tests are performed in a health-care provider's office, clinic, or hospital with local anesthesia.

Leak Point Pressure Measurement

This urodynamic test measures pressure at the point of leakage during a cystometric test. While the bladder is being filled for the cystometric test, it may suddenly contract and squeeze some water out without warning. The manometer measures the pressure inside the bladder when this leakage occurs. This reading may provide information about the kind of bladder problem that exists. The person may be asked to apply abdominal pressure to the bladder by coughing, shifting position, or trying to exhale while holding the nose and mouth. These actions help the health-care provider evaluate the sphincters.

Pressure Flow Study

A pressure flow study measures the bladder pressure required to urinate and the flow rate a given pressure generates. After the cystometric test, the person empties the bladder, during which time a manometer is used to measure bladder pressure and flow rate. This pressure flow study helps identify bladder outlet blockage that men may experience with prostate enlargement. Bladder outlet blockage is less common in women, but can occur with a cystocele or, rarely, after a surgical procedure for urinary incontinence. Pressure flow studies are performed in a health-care provider's office, clinic, or hospital with local anesthesia.

Electromyography

Electromyography uses special sensors to measure the electrical activity of the muscles and nerves in and around the bladder and the sphincters. If the health-care provider thinks the urinary problem is related to nerve or muscle damage, the person may be given an electromyography. The sensors are placed on the skin near the urethra and rectum or on a urethral or rectal catheter. Muscle and nerve activity is recorded on a machine. The patterns of the nerve impulses show whether the messages sent to the bladder and sphincters are coordinated correctly. Electromyography is performed by a specially trained technician in a health-care provider's office, outpatient clinic, or hospital. Anesthesia is not needed if sensors are placed on the skin. Local anesthesia is needed if sensors are placed on a urethral or rectal catheter.

Video Urodynamic Tests

Video urodynamic tests take pictures and videos of the bladder during filling and emptying. The imaging equipment may use x-rays or ultrasound. If x-ray equipment is used, the bladder will be filled with a special fluid, called "contrast medium," that shows up on x-rays. X-rays are performed by an x-ray technician in a health-care provider's office, outpatient facility, or hospital; anesthesia is not needed. If ultrasound equipment is used, the bladder is filled with warm water and harmless sound waves are used to create a picture of the bladder. The pictures and videos show the size and shape of the bladder and help the health-care provider understand the problem. Bladder ultrasounds are performed in a health-care provider's office, radiology center, or hospital by a specially trained technician and interpreted by a doctor, usually a radiologist. Although anesthesia is not needed for the ultrasound, local anesthesia is needed to insert the catheter to fill the bladder.

WHAT HAPPENS AFTER URODYNAMIC TESTS

After having urodynamic tests, a person may feel mild discomfort for a few hours when urinating. Drinking an 8-ounce glass of water every half-hour for 2 hours may help to reduce the discomfort. The health-care provider may recommend taking a warm bath or holding a warm, damp washcloth over the urethral opening to relieve the discomfort.

An antibiotic may be prescribed for 1 or 2 days to prevent infection, but not always. People with signs of infection – including pain, chills, or fever – should call their health-care provider immediately.

HOW SOON WILL TEST RESULTS BE AVAILABLE?

Results for simple tests such as cystometry and uroflowmetry are often available immediately after the test. Results of other tests such as electromyography and video urodynamic tests may take a few days to come back. A health-care provider will talk with the patient about the results and possible treatments.

Section 45.7 | **Tracking Chronic Kidney Disease**

This section includes text excerpted from "Chronic Kidney Disease Tests and Diagnosis," National Institute of Diabetes and Digestive and Kidney Diseases (NIDDK), October 2016. Reviewed October 2021.

HOW CAN YOU TELL IF YOU HAVE KIDNEY DISEASE?

Early kidney disease usually does not have any symptoms. Testing is the only way to know how well your kidneys are working. Get checked for kidney disease if you have:

- Diabetes
- High blood pressure (HBP)

- Heart disease
- A family history of kidney failure

If you have diabetes, get checked every year. If you have HBP, heart disease, or a family history of kidney failure, talk with your health-care provider about how often you should get tested. The sooner you know you have kidney disease, the sooner you can get treatment to help protect your kidneys.

WHAT TESTS DO DOCTORS USE TO DIAGNOSE AND MONITOR KIDNEY DISEASE?

To check for kidney disease, health-care providers use:

- A blood test that checks how well your kidneys are filtering your blood, called "glomerular filtration rate" (GFR).
- A urine test to check for albumin. Albumin is a protein that can pass into the urine when the kidneys are damaged.

If you have kidney disease, your health-care provider will use the same two tests to help monitor your kidney disease and make sure your treatment plan is working.

Blood Test for Glomerular Filtration Rate

Your health-care provider will use a blood test to check your kidney function. The results of the test mean the following:

- A GFR of 60 or more is in the normal range. Ask your health-care provider when your GFR should be checked again.
- A GFR of less than 60 may mean you have kidney disease. Talk with your health-care provider about how to keep your kidney health at this level.
- A GFR of 15 or less is called "kidney failure." Most people below this level need dialysis or a kidney transplant. Talk with your health-care provider about your treatment options.

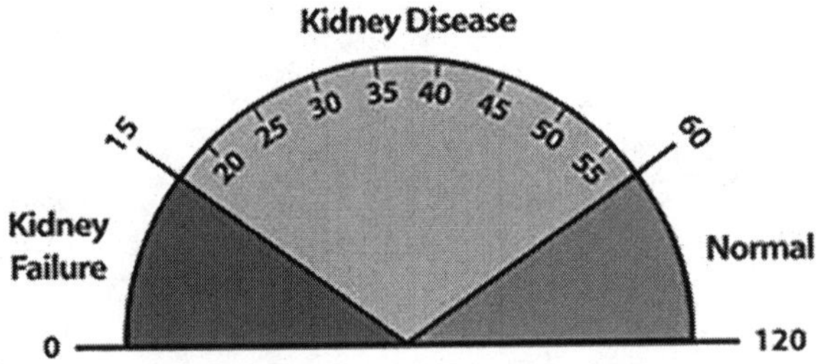

Figure 45.4. Glomerular Filtration Rate Kidney Results

Note: *GFR results show whether your kidneys are filtering at a normal level.*

You cannot raise your GFR, but you can try to keep it from going lower.

Creatinine. It is a waste product from the normal breakdown of muscles in your body. Your kidneys remove creatinine from your blood. Providers use the amount of creatinine in your blood to estimate your GFR. As kidney disease gets worse, the level of creatinine goes up.

Urine Test for Albumin

If you are at risk for kidney disease, your provider may check your urine for albumin.

Albumin is a protein found in your blood. A healthy kidney does not let albumin pass into the urine. A damaged kidney lets some albumin pass into the urine. The less albumin in your urine, the better. Having albumin in the urine is called "albuminuria."

A health-care provider can check for albumin in your urine in two ways:

- **Dipstick test for albumin.** A provider uses a urine sample to look for albumin in your urine. You collect the urine sample in a container in a health-care provider's office or lab. For the test, a provider places a strip of chemically treated paper, called a "dipstick," into the urine. The dipstick changes color if albumin is present in the urine.

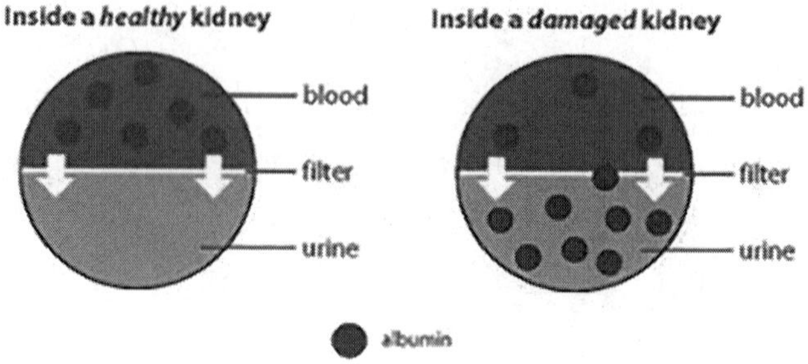

Figure 45.5. Healthy Kidney and Damaged Kidney

Note: *A healthy kidney does not let albumin pass into the urine. A damaged kidney lets some albumin pass into the urine.*

- **Urine albumin-to-creatinine ratio (UACR).** This test measures and compares the amount of albumin with the amount of creatinine in your urine sample. Providers use your UACR to estimate how much albumin would pass into your urine over 24 hours. A urine albumin result of:
  - 30 mg/g or less is normal
  - More than 30 mg/g may be a sign of kidney disease

If you have albumin in your urine, your provider may want you to repeat the urine test one or two more times to confirm the results. Talk with your provider about what your specific numbers mean for you.

If you have kidney disease, measuring the albumin in your urine helps your provider know which treatment is best for you. A urine albumin level that stays the same or goes down may mean that treatments are working.

HOW DO YOU KNOW IF YOUR KIDNEY DISEASE IS GETTING WORSE?

You can keep track of your test results over time. You can tell that your treatments are working if your:

- GFR stays the same
- Urine albumin stays the same or goes down

Your health-care provider will work with you to manage your kidney disease.

Chapter 46 | **Lung Disease Tests**

Chapter Contents

Section 46.1 | **Understanding Lung Function Tests**

This section includes text excerpted from "Lung Function Tests," MedlinePlus, National Institutes of Health (NIH), September 9, 2021.

WHAT ARE LUNG FUNCTION TESTS?

Lung function tests, also known as "pulmonary function tests," or "PFTs," are a group of tests that check to see if your lungs are working right. The tests look for:

- How much air your lungs can hold
- How well you move air in and out of your lungs
- How well the lungs move oxygen into your bloodstream. Your blood cells need oxygen to grow and stay healthy.

There are several types of lung function tests. They include:

- **Spirometry.** The most common type of lung function test. It measures how much and how quickly you can move air in and out of your lungs.
- **Lung volume test.** Also known as "body plethysmography." This test measures the amount of air you can hold in your lungs and the amount of air that remains after you exhale (breathe out) as much as you can.
- **Gas diffusion test.** This test measures how oxygen and other gases move from the lungs to the bloodstream.
- **Exercise stress test.** This test looks at how exercise affects lung function.

These tests may be used together or by themselves, depending on your specific symptoms or condition.

WHAT ARE THEY USED FOR?

Lung function tests are often used to:

- Find the cause of breathing problems
- Diagnose and monitor chronic lung diseases, including asthma, chronic obstructive pulmonary disease (COPD), and emphysema

- See if lung disease treatments are working
- Check lung function before surgery
- Check whether exposure to chemicals or other substances in the home or workplace have caused lung damage

WHY DO YOU NEED A LUNG FUNCTION TEST?

You may need this test if you:

- Have symptoms of a breathing problem such as shortness of breath, wheezing, and/or coughing
- Have a chronic lung disease
- Have been exposed to asbestos or other substances known to cause lung damage
- Have scleroderma, a disease that damages connective tissue
- Have sarcoidosis, a disease that causes damage to cells around the lungs, liver, and other organs
- Have a respiratory infection
- Had an abnormal chest x-ray
- Are scheduled for an operation such as abdominal or lung surgery

WHAT HAPPENS DURING LUNG FUNCTION TESTING

Below are the steps for the most common types of lung function tests.

For a spirometry test:

- You will sit in a chair and a soft clip will be put on your nose. This is done so you will breathe through your mouth, rather than your nose.
- You will be given a mouthpiece that is attached to a machine called a "spirometer."
- You will place your lips tightly around the mouthpiece, and breathe in and out as instructed by your provider.
- The spirometer will measure the amount and rate of air flow over a period of time.

For a lung volume (body plethysmography) test:

- You will sit in a clear, airtight room that looks like a telephone booth.
- As with a spirometry test, You will wear a nose clip and place your lips around a mouthpiece connected to a machine.
- You will breathe in and breathe out as instructed by your provider.
- The pressure changes inside the room help measure lung volume.

For a gas diffusion test:

- You will wear a mouthpiece connected to a machine.
- You will be asked to inhale (breathe in) a very small, nondangerous amount of carbon monoxide or other type of gas.
- Measurements will either be taken as you breathe in or as you breathe out.
- The test can show how effective your lungs are in moving gases to your bloodstream.

For an exercise test, you will:

- Ride a stationary bike or walk on a treadmill.
- You will be attached to monitors and machines that will measure blood oxygen, blood pressure, and heartbeat.
- This helps show how well your lungs perform during exercise.

WILL YOU NEED TO DO ANYTHING TO PREPARE FOR THE TESTS?

To prepare for a lung function test, you will need to take some steps to ensure your breathing is normal and unrestricted. These include:

- Do not eat a heavy meal before the test.
- Avoid food or drinks with caffeine.
- Do not smoke or do heavy exercise for six hours before the test.
- Wear loose, comfortable clothing.

- If you wear dentures, you will need to wear them during the test. They can help you form a tight seal around the mouthpiece.

ARE THERE ANY RISKS TO THE TESTS?

There is very little risk to having a lung function test. Some people may feel lightheaded or dizzy during the procedure. Also, some people may feel claustrophobic during a lung volume test. If you have questions or concerns about the tests, talk to your health-care provider.

WHAT DO THE RESULTS MEAN?

If any of your lung function test results were not normal, it may mean you have a lung disease. There are two main types of lung diseases that can be diagnosed with a lung function test:

- **Obstructive diseases.** These diseases cause airways to become narrow, making it hard for air to flow out of the lungs. Obstructive lung diseases include asthma, bronchitis, and emphysema.
- **Restrictive diseases.** In these diseases, the lungs or chest muscles are not able to expand enough. This reduces air flow and the ability to send oxygen into the bloodstream. Restrictive lung disorders include scleroderma, sarcoidosis, and pulmonary fibrosis.

If you have questions about your results, talk to your health-care provider.

IS THERE ANYTHING ELSE YOU NEED TO KNOW ABOUT LUNG FUNCTION TESTS?

In addition to your lung function tests, your health-care provider may order a blood oxygen level test. It is also known as an "arterial blood gases" (ABGs) test. This test measures the amount of oxygen and carbon dioxide in the blood.

Section 46.2 | **Cystic Fibrosis Tests**

This section includes text excerpted from "Cystic Fibrosis," National Heart, Lung, and Blood Institute (NHLBI), January 22, 2020.

WHAT IS CYSTIC FIBROSIS?

Cystic fibrosis (CF) is a genetic condition that affects a protein in the body. People who have cystic fibrosis have a faulty protein that affects the body's cells, tissues, and the glands that make mucus and sweat.

Mucus is normally slippery and protects the linings of the airways, digestive tract, and other organs and tissues. People who have cystic fibrosis make thick, sticky mucus that can build up and lead to blockages, damage, or infections in the affected organs. Inflammation also causes damage to organs such as the lungs and pancreas.

Some people who have cystic fibrosis have few or no signs or symptoms, while others experience severe symptoms or life-threatening complications. Symptoms of cystic fibrosis depend on which organs are affected and the severity of the condition. The most serious and common complications of cystic fibrosis are problems with the lungs, also known as "pulmonary" or "respiratory problems," which may include serious lung infections. People who have cystic fibrosis often also have problems maintaining good nutrition, because they have a hard time absorbing the nutrients from food. This is a problem that can delay growth.

Your doctor may recommend treatments to improve lung function and prevent or manage complications. Early treatment can improve your quality of life and help you live longer.

CAUSES OF CYSTIC FIBROSIS

Cystic fibrosis is an inherited disease caused by mutations in a gene called the "cystic fibrosis transmembrane conductance regulator (*CFTR*) gene." The *CFTR* gene provides instructions for the CFTR protein. The CFTR protein is located in every organ of the body that makes mucus, including the lungs, liver, pancreas, and intestines, as well as sweat glands. The CFTR protein has also been found in other cells in the body, such as cells of the heart and the immune system. The mutations in the *CFTR* gene cause the CFTR protein to not work properly. This causes thick, sticky mucus and blockages in the lungs and digestive system.

Normally, mucus coats tiny hair-like structures called "cilia" in the airways of your lungs, which sweep the mucus particles up to the nose and mouth where your body can get rid of them. In people who have cystic fibrosis, this process does not work properly.

What Gene Mutations Cause Cystic Fibrosis?

There are almost 2,000 known disease-causing mutations of the *CFTR* gene. Different mutations have different effects on how the CFTR protein is made and how it works. In the most common gene mutation, part of the *CFTR* gene is missing, resulting in a protein that does not work properly.

Normally, the CFTR protein controls the movement of ions from inside the cell to outside the cell. In people who have cystic fibrosis, the mutated gene causes the protein to not work properly, which, in turn, affects the movement of sodium and water. When this happens, the sweat glands make sweat that is saltier than it is in people who do not have cystic fibrosis. Also, there is less water in the mucus, which makes the mucus thick and sticky. The thick mucus creates blockages in the lungs and digestive system.

How Is Cystic Fibrosis Inherited?

Every person inherits two *CFTR* genes, one gene from each parent. Children who inherit a *CFTR* gene with a mutation from both parents will have cystic fibrosis. When a mutated *CFTR* gene is inherited from only one parent and a normal *CFTR* gene is inherited from the other, the person will be a cystic fibrosis carrier. CF carriers are generally healthy, but they can pass the mutated *CFTR* gene on to their children.

The Figure 46.1 shows how two parents who are both CF carriers can pass a *CFTR* gene mutation on to their children.

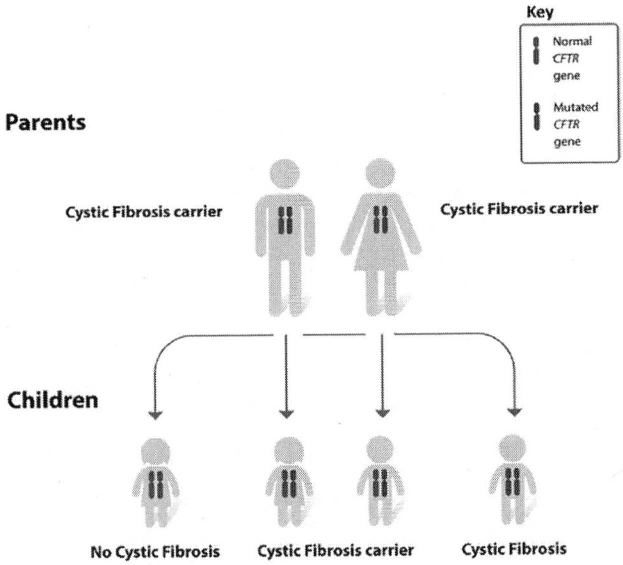

Figure 46.1. Cystic Fibrosis Carrier

Note: *Figure 46.1 shows how* CFTR *genes are inherited. A person inherits two copies of the* CFTR *gene, one from each parent. If each parent has a normal* CFTR *gene and a mutated* CFTR *gene, each child has a 25 percent chance of inheriting two normal genes, a 50 percent chance of inheriting one normal gene and one gene with a mutation and being a cystic fibrosis carrier, and a 25 percent chance of inheriting two genes with mutations and having cystic fibrosis.*

Note: Treatment will discuss medicines, supplements, and lifestyle changes that your doctors may recommend if you are diagnosed with cystic fibrosis.

SCREENING AND PREVENTION OF CYSTIC FIBROSIS

Genetic testing may be performed to look for carriers, as well as to screen relatives of people who have cystic fibrosis. Genetic testing may also be used as prenatal screening tool to look for a mutated *CFTR* gene. All newborns in the United States are now screened for cystic fibrosis. Since universal screening for cystic fibrosis began relatively recently, there are still young people and adults who have not been screened.

Carrier Screening to Detect CFTR Mutations

Genetic testing can tell you if you carry a mutation of the *CFTR* gene. This is called "carrier testing." People who have inherited a mutation of the *CFTR* gene from one parent are cystic fibrosis carriers. People who have inherited a mutation of the *CFTR* gene from both parents will have cystic fibrosis. Genetic testing looks at your DNA from a blood or saliva sample, or cells from the inside of your cheek.

The standard test to check for possible cystic fibrosis carriers looks for 23 of the most common disease-causing gene mutations. If you have a positive test, there is a 99 percent chance you are a carrier. However, if you have a negative test, there is still a small chance that you could carry a *CFTR* mutation that did not show up on the test.

Siblings of a person who has cystic fibrosis may want to be tested for cystic fibrosis whether or not they have symptoms. Other relatives, such as first cousins and half-siblings, may be tested if they have symptoms, or if the family is concerned that the individual may have cystic fibrosis.

After a positive screening test, the diagnosis should be confirmed with further testing.

Prenatal Screening

Couples who are planning to have children may want to be tested to see if they are cystic fibrosis carriers. Genetic testing, such as the carrier screening described above, may be done before or during pregnancy. Often, the mother is tested first. However, if you are already pregnant, you and your partner may choose to be tested at the same time. If the father has a family history of cystic fibrosis, he may be tested first. Similar to standard genetic testing, prenatal screening uses a sample of blood, saliva, or cells from the inside of your cheek to check your DNA.

If one partner is a carrier for a cystic fibrosis gene mutation, then the next step is to test the partner if this has not been done. If both parents are cystic fibrosis carriers, then prenatal diagnostic testing may be performed to see whether your unborn baby has cystic fibrosis or is a carrier.

Newborn Screening

When a child has cystic fibrosis, it is very important to diagnose it early to help prevent complications. Newborn screening for cystic fibrosis is performed during a baby's first two to three days of life. A few drops of blood from a heel prick are placed on a special card and analyzed in labs.

The type of newborn screening that is performed varies from state to state. Every state and the District of Columbia begins with a blood test to check for levels of a chemical made by the pancreas called "immunoreactive trypsinogen" (IRT). In people who have cystic fibrosis, IRT tends to be high. However, most babies with high levels of IRT do not have cystic fibrosis. IRT may also be high if the baby is premature, had a stressful delivery, or is a carrier of cystic fibrosis.

Some states test only IRT for cystic fibrosis newborn screening. Other states test IRT and also perform DNA testing. In states that test both IRT and DNA, if IRT is high, then the hospital will test the baby's DNA for some of the gene mutations that cause cystic fibrosis.

After a positive screening test, the diagnosis should be confirmed with further testing.

Prevention Strategies

There is no way to prevent whether or not you have cystic fibrosis. Couples who are planning to have children and know that they are at risk of having a child with cystic fibrosis may want to meet with a genetic counselor. A genetic counselor can answer questions about the risk and explain the choices that are available.

SIGNS, SYMPTOMS, AND COMPLICATIONS OF CYSTIC FIBROSIS

Signs and Symptoms

Symptoms of cystic fibrosis depend on which organs are affected and the severity of the condition. Most patients who have cystic fibrosis have noticeable symptoms. Some patients have few or no signs or symptoms, while others experience severe symptoms or life-threatening complications. Symptoms may also change over time. The most common complications of cystic fibrosis affect the lungs and pancreas.

Cystic fibrosis most commonly affects the lungs. Some people who have cystic fibrosis may have wheezing and a cough that may produce mucus or blood.

Other signs and symptoms depend on the organs affected and may include:

- Blockage of the intestine in a baby soon after birth
- Clubbing of fingers and toes due to less oxygen getting to the hands and feet
- Fever, which may include night sweats
- Gastrointestinal symptoms, such as severe abdominal pain, chronic diarrhea, or constipation
- Jaundice, or yellow skin, for an abnormally long time after birth
- Low body mass index (BMI) or being underweight
- Muscle and joint pain
- Delayed growth or puberty
- Salty skin and saltier than normal sweat
- Sinus infections

Complications

Cystic fibrosis affects many parts and systems of the body. Complications will depend on the affected organs and the severity of disease. People who have cystic fibrosis produce thick, sticky mucus that causes problems in the lungs and digestive system. The buildup of mucus in the lungs makes it easy for bacteria to grow and often leads to serious lung infections. People who have cystic fibrosis often have problems with nutrition, too, because their pancreas does not work properly.

Possible complications of cystic fibrosis include:

- Allergic bronchopulmonary aspergillosis (ABPA), which is an allergic reaction in the lungs to the fungus Aspergillus.
- Bronchiectasis, a widening of the airways in the lungs caused by chronic inflammation or obstruction of the airways. This is a common complication of cystic fibrosis.

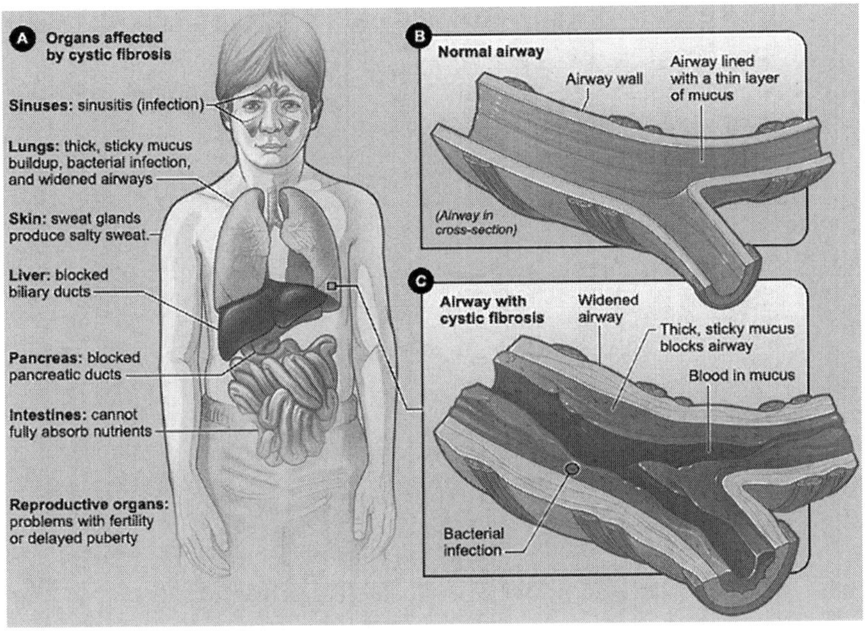

Figure 46.2. Organs Affected by Cystic Fibrosis

Note: *Figure A shows the organs that may be affected by cystic fibrosis. People who have cystic fibrosis may have sinusitis or infections of the sinus. The lungs have a buildup of thick, sticky mucus, which may lead to infections and widened airways. The sweat glands in the skin produce sweat that is saltier than normal. In the liver, the biliary ducts may be blocked. This may cause liver damage and cirrhosis. The pancreas is also affected by cystic fibrosis, resulting in blocked pancreatic ducts. This may lead to diabetes and poor absorption of nutrients in the intestines from lack of pancreatic enzymes. Reproductive organs may also be affected by cystic fibrosis, such as in problems with fertility and delayed puberty. Figure B shows a cross-section of a normal airway and the thin layer of mucus lining the wall. Figure C shows an airway with cystic fibrosis. The widened airway is blocked by thick, sticky mucus that contains blood and bacteria.*

- Cancers of the digestive tract, including the esophagus, stomach, small bowel, large bowel, liver, and pancreas
- Collapsed lung, called "pneumothorax," resulting in air in the space between your lung and chest wall
- Diabetes due to damage to the pancreas. The pancreas is where insulin is made.
- Fertility problems
- Gastrointestinal complications, such as distal intestinal obstruction syndrome (DIOS), in which your intestine

becomes blocked by very thick intestinal contents. Another possible complication is rectal prolapse, in which part of the rectum sticks out through the anus.
- Heart failure because of lung damage
- Hemoptysis
- Kidney problems due to diabetes and some antibiotics, or kidney stones
- Liver disease or failure caused by blockage of the bile ducts in the liver, which leads to bile damaging your liver. This may lead to cirrhosis and a need for a liver transplant.
- Lung infections that may come back or be difficult to treat
- Malnutrition because the pancreas may not make enough enzymes to help digest and absorb nutrients from food
- Mental-health problems, such as depression and anxiety
- Muscle and bone complications, including low bone density and osteoporosis, joint pain and arthritis, and muscle pains
- Pancreatitis and low levels of pancreatic enzymes leading to nutritional deficiencies, including low levels of vitamins A, D, E, and K
- Pulmonary exacerbations, which are episodes of worsening cough, shortness of breath, and mucus production caused by airway inflammation and blockage from an increase in bacteria in your airways and lungs. These episodes may also cause fatigue, loss of appetite, and weight loss.
- Salt loss syndrome, in which your body quickly loses salt, or sodium and chloride, causing electrolyte and other imbalances.
- Urinary incontinence, or loss of bladder control

NOTE

- Diagnosis will discuss tests and procedures used to detect signs of cystic fibrosis and help rule out other conditions that may mimic cystic fibrosis.

- Treatment will discuss treatment-related complications or side effects.

DIAGNOSIS OF CYSTIC FIBROSIS

Your doctor may diagnose cystic fibrosis based on your signs and symptoms and results from certain tests, such as genetic and sweat tests that are done to confirm screening tests.

Diagnostic Tests and Procedures

To diagnose cystic fibrosis, your doctor may recommend some of the following tests and procedures:

- **Genetic testing to detect mutated *CFTR* genes.** This test can confirm a positive cystic fibrosis screening test and sweat test. If genetic testing is done as part of newborn or other screening, it may not be repeated during the newborn stage. Genetic testing is described in more detail in Screening and Prevention.
- Prenatal diagnostic tests to diagnose cystic fibrosis in an unborn baby, using mutated *CFTR* genes. This is done with procedures that take either a sample of amniotic fluid, the liquid in the sac surrounding your unborn baby, or tissue from the placenta. Cells from these samples are checked for gene mutations. Infants with positive prenatal testing for cystic fibrosis will be further tested after birth to confirm the diagnosis of cystic fibrosis.
- Sweat test for high sweat chloride to see if you have high levels of chloride in your sweat. The sweat test is the standard test for diagnosing cystic fibrosis. It may be used if you have symptoms that may indicate cystic fibrosis, or to confirm a positive diagnosis from a screening of your newborn baby. A normal sweat chloride test alone does not mean you do not have cystic fibrosis. Lower levels of chloride may indicate the need for further testing to diagnose or rule out cystic fibrosis.

Table 46.1. Test Results of Sweat Chloride

Chloride Level of mmol/L	Result
60 or Greater	Cystic fibrosis diagnosis
30 to 59	Unclear diagnosis; further testing needed
Less than 30	Cystic fibrosis unlikely

Table 46.1 shows how much chloride in a person's sweat sample must be present in order to determine whether the diagnosis for cystic fibrosis is positive, unclear, or unlikely. A chloride level of 60 millimoles per liter (mmol/L) or greater indicates cystic fibrosis. A chloride level of 30 to 59 mmol/L indicates a diagnosis of cystic fibrosis is unclear, and that further testing is needed. A chloride level of less than 30 mmol/L indicates a diagnosis of cystic fibrosis is unlikely.

HOW IS A SWEAT CHLORIDE TEST PERFORMED?

The sweat test detects a higher amount of chloride – a component of salt that is made of sodium and chloride – in the sweat of people who have cystic fibrosis. In order to make sweat for this test, a colorless, odorless chemical and a little electrical stimulation are applied to a small area of an arm or leg. The sweat is collected and sent to a hospital lab for testing.

TREATMENT OF CYSTIC FIBROSIS

While there is not yet a cure for cystic fibrosis, advances in treatment are helping people live longer, healthier lives. To better manage your condition, you or your child will work with cystic fibrosis specialists. In newborns with a positive screening result, treatment may begin while the diagnosis is being confirmed. Treatment for cystic fibrosis is focused on airway clearance, medicines to improve the function of the faulty CFTR protein and prevent complications, and surgery, if needed.

Your Health-Care Team

Your health-care team will likely include a cystic fibrosis specialist. This is a doctor who is familiar with the complex nature of cystic fibrosis. Your doctor may work with a medical team that specializes in cystic fibrosis, often at major medical centers. The United States has more than 100 CF Care Centers, with medical teams that include:

- Doctors specializing in the lungs, diabetes, and the digestive system
- Genetic counselors
- Nurses
- Nutritionists and dietitians
- Pharmacists
- Physical therapists
- Psychologists
- Respiratory therapists
- Social workers

Airway Clearance Techniques

Airway clearance techniques help loosen lung mucus so it can be cleared, reducing infections and improving breathing. The techniques include special ways of breathing and coughing, devices used by mouth and therapy vests that use vibrations to loosen mucus, and chest physical therapy. These techniques are often used along with medicines such as bronchodilators and mucus thinners.

Medicines

Medicines to treat cystic fibrosis include those used to maintain and improve lung function, fight infections, clear mucus and help breathing, and work on the faulty CFTR protein. Your doctor may prescribe some of the following medicines to treat cystic fibrosis:

- Antibiotics to prevent or treat lung infections and improve lung function. Your doctor may prescribe oral, inhaled, or intravenous (IV) antibiotics.
- Anti-inflammatory medicines, such as ibuprofen or corticosteroids, to reduce inflammation. Inflammation causes many of the changes in cystic fibrosis, such as lung disease. Ibuprofen is especially beneficial for children, but side effects can include kidney and stomach problems. Corticosteroids can cause bone thinning and increased blood sugar and blood pressure.
- Bronchodilators to relax and open airways. These treatments are taken by inhaling them.

- CFTR modulators that improve the function of the faulty CFTR protein. They improve lung function and help prevent lung problems and other complications. Examples include ivacaftor and lumacaftor and a triple combination medicine. The combination medicine is the first approved treatment that may help up to 90 percent of people who have cystic fibrosis. It is currently approved to use in adults and children older than 12 years.
- Mucus thinners to make it easier to clear the mucus from your airways. These treatments are taken by inhaling them.

Surgery

Surgery may be an option for people with advanced conditions.

Chapter 47 | COVID-19

Chapter Contents

Section 47.1 | About COVID-19

This section includes text excerpted from "COVID-19: Frequently Asked Questions," Centers for Disease Control and Prevention (CDC), October 21, 2021.

WHAT IS COVID-19?

Coronavirus disease (COVID-19) is a disease caused by a virus called "severe acute respiratory syndrome coronavirus 2" (SARS-CoV-2). Most people with COVID-19 have mild symptoms, but some people can become severely ill. Although most people with COVID-19 get better within weeks of illness, some people experience post-COVID conditions. Post-COVID conditions are a wide range of new, returning, or ongoing health problems people can experience more than four weeks after first being infected with the virus that causes COVID-19. Older people and those who have certain underlying medical conditions are more likely to get severely ill from COVID-19. Vaccines against COVID-19 are safe and effective.

HOW DOES THE VIRUS SPREAD?

COVID-19 spreads when an infected person breathes out droplets and very small particles that contain the virus. These droplets and particles can be breathed in by other people or land on their eyes, noses, or mouth. In some circumstances, they may contaminate surfaces they touch. People who are closer than 6 feet from the infected person are most likely to get infected.

COVID-19 is spread in three main ways:

- Breathing in air when close to an infected person who is exhaling small droplets and particles that contain the virus.
- Having these small droplets and particles that contain virus land on the eyes, nose, or mouth, especially through splashes and sprays like a cough or sneeze.

- Touching eyes, nose, or mouth with hands that have the virus on them.

SYMPTOMS OF COVID-19

People with COVID-19 have had a wide range of symptoms reported – ranging from mild symptoms to severe illness. Symptoms may appear 2 to 14 days after exposure to the virus. Anyone can have mild to severe symptoms. People with these symptoms may have COVID-19:

- Fever or chills
- Cough
- Shortness of breath or difficulty breathing
- Fatigue
- Muscle or body aches
- Headache
- New loss of taste or smell
- Sore throat
- Congestion or runny nose
- Nausea or vomiting
- Diarrhea

This list does not include all possible symptoms. Older adults and people who have severe underlying medical conditions like heart or lung disease or diabetes seem to be at higher risk for developing more serious complications from COVID-19 illness.

Section 47.2 | **Test for Current Infection**

This section includes text excerpted from "COVID-19: Test for Current Infection," Centers for Disease Control and Prevention (CDC), August 2, 2021.

VIRAL TESTS ARE USED TO LOOK FOR CURRENT INFECTION

A viral test checks specimens from your nose or your mouth to find out if you are currently infected with the virus that causes coronavirus disease (COVID-19). Viral tests can be performed in a laboratory, at a testing site, or at home or anywhere else. Two types of viral tests are used: nucleic acid amplification tests (NAATs) and antigen tests.

WHO SHOULD GET TESTED?

The following people should get tested for COVID-19:

- People who have symptoms of COVID-19.
- People who have had a known exposure to someone with suspected or confirmed COVID-19.
- People who are fully vaccinated should get tested 3 to 5 days after exposure, and wear a mask in public indoor settings for 14 days or until they receive a negative test result.
- People who are not fully vaccinated should quarantine and be tested immediately after being identified, and, if negative, tested again in 5 to 7 days after last exposure or immediately if symptoms develop during quarantine.
- People not fully vaccinated with COVID-19 vaccine who are prioritized for expanded community screening for COVID-19.
- People not fully vaccinated with COVID-19 vaccine who have been asked or referred to get testing by their school, workplace, health-care provider, state, tribal, local or territorial health department.

WHO DOES NOT NEED TO BE TESTED

The following people who have been exposed to someone with COVID-19 do not need to get tested if they do not have COVID-19 symptoms:

- People who have tested positive for COVID-19 within the past 3 months and recovered, as long as they do not develop new symptoms, do not need to get tested.

COVID-19 VIRAL TESTING TOOL

The COVID-19 Viral Testing Tool is an interactive web tool designed to help both health-care providers and individuals understand COVID-19 testing options. This tool helps health-care providers quickly access the most relevant, actionable information to determine what type(s) of COVID-19 testing they should recommend to patients. The tool helps individuals determine what type of test they should seek. After test results are in, the tool can help interpret test results and guide next steps.

The online, mobile-friendly tool asks a series of questions, and provides recommended actions and resources based on the user's responses.

HOW TO GET A VIRAL TEST

- Visit your state, tribal, local, or territorial health department's website to look for the latest local information on testing.
- Visit your health-care or public-health department clinic provider to get a self-collection kit or self-test.
- You and your health-care provider might consider either self-collection kit or a self-test if you have symptoms of COVID-19 and cannot get tested by a health-care provider.

POSITIVE VIRAL TEST

If you test positive for the virus that causes COVID-19, take the following steps to protect others regardless of your COVID-19 vaccination status: Isolate at home and isolate away from others for at least 10 days.

- If you do not have any symptoms, you should still isolate at home for at least 10 days.
- If you develop symptoms, continue to isolate for at least 10 days after symptoms began as long as symptoms have improved, and no fever is present for at least 24 hours without use of fever-reducing medications.
- Most people have mild COVID-19 illness and can recover at home without medical care.
- Contact your health-care provider as soon as possible if you are more likely to get very sick because of being an

older adult or having underlying medical conditions or if your symptoms get worse.

Talk to your health-care provider or local health department to find out how long to isolate if you:

- Are severely ill with COVID-19 or have a weakened immune system;
- Had a positive test result followed by a negative result; or
- Test positive for many weeks after the initial result.

NEGATIVE VIRAL TEST

If you test negative for the virus that causes COVID-19, the virus was not detected.

If you have symptoms of COVID-19:

- You may have received a false negative test result and still might have COVID-19. You should isolate away from others.
- Contact your health-care provider about your symptoms, especially if they worsen, about follow-up testing, and how long to isolate.

If you do not have symptoms of COVID-19, and you were exposed to a person with COVID 19:

- You are likely not infected, but you still may get sick.
- Self-quarantine at home for 14 days after your exposure.
- Persons who are fully vaccinated with COVID-19 vaccine do not need to self-quarantine at home
- For residents of nonhealthcare congregate settings (e.g., correctional and detention facilities, group homes) and employees of residential congregate settings and high-density workplaces (e.g., meat and poultry processing and manufacturing plants), refer to the Centers for Disease Control and Prevention's (CDC) recommendations for fully vaccinated people.

- Contact your local health department regarding options to reduce the length of quarantine. If symptoms develop during home quarantine:
  - Contact your health-care provider about follow-up testing; and
  - Isolate at home separated away from others.

If you do not have symptoms of COVID-19 and do not have a known exposure to a person with COVID-19:

- You do not need to self-quarantine.

Section 47.3 | Test for Past Infection

This section includes text excerpted from "COVID-19: Test for Past Infection," Centers for Disease Control and Prevention (CDC), July 15, 2021.

Antibody or serology tests look for antibodies in your blood that fight the virus that causes coronavirus disease (COVID-19).

- Antibodies are proteins created by your immune system that help you fight off infections. They are made after you have been infected or have been vaccinated against an infection.
- Vaccination is a safe, effective way to teach your body to create antibodies.
- Antibodies can protect you from getting those infections for some period of time afterward. How long this protection lasts is different for each disease and each person.
- Antibody tests should generally not be used to diagnose a current infection with the virus that causes COVID-19. An antibody test may not show if you have a current infection because it can take 1 to 3 weeks after the infection for your body to make antibodies.

HOW TO GET AN ANTIBODY TEST

Decisions about testing are made by state or local health departments or health-care professionals.

Antibody tests for COVID-19 are available through health-care professionals and laboratories. Check with your health-care professional to see if they offer antibody tests and whether you should get one.

WHAT DO YOUR RESULTS MEAN?

If You Test Positive

- A positive antibody test result shows you may have antibodies from a previous infection or from vaccination for the virus that causes COVID-19.
- Some antibodies made for the virus that causes COVID-19 provide protection from getting infected. The CDC is evaluating antibody protection and how long protection from antibodies might last. Cases of reinfection and infection after vaccination have been reported, but remain rare. But, getting vaccinated, even if you have already had COVID-19, can help your body make more of these antibodies.
- You may test positive for antibodies even if you have never had symptoms of COVID-19 or have not yet received a COVID-19 vaccine. This can happen if you had an infection without symptoms, which is called an "asymptomatic infection."
- Sometimes a person can test positive for SARS-CoV-2 antibodies when they do not actually have those specific antibodies. This is called a "false positive."
- Talk with your health-care professional about your test result and the type of test you took to understand what your result means. Your health-care professional may suggest you take a second type of antibody test to see if the first test was accurate.

If You Test Negative

- You may not have COVID-19 antibodies. This could be because you have not had an infection with the virus that causes COVID-19 or have not received a COVID-19 vaccine.

- Antibody testing is not currently recommended to determine if you are immune to COVID-19 following COVID-19 vaccination.
- Some antibody tests will only detect antibodies from infection, not from vaccination with the virus that causes COVID-19.
- You could have a current infection, been recently infected, or been recently vaccinated. It typically takes 1 to 3 weeks after infection or vaccination for your body to make antibodies. If you are infected, you may get sick and spread the virus before you develop antibodies.
- Some people may take even longer to develop antibodies, and a small portion of people who are infected or vaccinated may never develop antibodies.
- Sometimes people test negative for SARS-CoV-2 antibodies when they have those specific antibodies. This is called a "false negative."
- Talk with your health-care professional about your test result and the type of test you took to understand what your result means.

If you have symptoms of COVID-19, you should get a viral test to detect a current infection, even if you were previously infected or vaccinated.

Section 47.4 | **Contact Tracing**

This section includes text excerpted from "COVID-19: Contact Tracing," Centers for Disease Control and Prevention (CDC), October 19, 2021.

Contact tracing is key to slowing the spread of coronavirus disease (COVID-19) and helps protect you, your family, and your community.

CONTACT TRACING SLOWS THE SPREAD OF COVID-19

Contact tracing helps protect you, your family, and your community by:

- Helping people diagnosed with COVID-19 get referrals for services and resources they may need to safely isolate.
- Notifying people who have come into close contact with someone diagnosed with COVID-19 about their exposure.
- Helping people who were exposed to COVID-19 know what steps to take, depending on their vaccination status. Follow-up may include testing and quarantine for unvaccinated or not fully vaccinated people, and testing and wearing a mask for fully vaccinated.

Discussions with public health workers are confidential. This means that your personal and medical information will be kept private and only shared with those who may need to know, like your health-care provider.

WHAT YOU CAN EXPECT TO HAPPEN

Table 47.1. What to Do If You Come Into Close Contact with Someone Diagnosed with COVID-19

	If You Come Into Close Contact with Someone with COVID-19 and You Are Unvaccinated or Not Fully Vaccinated	**If You Come Into Close Contact with Someone with COVID-19 and You Are Fully Vaccinated**	**If You Come Into Close Contact with Someone with COVID-19 and You Have Tested Positive for the Virus That Causes COVID-19 within the past 90 Days and Recovered (Regardless of Vaccination Status)**
You should get tested	You should get tested immediately after finding out you are a close contact. If you need help, health department staff can provide information about the best time to get a vaccine and resources for COVID-19 testing and vaccination your area. If your test result is negative, get tested again 5–7 days after your last exposure or immediately if symptoms develop. If your test result is positive, you have COVID-19 and should isolate for 10 days.	If you are fully vaccinated and become infected, you can spread the virus to others. Get tested immediately if you develop symptoms. Even if you don't have symptoms, you should get tested 5–7 days after your exposure. If you need help, health department staff can provide information about the best time to get a vaccine and resources for COVID-19 testing in your area. If your test result is positive, you have COVID-19 and should isolate for 10 days.	If you develop symptoms, consult with a health-care professional for testing recommendations.
You should monitor your symptoms	Monitor your symptoms. If you have an emergency warning sign (including trouble breathing), seek emergency medical care immediately. Get tested immediately if you develop symptoms.	Monitor your symptoms. If you have an emergency warning sign (including trouble breathing), seek emergency medical care immediately. Get tested immediately if you develop symptoms.	Monitor your symptoms. If you have an emergency warning sign (including trouble breathing), seek emergency medical care immediately. If you develop symptoms, consult with a health-care professional for testing recommendations

Table 47.1. Continued

	If You Come Into Close Contact with Someone with COVID-19 and You Are Unvaccinated or Not Fully Vaccinated	**If You Come Into Close Contact with Someone with COVID-19 and You Are Fully Vaccinated**	**If You Come Into Close Contact with Someone with COVID-19 and You Have Tested Positive for the Virus That Causes COVID-19 within the past 90 Days and Recovered (Regardless of Vaccination Status)**
You should wear a mask	As a close contact, you should wear a mask correctly and consistently at all times.	As a close contact, you should wear a mask indoors in public for 14 days following exposure or until your test result is negative.	As a close contact, you should wear a mask indoors in public for 14 days following exposure.
You should minimize contact with others	As a close contact, you should stay home and away from others (quarantine) for 14 days from the date of your last known exposure to a person with COVID-19 and follow the quarantine steps.	As a close contact, you do not need to quarantine. You should wear a mask indoors in public for 14 days following exposure or until your test result is negative.	As a close contact, you do not need to quarantine. You should wear a mask indoors in public for 14 days following exposure.
You may get a call from a health-care worker or your close contact	A public health worker, other professional, or the person you came into close contact with, may tell you that you are a close contact and have been exposed to COVID-19.	A public health worker, other professional, or the person you came into close contact with, may tell you that you are a close contact and have been exposed to COVID-19.	A public health worker, other professional, or the person you came into close contact with, may tell you that you are a close contact and have been exposed to COVID-19.

Section 47.5 | **Point of Care- and Rapid-Testing**

This section includes text excerpted from "COVID-19: Guidance for SARS-CoV-2 Point-of-Care and Rapid Testing," Centers for Disease Control and Prevention (CDC), July 8, 2021.

Point-of-care tests are diagnostic tests performed at or near the place where a specimen is collected, and they provide results within minutes rather than hours. These may be nucleic acid amplification test (NAAT,) antigen, or antibody tests.

Rapid point-of-care tests provide results within minutes (depending on the test) and are used to diagnose current or detect past severe acute respiratory syndrome coronavirus 2 (SARS-CoV-2) infections in various settings, such as:

- Physician offices
- Urgent care facilities
- Pharmacies
- School health clinics
- Long-term care facilities and nursing homes
- Temporary locations, such as drive-through sites managed by local organizations

REGULATORY REQUIREMENTS FOR POINT OF CARE- AND RAPID-TESTING/ TESTS

There are four different types of Clinical Laboratory Improvement Amendments (CLIA) certificates (www.cms.gov/Regulations-and-Guidance/Legislation/CLIA/Downloads/TYPES_OF_CLIA_CERTIFICATES.pdf), any one of which is appropriate for point-of-care testing. A CLIA Certificate of Waiver is appropriate for SARS-CoV-2 point-of-care testing and can be obtained as follows:

- Complete an application (Form CMS-116) (www.cms.gov/Medicare/CMS-Forms/CMS-Forms/Downloads/CMS116.pdf), available on the CMS CLIA website (www.cms.gov/Regulations-and-Guidance/Legislation/CLIA) or from a local State Agency.
- Send the completed application to the address of the local State Agency (www.cms.gov/Regulations-and-Guidance/Legislation/CLIA/

State_Agency_and_Regional_Office_CLIA_Contacts) for the state where testing will be performed.
- Pay the CLIA Certificate of Waiver fee, following instructions provided by the State Agency.

Laboratories or point-of-care testing sites that have applied for a CLIA Certificate of Waiver to perform SARS-CoV-2 point-of-care testing can begin testing and reporting SARS-CoV-2 results as soon as they have submitted their application to the State Agency, as long as they meet any additional state licensure requirements that apply. A noncertified point-of-care testing site will be treated as operating under a Certificate of Waiver while their application is being processed. The point-of-care testing site must keep its certificate information current. The State Agency should be notified of any changes to the laboratory or testing site ownership, name, address, or director within 30 days.

During the COVID-19 public-health emergency, CMS allows a laboratory or testing site to use its existing Certificate of Waiver to operate a temporary COVID-19 testing site in an off-site location, such as a nursing home or drive-through location. A temporary COVID-19 testing site can only perform CLIA-waived or FDA-authorized point-of-care tests for SARS-CoV-2 and must be under the direction of the existing laboratory or testing site director.

TESTS THAT CAN BE USED FOR POINT OF CARE- AND RAPID-SARS-COV-2 TESTING

Refer to the U.S. Food and Drug Administration (FDA) website for a list of the SARS-CoV-2 point of care- and rapid-tests that have received Emergency Use Authorization (EUA) (www.fda.gov/medical-devices/coronavirus-disease-2019-covid-19-emergency-use-authorizations-medical-devices/in-vitro-diagnostics-euas). Tests that have been authorized for use in a point-of-care setting will have a W, for Waived, in the Authorized Settings column of the FDA table. The laboratory or testing site must use a test authorized for point-of-care use by the FDA and must follow the manufacturer's instructions for each test. The instructions for use provide specific information on how to perform the test, which specimens can be used, and the people who may be tested. All of the FDA-authorized tests for current SARS-CoV-2 infection are for use on symptomatic people. However, CMS has indicated (www.cms.gov/files/document/clia-sars-cov-2-point-care-test-enforcement-discretion.pdf) that CLIA will temporarily allow CLIA-certified laboratories and other testing sites to use SARS-CoV-2 point of care- and rapid-antigen tests on asymptomatic people for the duration of the COVID-19 public health emergency.

REPORTING REQUIREMENTS FOR POINT OF CARE- AND RAPID-TESTING/ TESTS

A CLIA-certified laboratory or testing site must report all SARS-CoV-2 diagnostic and screening test results for current or past infections to the person who was tested or that person's healthcare provider. Depending on the test manufacturer's instructions for use, which can be found on FDA's EUA website (www.fda.gov/medical-devices/coronavirus-disease-2019-covid-19-emergency-use-authorizations-medical-devices/in-vitro-diagnostics-euas), the laboratory or testing site may be required to report a negative test result as a "presumptive negative."

A CLIA-certified laboratory or testing site must also report all COVID-19 test results to their respective state, tribal, local (www.naccho.org/membership/lhd-directory), and territorial health department's website (www.cdc.gov/publichealthgateway/healthdirectories/index.html) in accordance with the Coronavirus Aid, Relief, and Economic Security (CARES) Act; refer to the CMS interim final rule for regulatory reporting requirements (www.govinfo.gov/content/pkg/FR-2020-09-02/pdf/2020-19150.pdf).

CMS-certified long-term care (LTC) facilities can submit point-of-care SARS-CoV-2 testing data, including antigen testing data, to CDC's National Healthcare Safety Network (NHSN). This CDC- and CMS-preferred pathway to submit data to CDC's NHSN applies only to CMS-certified LTC facilities. Test data submitted to NHSN will be reported to appropriate state and local health departments using standard electronic laboratory messages. Other types of LTC facilities can also report testing data in NHSN for self-tracking or to fulfill state or local reporting requirements, if any. While NHSN is the Centers for Disease Control and Prevention (CDC)- and Centers for Medicare & Medicaid Services (CMS)-preferred pathway, Medicare and Medicaid-certified LTC facilities can submit data through the other mechanisms described in the Current Methods of Submission section of HHS Laboratory Reporting Guidance (www.hhs.gov/sites/default/files/covid-19-laboratory-data-reporting-guidance.pdf) to meet the reporting requirements.

SPECIMEN COLLECTION AND HANDLING OF POINT-OF-CARE AND RAPID TESTS

Each point-of-care test has been authorized for use with certain specimen types and should only be used with those specimen types. Proper specimen collection and handling are critical for all COVID-19 testing, including those tests performed in point-of-care settings. A specimen that is not collected or handled correctly can lead to inaccurate or unreliable test results.

For personnel collecting specimens or working within 6 feet of patients suspected to be infected with SARS-CoV-2, maintain proper infection control and use recommended personal protective equipment (PPE), which could include an N95 or higher-level respirator (or face mask if a respirator is not available), eye protection, gloves, and a lab coat or gown.

For personnel handling specimens but not directly involved in the collection (e.g., self-collection) and not working within 6 feet of the patient, follow Standard Precautions. It is recommended that personnel wear well-fitting cloth masks, facemasks, or respirators at all times while at the point-of-care site where the testing is being performed.

Disinfect surfaces within 6 feet of the specimen collection and handling area before, during, and after testing and at these times:

- Before testing begins each day
- Between each specimen collection
- At least hourly during testing
- When visibly soiled
- In the event of a specimen spill or splash
- At the end of every testing day

CDC Recommends the Following Practices When Performing Point-of-Care Tests

BEFORE THE TEST

- Perform a risk assessment to identify what could go wrong, such as breathing in infectious material or touching contaminated objects and surfaces. Then
    - Implement appropriate control measures to prevent these potentially negative outcomes from happening.
- Use a new pair of gloves each time a specimen is collected from a different person. If specimens are tested in batches, also change gloves before putting a new specimen into a testing device. Doing so will help to avoid cross-contamination.
- Do not reuse used test devices, reagent tubes, solutions, swabs, lancets, or fingerstick collection devices.
- Store reagents, specimens, kit contents, and test devices according to the manufacturer's instructions found in the package insert.
- Discard tests and test components that have exceeded the expiration date or show signs of damage or discoloration (such as reagents showing any signs of alteration).
- Do not open reagents, test devices, and cassettes until the test process is about to occur. Refer to the manufacturer's instructions to see how long a reagent, test device, or cassette can be used after opening.
- Label each specimen with appropriate information to definitively connect that specimen to the correct person being tested.
- When transferring specimens from a collection area to a testing area, follow the instructions for the point-of-care test used.

DURING THE TEST

- Follow all of the manufacturer's instructions for performing the test in the exact order specified.
- Perform regular quality control and instrument calibration, as applicable, according to the manufacturer's

instructions. If quality control or calibration fails, identify and correct issues before proceeding with patient testing.
- When processing multiple specimens successively in batches, ensure proper timing for each specimen and each step of the testing process, as specified by the test manufacturer. To avoid cross-contamination, change gloves before putting a new specimen into a testing device.

AFTER THE TEST

- Read and record results only within the amount of time specified in the manufacturer's instructions. Do not record results from tests that have not been read within the manufacturer's specified timeframe.
- Decontaminate the instrument after each use. Follow the manufacturer's recommendations for using an approved disinfectant, including proper dilution, contact time, and safe handling.
- Handle laboratory waste from testing SARS-CoV-2 specimens in the same manner as all other biohazardous waste in the laboratory. Currently, there is no evidence to suggest that laboratory waste needs additional packaging or disinfection procedures.

Chapter 48 | Cancer Screening Tests

Chapter Contents

Section 48.1 | **Cancer Screening Overview**

This section includes text excerpted from "Cancer Screening Overview (PDQ®) – Patient Version," National Cancer Institute (NCI), August 19, 2020.

WHAT IS CANCER SCREENING?

Cancer screening is looking for cancer before a person has any symptoms.

Screening tests can help find cancer at an early stage, before symptoms appear. When abnormal tissue or cancer is found early, it may be easier to treat or cure. By the time symptoms appear, the cancer may have grown and spread. This can make the cancer harder to treat or cure.

It is important to remember that when your doctor suggests a screening test, it does not always mean she or he thinks you have cancer. Screening tests are done when you have no cancer symptoms.

TYPES OF SCREENING TESTS

There are different kinds of screening tests.

Screening tests include the following:

- **Physical exam and history.** An exam of the body to check general signs of health, including checking for signs of disease, such as lumps or anything else that seems unusual. A history of the patient's health habits and past illnesses and treatments will also be taken.
- **Laboratory tests.** Medical procedures that test samples of tissue, blood, urine, or other substances in the body.
- **Imaging procedures.** Procedures that make pictures of areas inside the body.
- **Genetic tests.** A laboratory test in which cells or tissue are analyzed to look for changes in genes or chromosomes. These changes may be a sign that a person has or is at risk of having a specific disease or condition.

RISKS OF SCREENING TESTS

Screening tests have risks.

Not all screening tests are helpful and most have risks. It is important to know the risks of the test and whether it has been proven to decrease the chance of dying from cancer.

Some screening tests can cause serious problems.

Some screening procedures can cause bleeding or other problems. For example, colon cancer screening with sigmoidoscopy or colonoscopy can cause tears in the lining of the colon.

- **False-positive test results are possible.** Screening test results may appear to be abnormal even though there is no cancer. A false-positive test result (one that shows there is cancer when there really is not) can cause anxiety and is usually followed by more tests and procedures, which also have risks.
- **False-negative test results are possible.** Screening test results may appear to be normal even though there is cancer. A person who receives a false-negative test result (one that shows there is no cancer when there really is) may delay seeking medical care even if there are symptoms.

Finding the cancer may not improve the person's health or help the person live longer.

Some cancers never cause symptoms or become life-threatening, but if found by a screening test, the cancer may be treated. There is no way to know if treating the cancer would help the person live longer than if no treatment were given. In both teenagers and adults, there is a rare risk of attempted or actual suicide in the first year after being diagnosed with cancer. Also, treatments for cancer have side effects.

For some cancers, finding and treating the cancer early does not improve the chance of a cure or help the person live longer.

INFORMED AND SHARED DECISION-MAKING

It is important that you understand the benefits and harms of screening tests and make an informed choice about which screening tests are right for you.

Before having any screening test, it is important that you discuss the test with your doctor or other health-care provider. Every screening test has both benefits and harms. Your health-care provider should talk to you about the benefits and harms of a screening test and include you in the decision about whether the screening test is right for you. This is called "informed and shared decision-making."

- Your health-care provider will talk to you about the possible benefits, harms, and unknowns of a screening test. This may include information about the benefits of finding a cancer early or the harms related to false test results, overdiagnosis, and overtreatment. Your health-care provider may also give you information in a leaflet, booklet, video, website, or other material.
- After you understand the benefits and harms of a screening test, you can decide whether or not you want to have the screening test based on what is best for you. Sometimes the harms and benefits are closely matched and the decision about whether to have a screening test is hard to make.
- Your health-care provider will write your decision down in your medical record and order the screening test, if that was your decision.

GOALS OF SCREENING TESTS

Screening tests have many goals.

A screening test that works the way it should and is helpful does the following:

- Finds cancer before symptoms appear.
- Screens for a cancer that is easier to treat and cure when found early.
- Has few false-negative test results and false-positive test results.
- Decreases the chance of dying from cancer.

Screening tests usually do not diagnose cancer. If a screening test result is abnormal, more tests may be done to check for cancer. For example, a screening mammogram may find a lump in the breast. A lump may be cancer or something else. More tests need to be done to find out if the lump is cancer. These are called "diagnostic tests." Diagnostic tests may include a biopsy, in which cells or tissues are removed so a pathologist can check them under a microscope for signs of cancer.

WHO NEEDS TO BE SCREENED

Certain screening tests may be suggested only for people who have a high risk for certain cancers.

Anything that increases the chance of cancer is called a "cancer risk factor." Having a risk factor does not mean that you will get cancer; not having risk factors does not mean that you will not get cancer.

Some screening tests are used only for people who have known risk factors for certain types of cancer. People known to have a higher risk of cancer than others include those who have any of the following:

- A personal history of cancer.
- A family history of cancer.
- Certain gene mutations (changes) that have been linked to cancer.
- Exposure to cancer-causing agents such as tobacco smoke or workplace chemicals.
- A blood clot that develops for no known reason.
- Older age.
- People who have a high risk of cancer may need to be screened more often or at an earlier age than other people.

HOW CANCER RISK IS MEASURED

Cancer risk is measured in different ways. The findings from surveys and studies about cancer risk are studied and the results are explained in different ways. Some of the ways risk is explained include absolute risk, relative risk, and odds ratios.

- **Absolute risk.** This is the risk a person has of developing a disease, in a given population (e.g., the entire U.S. population) over a certain period of time. Researchers estimate the absolute risk by studying a large number of people that are part of a certain population (e.g., women in a given age group). Researchers count the number of people in the group who get a certain disease over a certain period of time. For example, a group of 100,000 women between the ages of 20 and 29 are observed for one year, and 4 of them get breast cancer during that time. This means that the one-year absolute risk of breast cancer for a woman in this age group is 4 in 100,000, or 4 chances in 100,000.

- **Relative risk.** This is often used in research studies to find out whether a trait or a factor can be linked to the risk of a disease. Researchers compare two groups of people who are a lot alike. However, the people in one of the groups must have the trait or factor being studied (they have been "exposed"). The people in the other group do not have it (they have not been exposed). To figure out relative risk, the percentage of people in the exposed group who have the disease is divided by the percentage of people in the unexposed group who have the disease. Relative risks can be:
    - **Larger than 1.** The trait or factor is linked to an increase in risk.
    - **Equal to 1.** The trait or factor is not linked to risk.
    - **Less than 1.** The trait or factor is linked to a decrease in risk.

Relative risks are also called "risk ratios."

- **Odds ratio.** In some types of studies, researchers do not have enough information to figure out relative risks. They use something called an "odds ratio" instead. An odds ratio can be an estimate of relative risk. One type of study that uses an odds ratio instead of relative risk is called a "case-control study." In a case-control study, two groups of people are compared.

However, the individuals in each group are chosen based on whether or not they have a certain disease. Researchers look at the odds that the people in each group were exposed to something (a trait or factor) that might have caused the disease. Odds describes the number of times the trait or factor was present or happened, divided by the number of times it was not present or did not happen. To get an odds ratio, the odds for one group are divided by the odds for the other group. Odds ratios can be:

- **Larger than 1.** The trait or factor is linked to an increase in risk.
- **Equal to 1.** The trait or factor is not linked to risk.
- **Less than 1.** The trait or factor is linked to a decrease in risk.

Looking at traits and exposures in people with and without cancer can help find possible risk factors. Knowing who is at an increased risk for certain types of cancer can help doctors decide when and how often they should be screened.

DOES SCREENING HELP PEOPLE LIVE LONGER?

Finding some cancers at an early stage (before symptoms appear) may help decrease the chance of dying from those cancers.

For many cancers, the chance of recovery depends on the stage (the amount or spread of cancer in the body) of the cancer when it was diagnosed. Cancers that are diagnosed at earlier stages are often easier to treat or cure.

Studies of cancer screening compare the death rate of people screened for a certain cancer with the death rate from that cancer in people who were not screened. Some screening tests have been shown to be helpful both in finding cancers early and in decreasing the chance of dying from those cancers. These include mammograms for breast cancer and sigmoidoscopy and fecal occult blood testing for colorectal cancer. Other tests are used because they have been shown to find a certain type of cancer in some people before symptoms appear, but they have not been proven to decrease the risk of dying from that cancer. If a cancer is fast-growing and spreads quickly, finding it early may not help the person survive the cancer.

Screening studies are done to see whether deaths from cancer decrease when people are screened.

When collecting information on how long cancer patients live, some studies define survival as living 5 years after the diagnosis. This is often used to measure how well cancer treatments work. However, to see if screening tests are useful, studies usually look at whether deaths from the cancer decrease in people who were screened. Over time, signs that a cancer screening test is working include:

- An increase in the number of early-stage cancers found
- A decrease in the number of late-stage cancers found
- A decrease in the number of deaths from the cancer

The number of deaths from cancer is lower today than it was in the past. It is not always clear if this is because screening tests found the cancers earlier or because cancer treatments have gotten better, or both. The Surveillance, Epidemiology, and End Results (SEER) Program of the National Cancer Institute collects and reports information on survival times of people with cancer in the United States. This information is studied to see if finding cancer early affects how long these people live.

Certain factors may cause survival times to look like they are getting better when they are not.

These factors include lead-time bias, overdiagnosis, and healthy screenee bias.

Lead-Time Bias

Survival time for cancer patients is usually measured from the day the cancer is diagnosed until the day they die. Patients are often diagnosed after they have signs and symptoms of cancer. If a screening test leads to a diagnosis before a patient has any symptoms, the patient's survival time is increased because the date of diagnosis is earlier. This increase in survival time makes it seem as though screened patients are living longer when that may not be happening. This is called "lead-time bias." It could be that the only reason the survival time appears to be longer is that the date of diagnosis is earlier for the screened patients. But, the screened patients may die at the same time they would have without the screening test.

Overdiagnosis

Sometimes, screening tests find cancers that do not matter because they would have gone away on their own or never caused any symptoms. These cancers would never have been found if not for the screening test (for example, a computed tomography (CT) scan). Finding these cancers is called "overdiagnosis." Overdiagnosis can make it seem like more people are surviving cancer longer, but in reality, these are people who would not have died from cancer anyway.

Healthy Screenee Bias

People who choose to have screening tests are often more health conscious than the general public and tend to make other healthy choices in their lives. People with early-stage cancer found by screening may live longer than people who do not get screened. They may live longer because of the benefits of their healthy lifestyle rather than screening. This is sometimes called "healthy screenee bias."

Section 48.2 | Bladder and Other Urothelial Cancers

This section includes text excerpted from "Bladder and Other Urothelial Cancers Screening (PDQ®) – Patient Version," National Cancer Institute (NCI), July 30, 2021.

Bladder and other urothelial cancers are diseases in which malignant (cancer) cells form in the urothelium.

The bladder is a hollow organ in the lower part of the abdomen. It is shaped like a small balloon and has a muscle wall that allows it to get larger or smaller to store urine made by the kidneys. There are two kidneys, one on each side of the backbone, above the waist. Tiny tubules in the kidneys filter and clean the blood. They take out waste products and make urine. The urine passes from each kidney through a long tube called a "ureter" into the bladder. The bladder holds the urine until it passes through the urethra and leaves the body.

The urothelium is a layer of tissue that lines the urethra, bladder, ureters, prostate, and renal pelvis. Cancer that begins in the urothelium of the bladder is much more common than cancer that begins in the urothelium of the urethra, ureters, prostate, or renal pelvis. Because it is the most common form of urothelial cancer, bladder cancer is the focus of this summary.

There are three types of cancer that begin in the urothelial cells of the bladder. These cancers are named for the type of cells that become malignant (cancerous):

- **Transitional cell carcinoma.** Cancer that begins in cells in the innermost layer of the bladder urothelium. These cells are able to stretch when the bladder is full and shrink when it is emptied. Most bladder cancers begin in the transitional cells.
- **Squamous cell carcinoma.** Cancer that forms in squamous cells (thin, flat cells that line the bladder). Cancer may form after long-term infection or irritation.
- **Adenocarcinoma.** Cancer that begins in glandular cells. Glandular cells in the bladder urothelium make substances such as mucus.

In the United States, bladder cancer occurs more often in men than in women, and more often in white individuals than in Black individuals. Rates of bladder cancer have stayed about the same since the 1970s, although more recently (2008 to 2017), bladder cancer rates have been decreasing slightly each year. Deaths from bladder cancer decreased in all races and sexes between 1975 and 2017.

Anything that increases your chance of getting a disease is called a "risk factor." Having a risk factor does not mean that you will get cancer; not having risk factors does not mean that you will not get cancer. Talk to your doctor if you think you may be at risk for bladder cancer.

Risk factors for bladder cancer include the following:

- Using tobacco, especially smoking cigarettes.
- Having a family history of bladder cancer.
- Having certain changes in the genes that are linked to bladder cancer.
- Being exposed to paints, dyes, metals, or petroleum products in the workplace.
- Past treatment with radiation therapy to the pelvis or with certain anticancer drugs, such as cyclophosphamide or ifosfamide.
- Taking *Aristolochia fangchi*, a Chinese herb.
- Drinking water from a well that has high levels of arsenic.
- Drinking water that has been treated with chlorine.
- Having a history of bladder infections, including bladder infections caused by *Schistosoma haematobium.*
- Using urinary catheters for a long time.

Older age is a risk factor for most cancers. The chance of getting cancer increases as you get older.

SCREENING FOR BLADDER AND OTHER UROTHELIAL CANCERS

Tests Are Used to Screen for Different Types of Cancer When a Person Does Not Have Symptoms.

Scientists study screening tests to find those with the fewest harms and most benefits. Cancer screening trials also are meant to show whether early detection (finding cancer before it causes symptoms) helps a person live longer or decreases a person's chance of dying from the disease. For some types of cancer, the chance of recovery is better if the disease is found and treated at an early stage.

There is no standard or routine screening test for bladder cancer.

Hematuria Tests Have Been Studied as a Way to Screen for Bladder Cancer

Hematuria (red blood cells in the urine) may be caused by cancer or by other conditions. A hematuria test is used to check for blood in a sample of urine by viewing it under a microscope or using a special test strip. The test may be repeated over time.

Two Tests May Be Used to Screen for Bladder Cancer in Patients Who Have Had Bladder Cancer in the Past

CYSTOSCOPY

Cystoscopy is a procedure to look inside the bladder and urethra to check for abnormal areas. A cystoscope (a thin, lighted tube) is inserted through the urethra into the bladder. Tissue samples may be taken for biopsy.

URINE CYTOLOGY

Urine cytology is a laboratory test in which a sample of urine is checked under a microscope for abnormal cells.

RISKS OF SCREENING FOR BLADDER AND OTHER UROTHELIAL CANCERS

Decisions about screening tests can be difficult. Not all screening tests are helpful and most have risks. Before having any screening test, you may want to discuss the test with your doctor. It is important to know the risks of the test and whether it has been proven to reduce the risk of dying from cancer.

False-Positive Test Results Can Occur

Screening test results may appear to be abnormal even though no cancer is present. A false-positive test result (one that shows there is cancer when there really is not) can cause anxiety and is usually followed by more tests (such as cystoscopy or other invasive procedures), which also have risks. False-positive results often occur with hematuria testing; blood in the urine is usually caused by conditions other than cancer.

False-Negative Test Results Can Occur

Screening test results may appear to be normal even though bladder cancer is present. A person who receives a false-negative test result (one that shows there is no cancer when there really is) may delay seeking medical care even if there are symptoms.

Your doctor can advise you about your risk of bladder cancer and your need for screening tests.

Section 48.3 | **Breast Cancer**

This section includes text excerpted from "Breast Cancer Screening (PDQ®) – Patient Version," National Cancer Institute (NCI), August 4, 2021.

Breast cancer is a disease in which malignant (cancer) cells form in the tissues of the breast.

The breast is made up of lobes and ducts. Each breast has 15 to 20 sections called "lobes," which have many smaller sections called "lobules." Lobules end in dozens of tiny bulbs that can produce milk. The lobes, lobules, and bulbs are linked by thin tubes called "ducts."

Each breast also has blood vessels and lymph vessels. The lymph vessels carry an almost colorless, watery fluid called "lymph." Lymph vessels carry lymph between lymph nodes. Lymph nodes are small, bean-shaped structures that filter lymph and store white blood cells that help fight infection and disease. Groups of lymph nodes are found near the breast in the axilla (under the arm), above the collarbone, and in the chest.

Breast cancer is the second leading cause of death from cancer in American women.

Women in the United States get breast cancer more than any other type of cancer except for skin cancer.

Breast cancer is more likely to occur as a woman ages. It occurs more often in white women than in Black women, but Black women die from breast cancer more often than white women.

Breast cancer rarely occurs in men. Because men with breast cancer usually have a lump that can be felt, screening tests are not likely to be helpful.

SCREENING FOR BREAST CANCER

Tests Are Used to Screen for Different Types of Cancer When a Person Does Not Have Symptoms

Scientists study screening tests to find those with the fewest harms and most benefits. Cancer screening trials also are meant to show whether early detection (finding cancer before it causes symptoms) helps a person live longer or decreases a person's chance of dying from the disease. For some types of cancer, the chance of recovery is better if the disease is found and treated at an early stage.

Mammography Is the Most Common Screening Test for Breast Cancer

A mammogram is a picture of the inside of the breast. Mammography may find tumors that are too small to feel. It may also find ductal carcinoma in situ (DCIS). In DCIS, abnormal cells line the breast duct, and in some women may become invasive cancer.

There are three types of mammograms:

- Film mammography is an x-ray picture of the breast.
- Digital mammography is a computer picture of the breast.
- Digital breast tomosynthesis (DBT) uses x-rays to take a series of pictures of the breast from many different angles. A computer is used to make 3-D pictures of the breast from these x-rays.

DBT was approved by the U.S. Food and Drug Administration (FDA) in 2018 and is now used in three out of four facilities. One study found that DBT reduced false-positive test results (one that shows there is cancer when there really is not) and was likely to reduce breast cancer deaths. More studies are being done to provide information on digital mammography compared to DBT.

Mammography is less likely to find breast tumors in women with dense breast tissue. Because both tumors and dense breast tissue appear white on a mammogram, it can be harder to find a tumor when there is dense breast tissue. Younger women are more likely to have dense breast tissue.

Many factors affect whether mammography is able to detect (find) breast cancer:

- The age and weight of the patient.
- The size and type of tumor.
- Where the tumor has formed in the breast.
- How sensitive the breast tissue is to hormones.
- How dense the breast tissue is.
- The timing of the mammography within the woman's menstrual cycle.
- The quality of the mammogram picture.
- The skill of the radiologist in reading the mammogram.

Women aged 50 to 69 years who have screening mammograms have a lower chance of dying from breast cancer than women who do not have screening mammograms.

Fewer women are dying of breast cancer in the United States, but it is not known whether the lower risk of dying is because the cancer was found early by screening or whether the treatments were better.

Magnetic Resonance Imaging May Be Used to Screen Women Who Have a High Risk of Breast Cancer.

MRI is a procedure that uses a magnet, radio waves, and a computer to make a series of detailed pictures of areas inside the body. This procedure is also called "nuclear magnetic resonance imaging" (NMRI). MRI does not use any x-rays and the woman is not exposed to radiation.

MRI may be used as a screening test for women who have a high risk of breast cancer. Factors that put women at high risk include the following:

- Certain gene changes, such as changes in the *BRCA1* or *BRCA2* genes.
- A family history (first degree relative, such as a mother, daughter or sister) with breast cancer.
- Certain genetic syndromes, such as Li-Fraumeni or Cowden syndrome.

An MRI is more likely than mammography to find a breast mass that is not cancer.

Women with dense breasts who have supplemental screening (e.g., an MRI) show higher rates of breast cancer detection, but there is limited evidence about whether this leads to better health outcomes.

Whether a Woman Should Be Screened for Breast Cancer and the Screening Test to Use Depends on Certain Factors.

Women with risk factors for breast cancer, such as certain changes in the *BRCA1* or *BRCA2* gene or certain genetic syndromes may be screened at a younger age and more often.

Women who have had radiation treatment to the chest, especially at a young age, may start routine breast cancer screening at an earlier age. The benefits and risks of mammograms and MRIs for these women have not been studied.

Breast cancer screening has not been shown to benefit the following women:

- Elderly women who, if diagnosed with breast cancer through screening, will usually die of other causes. Screening mammograms for those aged 66 to 79 years may find cancer in a very small percentage of women, but most of these cancers are low risk.
- In women with an average risk of developing breast cancer, screening mammography before age 40 has not shown any benefit.
- In women who are not expected to live for a long time and have other diseases or conditions, finding and treating early stage breast cancer may reduce their quality of life without helping them live longer.

Other Screening Tests Have Been or Are Being Studied in Clinical Trials.

Studies have been done to find out if the following breast cancer screening tests are useful in finding breast cancer or helping women with breast cancer live longer.

BREAST EXAM

A clinical breast exam is an exam of the breast by a doctor or other health professional. She or he will carefully feel the breasts and under the arms for lumps or anything else that seems unusual. It is not known if having clinical breast exams decreases the chance of dying from breast cancer.

Breast self-exams may be done by women or men to check their breasts for lumps or other changes. If you feel any lumps or notice any other changes in your breasts, talk to your doctor. Doing regular breast self-exams has not been shown to decrease the chance of dying from breast cancer.

THERMOGRAPHY

Thermography is a procedure in which a special camera that senses heat is used to record the temperature of the skin that covers the breasts. Tumors can cause temperature changes that may show up on the thermogram.

There have been no randomized clinical trials of thermography to find out how well it detects breast cancer or the harms of the procedure.

TISSUE SAMPLING

Breast tissue sampling is taking cells from breast tissue to check under a microscope. Breast tissue sampling as a screening test has not been shown to decrease the risk of dying from breast cancer.

HARMS OF BREAST CANCER SCREENING

Not all breast cancers will cause death or illness in a woman's lifetime, so they may not need to be found or treated.

Decisions about screening tests can be difficult. Not all screening tests are helpful and most have harms. Before having any screening test, you may want to discuss the test with your doctor. It is important to know the harms of the test and whether it has been proven to reduce the risk of dying from cancer.

The Harms of Mammography Include the Following

FALSE-POSITIVE TEST RESULTS CAN OCCUR

Screening test results may appear to be abnormal even though no cancer is present. A false-positive test result (one that shows there is cancer when there really is not) is usually followed by more tests (such as biopsy), which also have risks.

When a breast biopsy result is abnormal, getting a second opinion from a different pathologist may confirm a correct breast cancer diagnosis.

Most abnormal test results turn out not to be cancer. False-positive results are more common in the following:

- Younger women (under age 50).
- Women who have had previous breast biopsies.
- Women with a family history of breast cancer.
- Women who take hormones for menopause.

False-positive results are more likely the first time screening mammography is done than with later screenings. For every ten women who have a single mammogram, one will have a false-positive result. The chance of having a false-positive result goes up the more mammograms a woman has. Comparing a current mammogram with a past mammogram lowers the risk of a false-positive result.

The skill of the radiologist also can affect the chance of a false-positive result.

FALSE-POSITIVE RESULTS CAN LEAD TO EXTRA TESTING AND CAUSE ANXIETY

If a mammogram is abnormal, more tests may be done to diagnose cancer. Women can become anxious during the diagnostic testing.

Even if it is a false-positive test and cancer is not diagnosed, the result can lead to anxiety anywhere from a few days to years later.

Several studies show that women who feel anxiety after false-positive test results are more likely to schedule regular breast screening exams in the future.

FALSE-NEGATIVE TEST RESULTS CAN DELAY DIAGNOSIS AND TREATMENT

Screening test results may appear to be normal even though breast cancer is present. This is called a "false-negative test result." A woman who has a false-negative test result may delay seeking medical care even if she has symptoms. About one in five cancers are missed by mammography.

The chance of a false-negative test result is more common in women who:

- Are younger
- Have dense breast tissue
- Have cancer that is not dependent on hormones (estrogen and progesterone)
- Have cancer that is fast growing

FINDING BREAST CANCER MAY LEAD TO BREAST CANCER TREATMENT AND SIDE EFFECTS, BUT IT MAY NOT IMPROVE A WOMAN'S HEALTH OR HELP HER LIVE LONGER

Some breast cancers found only by screening mammography may never cause health problems or become life-threatening. Finding these cancers is called "overdiagnosis." When these cancers are found, having treatment may cause serious side effects and may not lead to a longer, healthier life.

MAMMOGRAPHY EXPOSES THE BREAST TO LOW DOSES OF RADIATION

Being exposed to high radiation doses is a risk factor for breast cancer. The radiation dose with a mammogram is very low. Women who start getting mammograms after age 50 have very little risk that the overall exposure to radiation from mammograms throughout their lives will cause harm. Women with large breasts or with breast implants may be exposed to slightly higher radiation doses during screening mammography.

THERE MAY BE PAIN OR DISCOMFORT DURING A MAMMOGRAM

During a mammogram, the breast is placed between two plates that are pressed together. Pressing the breast helps to get a better x-ray of the breast. Some women have pain or discomfort during a mammogram. The amount of pain may also depend on the following:

- The phase of the woman's menstrual cycle.
- The woman's anxiety level.
- How much pain the woman expected.

Talk to Your Doctor about Your Risk of Breast Cancer and Your Need for Screening Tests

Talk to your doctor or other care provider about your risk of breast cancer, whether a screening test is right for you, and the benefits and harms of the screening test. You should take part in the decision about whether you want to have a screening test, based on what is best for you.

Section 48.4 | Cervical Cancer

This section includes text excerpted from "Cervical Cancer Screening (PDQ®) – Patient Version," National Cancer Institute (NCI), August 27, 2021.

Cervical cancer is a disease in which malignant (cancer) cells form in the cervix.

The cervix is the lower, narrow end of the uterus (the hollow, pear-shaped organ where a fetus grows). The cervix leads from the uterus to the vagina (birth canal).

Cervical cancer usually develops slowly over time. Before cancer appears in the cervix, the cells of the cervix go through changes known as "dysplasia," in which cells that are not normal begin to appear in the cervical tissue. Later, cancer cells start to grow and spread more deeply into the cervix and to surrounding areas.

Screening for cervical cancer using the Pap test has decreased the number of new cases of cervical cancer and the number of deaths due to cervical cancer since 1950.

Cervical dysplasia occurs more often in women who are in their 20s and 30s. Death from cervical cancer is rare in women younger than 30 years and in women of any age who have regular screenings with the Pap test. The Pap test is used to detect cancer and changes that may lead to cancer. The chance of death from cervical cancer increases with age. In recent years, deaths from cervical cancer have been slightly higher in Black women younger than 50 years than in white women younger than 50 years. Deaths from cervical cancer are almost twice as likely in Black women older than 60 years than in white women older than 60 years.

Human papillomavirus (HPV) infection is the major risk factor for cervical cancer.

Although most women with cervical cancer have the human papillomavirus infection, not all women with an HPV infection will develop cervical cancer. Many different types of HPV can affect the cervix and only some of them cause abnormal cells that may become cancer. Some HPV infections go away without treatment.

HPV infections are spread mainly through sexual contact. Women who become sexually active at a young age and have many sexual partners are at increased risk for HPV infections.

Other risk factors for cervical cancer include:

- Giving birth to many children.
- Smoking cigarettes.
- Using oral contraceptives ("the pill").
- Having a weakened immune system.

SCREENING FOR CERVICAL CANCER

Tests Are Used to Screen for Different Types of Cancer When a Person Does Not Have Symptoms

Scientists study screening tests to find those with the fewest harms and most benefits. Cancer screening trials also are meant to show whether early detection (finding cancer before it causes symptoms) helps a person live longer or decreases a person's chance of dying from the disease. For some types of cancer, the chance of recovery is better if the disease is found and treated at an early stage.

Regular screening of women between the ages of 21 and 65 years with the Pap test decreases their chance of dying from cervical cancer.

A Pap Test Is Commonly Used to Screen for Cervical Cancer

A Pap test is a procedure to collect cells from the surface of the cervix and vagina. A piece of cotton, a brush, or a small wooden stick is used to gently scrape cells from the cervix and vagina. The cells are viewed under a microscope to find out if they are abnormal. This procedure is also called a "Pap smear." A new method of collecting and viewing cells has been developed, in which the cells are placed into a liquid before being placed on a slide. It is not known if the new method will work better than the standard method to reduce the number of deaths from cervical cancer.

After Certain Positive Pap Test Results, an HPV Test May Be Done

An HPV test is a laboratory test that is used to check DNA or RNA for certain types of HPV infection. Cells are collected from the cervix and DNA or RNA from the cells is checked to find out if there is an infection caused by a type of human papillomavirus that is linked to cervical cancer. This test may be done using the sample of cells removed during a Pap test. This test may also be done if the results of a Pap test show certain abnormal cervical cells. When both the HPV test and Pap test are done using cells from the sample removed during a Pap test, it is called a "Pap cotest" or "HPV cotest."

An HPV Test May Be Done with or without a Pap Test to Screen for Cervical Cancer

Screening women aged 30 and older with both the Pap test and the HPV test every 5 years finds more cervical changes that can lead to cancer than screening with the Pap test alone. Screening with both the Pap test and the HPV test lowers the number of cases of cervical cancer.

An HPV DNA test may be used without a Pap test for cervical cancer screening in women aged 25 years and older.

Samples for an HPV Test May Be Self-Collected

Samples for an HPV test may be collected by the patient using written instructions or in a clinic-based setting. The option for self-collection may improve access to cervical cancer screening, especially in communities with limited access to health-care providers.

RISKS OF CERVICAL CANCER SCREENING

Screening Tests Have Risks

Decisions about screening tests can be difficult. Not all screening tests are helpful and most have risks. Before having any screening test, you may want to discuss the test with your doctor. It is important to know the risks of the test and whether it has been proven to reduce the risk of dying from cancer.

The Risks of Cervical Cancer Screening Include the Following

UNNECESSARY FOLLOW-UP TESTS MAY BE DONE

In women younger than 21 years, screening with the Pap test may show changes in the cells of the cervix that are not cancer. This may lead to unnecessary follow-up tests and possibly treatment. Women in this age group have a very low risk of cervical cancer and it is likely that any abnormal cells will go away on their own.

FALSE-NEGATIVE TEST RESULTS CAN OCCUR

Screening test results may appear to be normal even though cervical cancer is present. A woman who receives a false-negative test result (one that shows there is no cancer when there really is) may delay seeking medical care even if she has symptoms.

FALSE-POSITIVE TEST RESULTS CAN OCCUR

Screening test results may appear to be abnormal even though no cancer is present. Also, some abnormal cells in the cervix never become cancer. When a Pap test shows a false-positive result (one that shows there is cancer when there really is not), it can cause anxiety and is usually followed by more tests and procedures (such as colposcopy, cryotherapy, or LEEP), which also have risks. The long-term effects of these procedures on fertility and pregnancy are not known.

The HPV test finds many infections that will not lead to cervical dysplasia or cervical cancer, especially in women younger than 30 years.

When both the Pap test and the HPV test are done, false-positive test results are more common.

Your Doctor Can Advise You about Your Risk for Cervical Cancer and Your Need for Screening Tests

Studies show that the number of cases of cervical cancer and deaths from cervical cancer are greatly reduced by screening with Pap tests. Many doctors recommend a Pap test be done every year. New studies have shown that after a woman has a Pap test and the results show no sign of abnormal cells, the Pap test can be repeated every two to three years.

The Pap test is not a helpful screening test for cervical cancer in the following groups of women:

- Women who are younger than 21 years.
- Women who have had a total hysterectomy (surgery to remove the uterus and cervix) for a condition that is not cancer.
- Women who are aged 65 years or older and have a Pap test result that shows no abnormal cells. These women are very unlikely to have abnormal Pap test results in the future.

The decision about how often to have a Pap test is best made by you and your doctor.

Section 48.5 | Colorectal Cancer

This section includes text excerpted from "Colorectal Cancer Screening (PDQ®) – Patient Version," National Cancer Institute (NCI), April 8, 2021.

Colorectal cancer is a disease in which malignant (cancer) cells form in the tissues of the colon or the rectum.

The colon and rectum are parts of the body's digestive system. The digestive system removes and processes nutrients (vitamins, minerals, carbohydrates, fats, proteins, and water) from foods and helps pass waste material out of the body. The digestive system is made up of the mouth, throat, esophagus, stomach, and the small and large intestines. The colon (large bowel) is the first part of the large intestine and is about 5 feet long. Together, the rectum and anal canal make up the last part of the large intestine and are 6-8 inches long. The anal canal ends at the anus (the opening of the large intestine to the outside of the body).

Cancer that begins in the colon is called "colon cancer," and cancer that begins in the rectum is called "rectal cancer." Cancer that begins in either of these organs may also be called "colorectal cancer."

Colorectal cancer is the third leading cause of death from cancer in the United States.

The number of new colorectal cancer cases and the number of deaths from colorectal cancer have both decreased slightly each year. However, in adults younger than 50 years, there has been a small increase in the number of new cases of colorectal cancer in recent years. Colorectal cancer is found more often in men than in women.

Different factors increase or decrease the risk of getting colorectal cancer.

Anything that increases your chance of getting a disease is called a "risk factor." Anything that decreases your chance of getting a disease is called a "protective factor."

SCREENING FOR COLORECTAL CANCER

Tests Are Used to Screen for Different Types of Cancer When a Person Does Not Have Symptoms

Scientists study screening tests to find those with the fewest harms and most benefits. Cancer screening trials also are meant to show whether early detection (finding cancer before it causes symptoms) helps a person live longer or decreases a person's chance of dying from the disease. For some types of cancer, the chance of recovery is better if the disease is found and treated at an early stage.

Studies show that some screening tests for colorectal cancer help find cancer at an early stage and may decrease the number of deaths from the disease.

Five Types of Tests Are Used to Screen for Colorectal Cancer

FECAL OCCULT BLOOD TEST

A fecal occult blood test (FOBT) is a test to check stool (solid waste) for blood that can only be seen with a microscope. A small sample of stool is placed on a special card or in a special container and returned to the doctor or laboratory for testing. Blood in the stool may be a sign of polyps, cancer, or other conditions.

There are two types of FOBTs:

- **Guaiac FOBT.** The sample of stool on the special card is tested with a chemical. If there is blood in the stool, the special card changes color.
- **Immunochemical FOBT.** A liquid is added to the stool sample. This mixture is injected into a machine that contains antibodies that can detect blood in the stool. If there is blood in the stool, a line appears in a window in the machine. This test is also called "fecal immunochemical test" or "FIT."

SIGMOIDOSCOPY

Sigmoidoscopy is a procedure to look inside the rectum and sigmoid (lower) colon for polyps, abnormal areas, or cancer. A sigmoidoscope is inserted through the rectum into the sigmoid colon. A sigmoidoscope is a thin, tube-like instrument with a light and a lens for viewing. It may also have a tool to remove polyps or tissue samples, which are checked under a microscope for signs of cancer.

COLONOSCOPY

Colonoscopy is a procedure to look inside the rectum and colon for polyps, abnormal areas, or cancer. A colonoscope is inserted through the rectum into the colon. A colonoscope is a thin, tube-like instrument with a light and a lens for viewing. It may also have a tool to remove polyps or tissue samples, which are checked under a microscope for signs of cancer.

VIRTUAL COLONOSCOPY

Virtual colonoscopy is a procedure that uses a series of x-rays called "computed tomography" (CT) to make a series of pictures of the colon. A computer puts the pictures together to create detailed images that may show polyps and anything else that seems unusual on the inside surface of the colon. This test is also called "computed tomography colonography" or "CTC."

Clinical trials are comparing virtual colonoscopy with other colorectal cancer screening tests. Some clinical trials are testing whether drinking a contrast material that coats the stool, instead of using laxatives to empty the colon, shows polyps clearly.

DNA STOOL TEST

This test checks DNA in stool cells for genetic changes that may be a sign of colorectal cancer.

Studies Have Shown That Screening for Colorectal Cancer Using Digital Rectal Exam Does Not Decrease the Number of Deaths from the Disease.

A digital rectal exam (DRE) is an exam of the rectum that may be done as part of a routine physical exam. A doctor or nurse inserts a lubricated, gloved finger into the lower part of the rectum to feel for lumps or anything else that seems unusual. Study results have shown that DRE does not work as a screening method for colorectal cancer.

RISKS OF COLORECTAL CANCER SCREENING

Screening Tests Have Risks

Decisions about screening tests can be difficult. Not all screening tests are helpful and most have risks. Different screening tests have different risks or harms. Screening tests may cause anxiety when you are thinking about or getting ready for the test or when there is a positive test result. Before having any screening test, you may want to discuss the test with your doctor. It is important to know the risks of the test and whether it has been proven to reduce the risk of dying from cancer.

Talk to your doctor about your risk for colorectal cancer and the need for screening tests.

FALSE-NEGATIVE TEST RESULTS CAN OCCUR

Screening test results may appear to be normal even though colorectal cancer is present. A person who receives a false-negative test result (one that shows there is no cancer when there really is) may delay seeking medical care even if there are symptoms.

FALSE-POSITIVE TEST RESULTS CAN OCCUR

Screening test results may appear to be abnormal even though no cancer is present. A false-positive test result (one that shows there is cancer when there really is not) can cause anxiety and is usually followed by more tests (such as biopsy), which also have risks.

The Following Colorectal Cancer Screening Tests Have Risks

RISK IN COLONOSCOPY

Serious problems caused by colonoscopy are rare, but can include tears in the lining of the colon and bleeding. These problems can be serious and need to be treated in a hospital. Tearing of the lining of the colon and bleeding occur more often when a biopsy or polypectomy is done.

Sedation is used to decrease the discomfort from the procedure. Sedation may cause heart and lung problems, such as irregular heartbeat, heart attack, or trouble breathing.

RISK IN SIGMOIDOSCOPY

There are fewer complications with a sigmoidoscopy than with a colonoscopy. Although tears in the lining of the colon and bleeding can occur, they are less common than with a colonoscopy. There is usually no sedation with sigmoidoscopy, lowering the risk of complications.

RISK IN VIRTUAL COLONOSCOPY

Virtual colonoscopy has fewer possible physical harms than either colonoscopy or sigmoidoscopy. The harms of being exposed to radiation from x-rays used in virtual colonoscopy are not known. Virtual colonoscopy often finds problems with organs other than the colon, including the kidneys, chest, liver, ovaries, spleen, and pancreas. Some of these findings lead to more testing, such as colonoscopy, that may not improve the patient's health.

RISK IN FECAL OCCULT BLOOD TEST OR DNA STOOL TEST

The results of an fecal occult blood test (FOBT) or DNA stool test may appear to be abnormal even though no cancer is found. A positive test result may lead to more testing, including colonoscopy.

Section 48.6 | **Esophageal Cancer**

This section includes text excerpted from "Esophageal Cancer Screening (PDQ®) – Patient Version," National Cancer Institute (NCI), July 30, 2021.

The esophagus is the hollow, muscular tube that moves food and liquid from the throat to the stomach. The wall of the esophagus is made up of several layers of tissue, including mucous membrane, muscle, and connective tissue. Esophageal cancer is a disease in which malignant (cancer) cells form in the tissues of the esophagus. Esophageal cancer starts in the inside lining of the esophagus and spreads outward through the other layers as it grows.

The two most common types of esophageal cancer are named for the type of cells that become malignant (cancerous):

- **Squamous cell carcinoma.** Cancer that forms in the thin, flat cells lining the inside of the esophagus.

This cancer is most often found in the upper and middle part of the esophagus, but can occur anywhere along the esophagus. This is also called "epidermoid carcinoma."

- **Adenocarcinoma.** Cancer that begins in glandular cells. Glandular cells in the lining of the esophagus produce and release fluids such as mucus. Adenocarcinomas usually form in the lower part of the esophagus, near the stomach.

Men are about three times more likely than women to have esophageal cancer. There are more new cases of esophageal adenocarcinoma each year and fewer new cases of squamous cell carcinoma. Although the rates of squamous cell carcinoma are declining overall, they remain much higher in Black men than in white men. The chance of developing esophageal cancer increases with age. White men develop esophageal cancer at higher rates than Black men in all age groups. In comparison, rates are higher in Black women through 69 years and higher in white women aged 70 years and older.

Anything that increases the chance of getting a disease is called a "risk factor." Having a risk factor does not mean that you will get cancer; not having risk factors does not mean that you will not get cancer. People who think they may be at risk should discuss this with their doctor.

Risk factors for squamous cell esophageal cancer include the following:

- Using tobacco
- Drinking a lot of alcohol
- Being malnourished (lacking nutrients and/or calories)
- Being infected with human papillomavirus (HPV)
- Having tylosis
- Having achalasia
- Having swallowed lye (a chemical found in some cleaning fluids)
- Drinking very hot liquids on a regular basis

Risk factors for esophageal adenocarcinoma include the following:

- Having gastroesophageal reflux disease (GERD)
- Having Barrett esophagus
- Having a history of using drugs that relax the lower esophageal sphincter (the ring of muscle that opens and closes the opening between the esophagus and the stomach)
- Being overweight

SCREENING FOR ESOPHAGEAL CANCER

Tests Are Used to Screen for Different Types of Cancer When a Person Does Not Have Symptoms

Scientists study screening tests to find those with the fewest harms and most benefits. Cancer screening trials also are meant to show whether early detection (finding cancer before it causes symptoms) helps a person live longer or decreases a person's chance of dying from the disease. For some types of cancer, the chance of recovery is better if the disease is found and treated at an early stage.

There Is No Standard or Routine Screening Test for Esophageal Cancer

Although there are no standard or routine screening tests for esophageal cancer, the following tests are being used or studied to screen for it:

ESOPHAGOSCOPY

A procedure to look inside the esophagus to check for abnormal areas. An esophagoscope is inserted through the mouth or nose and down the throat into the esophagus. An esophagoscope is a thin, tube-like instrument with a light and a lens for viewing. It may also have a tool to remove tissue samples, which are checked under a microscope for signs of cancer.

BIOPSY

The removal of cells or tissues so they can be viewed under a microscope by a pathologist to check for signs of cancer. Taking biopsy samples from several different areas in the lining of the lower part of the esophagus may detect early Barrett esophagus. This procedure may be used for patients who have risk factors for Barrett esophagus.

BRUSH CYTOLOGY

A procedure in which cells are brushed from the lining of the esophagus and viewed under a microscope to see if they are abnormal. This may be done during an esophagoscopy.

BALLOON CYTOLOGY

A procedure in which cells are collected from the lining of the esophagus using a deflated balloon that is swallowed by the patient. The balloon is then inflated and pulled out of the esophagus. Esophageal cells on the balloon are viewed under a microscope to see if they are abnormal.

CHROMOENDOSCOPY

A procedure in which a dye is sprayed onto the lining of the esophagus during esophagoscopy. Increased staining of certain areas of the lining may be a sign of early Barrett esophagus.

FLUORESCENCE SPECTROSCOPY

A procedure that uses a special light to view tissue in the lining of the esophagus. The light probe is passed through an endoscope and shines on the lining of the esophagus. The light given off by the cells lining the esophagus is then measured. Malignant tissue gives off less light than normal tissue.

RISKS OF ESOPHAGEAL CANCER SCREENING

Decisions about screening tests can be difficult. Not all screening tests are helpful and most have risks. Before having any screening test, you may want to discuss the test with your doctor. It is important to know the risks of the test and whether it has been proven to reduce the risk of dying from cancer.

The Risks of Esophageal Cancer Screening Tests Include the Following

FINDING ESOPHAGEAL CANCER MAY NOT IMPROVE HEALTH OR HELP A PERSON LIVE LONGER

Screening may not improve your health or help you live longer if you have advanced esophageal cancer or if it has already spread to other places in your body.

Some cancers never cause symptoms or become life-threatening, but if found by a screening test, the cancer may be treated. It is not known if treatment of these cancers will help you live longer than if no treatment were given, and treatments for cancer may have serious side effects.

FALSE-NEGATIVE TEST RESULTS CAN OCCUR

Screening test results may appear to be normal even though esophageal cancer is present. A person who receives a false-negative test result (one that shows there is no cancer when there really is) may delay seeking medical care even if there are symptoms.

FALSE-POSITIVE TEST RESULTS CAN OCCUR

Screening test results may appear to be abnormal even though no cancer is present. A false-positive test result (one that shows there is cancer when there really is not) can cause anxiety and is usually followed by more tests (such as biopsy), which also have risks.

SIDE EFFECTS MAY BE CAUSED BY THE TEST ITSELF

There are rare, but serious side effects that may occur with esophagoscopy and biopsy. These include the following:

- A small hole (puncture) in the esophagus
- Problems with breathing
- Heart attack
- Passage of food, water, stomach acid or vomit into the airway
- Severe bleeding that may need to be treated in a hospital

Section 48.7 | Lung Cancer

This section includes text excerpted from "Lung Cancer Screening (PDQ®) – Patient Version," National Cancer Institute (NCI), July 30, 2021.

Lung cancer is a disease in which malignant (cancer) cells form in the tissues of the lung.

The lungs are a pair of cone-shaped breathing organs inside the chest. The lungs bring oxygen into the body when breathing in and send carbon dioxide out of the body when breathing out. Each lung has sections called "lobes." The left lung has two lobes. The right lung, which is slightly larger, has three. A thin membrane called the "pleura" surrounds the lungs. Two tubes called "bronchi" lead from the trachea (windpipe) to the right and left lungs. The bronchi are sometimes involved in lung cancer. Small tubes called "bronchioles" and tiny air sacs called "alveoli" make up the inside of the lungs.

There are two types of lung cancer: small cell lung cancer and nonsmall cell lung cancer.

Lung cancer is the third most common type of nonskin cancer in the United States. Lung cancer is the leading cause of cancer death in men and in women.

Anything that increases your chance of getting a disease is called a "risk factor." Anything that decreases your chance of getting a disease is called a "protective factor."

Tobacco smoking is the most important risk factor for lung cancer. Cigarette, cigar, and pipe smoking all increase the risk of lung cancer. Tobacco smoking causes about 9 out of 10 cases of lung cancer in men and about 8 out of 10 cases of lung cancer in women. The best way to prevent lung cancer is to not smoke.

SCREENING FOR LUNG CANCER

Tests Are Used to Screen for Different Types of Cancer When a Person Does Not Have Symptoms

Scientists study screening tests to find those with the fewest harms and most benefits. Cancer screening trials also are meant to show whether early detection (finding cancer before it causes symptoms) helps a person live longer or decreases a person's chance of dying from the disease. For some types of cancer, the chance of recovery is better if the disease is found and treated at an early stage.

Three Screening Tests Have Been Studied to See If They Decrease the Risk of Dying from Lung Cancer

The following screening tests have been studied to see if they decrease the risk of dying from lung cancer:

- **Low-dose computed tomography (LDCT).** A procedure that uses low-dose radiation to make a series of very detailed pictures of areas inside the body using an x-ray machine that scans the body in a spiral path. This procedure is also called "spiral scan" or "helical scan."
- **Chest x-ray.** An x-ray of the organs and bones inside the chest. An x-ray is a type of energy beam that can go through the body and onto film, making a picture of areas inside the body.
- **Sputum cytology.** Sputum cytology is a procedure in which a sample of sputum (mucus that is coughed up from the lungs) is viewed under a microscope to check for cancer cells.

Screening with LDCT Scans Has Been Shown to Decrease the Risk of Dying from Lung Cancer in Heavy Smokers

The National Lung Screening Trial studied people aged 55 years to 74 years who had smoked at least 1 pack of cigarettes per day for 30 years or more. Participants were either current smokers or former smokers who had quit within the last 15 years. The trial used chest x-rays or LDCT scans to check for signs of lung cancer.

Screening with LDCT once a year for three years was better than chest x-rays at finding early-stage lung cancer and decreased the risk of dying from lung cancer in current and former heavy smokers.

Current smokers whose LDCT scan result shows possible signs of cancer may be more likely to quit smoking.

Screening with LDCT can cause possible harms, including:

- False-positive test results, which may lead to invasive procedures which are not needed
- Overdiagnosis of some lung cancers, though it is not clear how often this happens

Screening with Chest X-rays and/or Sputum Cytology Does Not Decrease the Risk of Dying from Lung Cancer

Chest x-ray and sputum cytology are two screening tests that have been used to check for signs of lung cancer. Screening with chest x-ray, sputum cytology, or both of these tests does not decrease the risk of dying from lung cancer.

RISKS OF LUNG CANCER SCREENING

Decisions about screening tests can be difficult. Not all screening tests are helpful and most have risks. Before having any screening test, you may want to discuss the test with your doctor. It is important to know the risks of the test and whether it has been proven to reduce the risk of dying from cancer.

The Risks of Lung Cancer Screening Tests Include the Following

FINDING LUNG CANCER MAY NOT IMPROVE HEALTH OR HELP YOU LIVE LONGER

Screening may not improve your health or help you live longer if you have lung cancer that has already spread to other places in your body.

When a screening test result leads to the diagnosis and treatment of a disease that may never have caused symptoms or become life-threatening, it is called "overdiagnosis." It is not known if treatment of these cancers would help you live longer than if no treatment were given, and treatments for cancer may have serious side effects. Harms of treatment may happen more often in people who have medical problems caused by heavy or long-term smoking.

FALSE-NEGATIVE TEST RESULTS CAN OCCUR

Screening test results may appear to be normal even though lung cancer is present. A person who receives a false-negative test result (one that shows there is no cancer when there really is) may delay seeking medical care even if there are symptoms.

FALSE-POSITIVE TEST RESULTS CAN OCCUR

Screening test results may appear to be abnormal even though no cancer is present. A false-positive test result (one that shows there is cancer when there really is not) can cause anxiety and is usually followed by more tests (such as biopsy), which also have risks. A biopsy to diagnose lung cancer can cause part of the lung to collapse. Sometimes surgery is needed to reinflate the lung. Harms of diagnostic tests may happen more often in patients who have medical problems caused by heavy or long-term smoking.

CHEST X-RAYS AND CT SCANS EXPOSE THE CHEST TO RADIATION

Radiation exposure from chest x-rays and low-dose CT scans may increase the risk of cancer. Younger people and people at low risk for lung cancer are more likely to develop lung cancer caused by radiation exposure from screening than to be spared death from lung cancer.

TALK TO YOUR DOCTOR ABOUT YOUR RISK FOR LUNG CANCER AND YOUR NEED FOR SCREENING TESTS

Talk to your doctor or other health-care provider about your risk for lung cancer, whether a screening test is right for you, and about the benefits and harms of the screening test. You should take part in the decision about whether a screening test is right for you.

Section 48.8 | **Oral Cavity, Pharyngeal, and Laryngeal Cancer**

This section includes text excerpted from "Oral Cavity, Pharyngeal, and Laryngeal Cancer Screening (PDQ®) – Patient Version," National Cancer Institute (NCI), October 8, 2021.

Oral cavity, pharyngeal, and laryngeal cancer are diseases in which malignant (cancer) cells form in the mouth and throat.

Oral cavity, pharyngeal, and laryngeal cancers usually form in the squamous cells (thin, flat cells lining the inside of the oral cavity, pharynx, and larynx).

Oral cavity cancer forms in any of these tissues of the oral cavity:

- The lips
- The front two thirds of the tongue
- The gingiva (gums)
- The buccal mucosa (the lining of the inside of the cheeks)
- The floor (bottom) of the mouth under the tongue
- The hard palate (the front of the roof of the mouth)
- The retromolar trigone (the small area behind the wisdom teeth)

Different factors increase or decrease the risk of oral cavity and nasopharyngeal cancers.

Anything that increases your chance of getting a disease is called a "risk factor." Anything that decreases your chance of getting a disease is called a "protective factor."

Being infected with Epstein-Barr virus (EBV) increases the risk of nasopharyngeal cancer

SCREENING FOR ORAL CAVITY, PHARYNGEAL, AND LARYNGEAL CANCER

Tests Are Used to Screen for Different Types of Cancer When a Person Does Not Have Symptoms

Scientists study screening tests to find those with the fewest harms and most benefits. Cancer screening trials also are meant to show whether early detection (finding cancer before it causes symptoms) helps a person live longer or decreases a person's chance of dying from the disease. For some types of cancer, the chance of recovery is better if the disease is found and treated at an early stage.

There Is No Standard or Routine Screening Test for Oral Cavity, Pharyngeal, and Laryngeal Cancer

No studies have shown that screening for oral cavity, pharyngeal, or laryngeal cancer would decrease the risk of dying from this disease.

A dentist or medical doctor may check the oral cavity during a routine checkup. The exam will include looking for lesions, including areas of leukoplakia (an abnormal white patch of cells) and erythroplakia (an abnormal red patch of cells). Leukoplakia and erythroplakia lesions on the mucous membranes may become cancerous.

If lesions are seen in the mouth, the following procedures may be used to find abnormal tissue that might become oral cavity cancer:

- **Toluidine blue stain.** A procedure in which lesions in the mouth are coated with a blue dye. Areas that stain darker are more likely to be cancer or become cancer.
- **Fluorescence staining.** A procedure in which lesions in the mouth are viewed using a special light. After the patient uses a fluorescent mouth rinse, normal tissue looks different from abnormal tissue when seen under the light.
- **Exfoliative cytology.** A procedure to collect cells from the oral cavity. A piece of cotton, a brush, or a small wooden stick is used to gently scrape cells from the lips, tongue, or mouth. The cells are viewed under a microscope to find out if they are abnormal.
- **Brush biopsy.** The removal of cells using a brush that is designed to collect cells from all layers of a lesion. The cells are viewed under a microscope to find out if they are abnormal.

More than half of oral cancers have already spread to lymph nodes or other areas by the time they are found.

Epstein-Barr virus (EBV) has been linked to nasopharyngeal cancer. Screening for nasopharyngeal cancer using the EBV antibody test or EBV DNA test has been studied. These are laboratory tests used to check the blood for EBV antibodies or EBV DNA. If EBV antibodies or DNA are found in the blood more tests may be done to check for nasopharyngeal cancer. No studies have shown that screening would decrease the risk of dying from this disease.

RISKS OF ORAL CAVITY, PHARYNGEAL, AND LARYNGEAL CANCER SCREENING

Decisions about screening tests can be difficult. Not all screening tests are helpful and most have risks. Before having any screening test, you may want to discuss the test with your doctor. It is important to know the risks of the test and whether it has been proven to reduce the risk of dying from cancer.

The Risks of Oral Cavity, Pharyngeal, and Laryngeal Cancer Screening Include the Following

FINDING ORAL CAVITY, PHARYNGEAL, OR LARYNGEAL CANCER MAY NOT IMPROVE HEALTH OR HELP A PERSON LIVE LONGER

Some cancers never cause symptoms or become life-threatening, but if found by a screening test, the cancer may be treated. Finding these cancers is called "overdiagnosis." It is not known if treatment of these cancers would help you live longer than if no treatment were given, and treatments for cancer, such as surgery and radiation therapy, may have serious side effects.

FALSE-NEGATIVE TEST RESULTS CAN OCCUR

Screening test results may appear to be normal even though oral cavity, pharyngeal, or laryngeal cancer is present. A person who receives a false-negative test result (one that shows there is no cancer when there really is) may delay seeking medical care even if there are symptoms.

FALSE-POSITIVE TEST RESULTS CAN OCCUR

Screening test results may appear to be abnormal even though no cancer is present. A false-positive test result (one that shows there is cancer when there really is not) can cause anxiety and is usually followed by more tests and procedures (such as biopsy), which also have risks.

MISDIAGNOSIS CAN OCCUR

A biopsy is needed to diagnose oral cavity, pharyngeal, and laryngeal cancer. Cells or tissues are removed from the oral cavity, pharynx, or larynx and viewed under a microscope by a pathologist to check for signs of cancer. When the cells are cancer and the pathologist reports them as not being cancer, the cancer is misdiagnosed. Cancer is also misdiagnosed when the cells are not cancer and the pathologist reports there is cancer. When cancer is misdiagnosed, treatment that is needed may not be given or treatment may be given that is not needed.

Section 48.9 | **Prostate Cancer**

This section includes text excerpted from "Prostate Cancer Screening (PDQ®) – Patient Version," National Cancer Institute (NCI), September 29, 2021.

The prostate is a gland in the male reproductive system located just below the bladder (the organ that collects and empties urine) and in front of the rectum (the lower part of the intestine). It is about the size of a walnut and surrounds part of the urethra (the tube that empties urine from the bladder). The prostate gland produces fluid that makes up part of semen.

As men age, the prostate may get bigger. A bigger prostate may block the flow of urine from the bladder and cause problems with sexual function. This condition is called "benign prostatic hyperplasia" (BPH), and although it is not cancer, surgery may be needed to correct it. The symptoms of benign prostatic hyperplasia or of other problems in the prostate may be similar to symptoms of prostate cancer.

Prostate cancer is a disease in which malignant (cancer) cells form in the tissues of the prostate. Prostate cancer is the most common nonskin cancer among men in the United States.

Prostate cancer is found mainly in older men. Although the number of men with prostate cancer is large, most men diagnosed with this disease do not die from it. Prostate cancer causes more deaths in men than any other cancer except lung cancer. Prostate cancer occurs more often in African-American men than in white men. African-American men with prostate cancer are more likely to die from the disease than white men with prostate cancer.

Anything that increases a person's chance of developing a disease is called a "risk factor." Anything that decreases your chance of getting a disease is called a "protective factor."

SCREENING FOR PROSTATE CANCER

Tests Are Used to Screen for Different Types of Cancer When a Person Does Not Have Symptoms

Scientists study screening tests to find those with the fewest harms and most benefits. Cancer screening trials also are meant to show whether early detection (finding cancer before it causes symptoms) helps a person live longer or decreases a person's chance of dying from the disease. For some types of cancer, the chance of recovery is better if the disease is found and treated at an early stage.

There Is No Standard or Routine Screening Test for Prostate Cancer

Although there are no standard or routine screening tests for prostate cancer, the following tests are being used or studied to screen for it:

DIGITAL RECTAL EXAM

Digital rectal exam (DRE) is an exam of the rectum. The doctor or nurse inserts a lubricated, gloved finger into the lower part of the rectum to feel the prostate for lumps or anything else that seems unusual.

PROSTATE-SPECIFIC ANTIGEN TEST

A prostate-specific antigen (PSA) test is a test that measures the level of PSA in the blood. PSA is a substance made mostly by the prostate that may be found in an increased amount in the blood of men who have prostate cancer. The level of PSA may also be high in men who have an infection or inflammation of the prostate or benign prostatic hyperplasia (BPH; an enlarged, but noncancerous, prostate).

A PSA test or a DRE may be able to detect prostate cancer at an early stage, but it is not clear whether early detection and treatment decrease the risk of dying from prostate cancer.

Studies are being done to find ways to make PSA testing more accurate for early cancer detection.

A Prostate Cancer Gene 3 (PCA3) RNA Test May Be Used for Certain Patients

If a man had a high PSA level and a biopsy of the prostate did not show cancer and the PSA level remains high after the biopsy, a prostate cancer gene 3 (*PCA3*) RNA test may be done. This test measures the amount of PCA3 RNA in the urine after a DRE. If the PCA3 RNA level is higher than normal, another biopsy may help diagnose prostate cancer.

RISKS OF PROSTATE CANCER SCREENING

Decisions about screening tests can be difficult. Not all screening tests are helpful and most have risks. Before having any screening test, you may want to discuss the test with your doctor. It is important to know the risks of the test and whether it has been proven to reduce the risk of dying from cancer.

The Risks of Prostate Screening Include the Following

FINDING PROSTATE CANCER MAY NOT IMPROVE HEALTH OR HELP A MAN LIVE LONGER

Screening may not improve your health or help you live longer if you have cancer that has already spread to the area outside of the prostate or to other places in your body.

Some cancers never cause symptoms or become life-threatening, but if found by a screening test, the cancer may be treated. Finding these cancers is called "overdiagnosis." It is not known if treatment of these cancers would help you live longer than if no treatment were given.

Treatments for prostate cancer, such as radical prostatectomy and radiation therapy, may have long-term side effects in many men. The most common side effects are erectile dysfunction and urinary incontinence.

Some studies of patients with newly diagnosed prostate cancer showed these patients had a higher risk of death from cardiovascular (heart and blood vessel) disease or suicide. The risk was greatest in the first weeks or months after diagnosis.

FOLLOW-UP TESTS, SUCH AS A BIOPSY, MAY BE DONE TO DIAGNOSE CANCER

If a PSA test is higher than normal, a biopsy of the prostate may be done. Complications from a biopsy of the prostate may include fever, pain, blood in the urine or semen, and urinary tract infection. Even if a biopsy shows that a patient does not have prostate cancer, he may worry more about developing prostate cancer in the future.

FALSE-NEGATIVE TEST RESULTS CAN OCCUR

Screening test results may appear to be normal even though prostate cancer is present. A man who receives a false-negative test result (one that shows there is no cancer when there really is) may delay seeking medical care even if he has symptoms.

FALSE-POSITIVE TEST RESULTS CAN OCCUR

Screening test results may appear to be abnormal even though no cancer is present. A false-positive test result (one that shows there is cancer when there really is not) can cause anxiety and is usually followed by more tests, (such as biopsy) which also have risks.

Your doctor can advise you about your risk for prostate cancer and your need for screening tests.

Section 48.10 | Skin Cancer

This section includes text excerpted from "Skin Cancer Screening (PDQ®) – Patient Version," National Cancer Institute (NCI), April 12, 2021.

The skin is the body's largest organ. It protects against heat, sunlight, injury, and infection. Skin also helps control body temperature and stores water, fat, and vitamin D. The skin has several layers, but the two main layers are the epidermis (top or outer layer) and the dermis (lower or inner layer). Skin cancer is a disease in which malignant (cancer) cells form in the tissues of the skin. Skin cancer begins in the epidermis, which is made up of three kinds of cells:

- **Squamous cells.** Thin, flat cells that form the top layer of the epidermis. Cancer that forms in squamous cells is called "squamous cell carcinoma" of the skin.
- **Basal cells.** Round cells under the squamous cells. Cancer that forms in basal cells is called "basal cell carcinoma."
- **Melanocytes.** Found in the lower part of the epidermis, these cells make melanin, the pigment that gives skin its natural color. When skin is exposed to the sun, melanocytes make more pigment and cause the skin to tan, or darken. Cancer that forms in melanocytes is called "melanoma."

There are two main types of skin cancer:

- Nonmelanoma skin cancer
  - Basal cell carcinoma
  - Squamous cell carcinoma (SCC)
- Melanoma

Basal cell carcinoma and squamous cell carcinoma of the skin, also called "nonmelanoma skin cancer," are the most common forms of skin cancer. Most basal cell and squamous cell skin cancers can be cured.

Melanoma is more likely to spread to nearby tissues and other parts of the body and can be harder to cure. Melanoma is easier to cure if the tumor is found before it spreads to the dermis (inner layer of skin). Melanoma is less likely to cause death when it is found and treated early.

In the United States, about 3 million cases of nonmelanoma skin cancer are diagnosed each year, and rates have likely been increasing in recent years. The number of cases of melanoma has been increasing for at least 40 years. Part of the reason for these increases may be that people have become more aware of skin cancer. They are more likely to have screening exams and do self-exams. As a result, they are more likely to be diagnosed with skin cancer.

From 2014 to 2018, the number of deaths from melanoma decreased slightly in all age groups.

The number of cases of childhood melanoma diagnosed in the United States is low, but increasing over time. The number of childhood deaths from melanoma has stayed about the same.

Anything that increases your chance of getting a disease is called a "risk factor." Anything that decreases your chance of getting a disease is called a "protective factor."

SCREENING FOR SKIN CANCER

Tests Are Used to Screen for Different Types of Cancer When a Person Does Not Have Symptoms

Scientists study screening tests to find those with the fewest harms and most benefits. Cancer screening trials also are meant to show whether early detection (finding cancer before it causes symptoms) helps a person live longer or decreases a person's chance of dying from the disease. For some types of cancer, the chance of recovery is better if the disease is found and treated at an early stage.

Screening for Skin Cancer May Include Examination by Both the Patient and the Health-Care Provider

A visual self-exam by the patient and a clinical examination by the health-care provider may be used to screen for skin cancer.

During a skin exam a doctor or nurse checks the skin for moles, birthmarks, or other pigmented areas that look abnormal in color, size, shape, or texture. Skin exams to screen for skin cancer have not been shown to decrease the number of deaths from the disease.

Regular skin checks by a doctor are important for people who have already had skin cancer. If you are checking your skin and find a worrisome change, you should report it to your doctor.

If an area on the skin looks abnormal, a biopsy is usually done. The doctor will remove as much of the suspicious tissue as possible with a local excision. A pathologist then looks at the tissue under a microscope to check for cancer cells. Because it is sometimes difficult to tell if a skin growth is benign (not cancer) or malignant (cancer), you may want to have the biopsy sample checked by a second pathologist.

Most melanomas in the skin can be seen by the naked eye. Usually, melanoma grows for a long time under the top layer of skin (the epidermis), but does not grow into the deeper layer of skin (the dermis). This allows time for skin cancer to be found early. Melanoma is easier to cure if it is found before it spreads.

Mobile phone applications ("apps") that evaluate skin lesions to detect skin cancer and malignant melanoma have been developed. However, these apps require further study in large-scale testing programs to find out if they are accurate and useful for skin cancer screening.

RISKS OF SKIN CANCER SCREENING

Screening Tests Have Risks

Decisions about screening tests can be difficult. Not all screening tests are helpful and most have risks. Before having any screening test, you may want to discuss the test with your doctor. It is important to know the risks of the test and whether it has been proven to reduce the risk of dying from cancer.

The Risks of Skin Cancer Screening Tests Include the Following

FINDING SKIN CANCER DOES NOT ALWAYS IMPROVE HEALTH OR HELP YOU LIVE LONGER

Screening may not improve your health or help you live longer if you have advanced skin cancer.

Some cancers never cause symptoms or become life-threatening, but if found by a screening test, the cancer may be treated. Treatments for cancer may have serious side effects.

FALSE-NEGATIVE TEST RESULTS CAN OCCUR

Screening test results may appear to be normal even though cancer is present. A person who receives a false-negative test result (one that shows there is no cancer when there really is) may delay getting medical care even if there are symptoms.

FALSE-POSITIVE TEST RESULTS CAN OCCUR

Screening test results may appear to be abnormal even though no cancer is present. A false-positive test result (one that shows there is cancer when there really is not) can cause anxiety and is usually followed by more tests (such as a biopsy), which also have risks.

A BIOPSY MAY CAUSE SCARRING

When a skin biopsy is done, the doctor will try to leave the smallest scar possible, but there is a risk of scarring and infection.

Talk to your doctor about your risk for skin cancer and your need for screening tests.

Section 48.11 | Testicular Cancer

This section includes text excerpted from "Testicular Cancer Screening (PDQ®) – Patient Version," National Cancer Institute (NCI), September 29, 2021.

Testicular cancer is a disease in which malignant (cancer) cells form in the tissues of one or both testicles.

The testicles are 2 egg-shaped glands inside the scrotum (a sac of loose skin that lies directly below the penis). The testicles are held within the scrotum by the spermatic cord. The spermatic cord also contains the vas deferens and vessels and nerves of the testicles.

The testicles are the male sex glands and make testosterone and sperm. Germ cells in the testicles make immature sperm. These sperm travel through a network of tubules (tiny tubes) and larger tubes into the epididymis (a long coiled tube next to the testicles). This is where the sperm mature and are stored.

Almost all testicular cancers start in the germ cells. The two main types of testicular germ cell tumors are seminomas and nonseminomas.

Testicular cancer is the most common cancer in men aged 15 to 34 years.

Testicular cancer is very rare, but it is the most common cancer found in men between the ages of 15 and 34. White men are four times more likely than Black men to have testicular cancer.

Testicular cancer can usually be cured.

Although the number of new cases of testicular cancer has doubled in the last 40 years, the number of deaths caused by testicular cancer has decreased greatly because of better treatments. Testicular cancer can usually be cured, even in late stages of the disease.

A condition called "cryptorchidism" (an undescended testicle) is a risk factor for testicular cancer.

Anything that increases the chance of getting a disease is called a "risk factor." Having a risk factor does not mean that you will get cancer; not having risk factors does not mean that you will not get cancer. Talk to your doctor if you think you may be at risk. Risk factors for testicular cancer include the following:

- Having cryptorchidism (an undescended testicle).
- Having a testicle that is not normal, such as a small testicle that does not work the way it should.
- Having testicular carcinoma in situ.
- Being a white man.
- Having a personal or family history of testicular cancer.
- Having Klinefelter syndrome.

Men who have cryptorchidism, a testicle that is not normal, or testicular carcinoma in situ have an increased risk of testicular cancer in one or both testicles, and need to be followed closely.

SCREENING FOR TESTICULAR CANCER

Tests Are Used to Screen for Different Types of Cancer When a Person Does Not Have Symptoms

Scientists study screening tests to find those with the fewest harms and most benefits. Cancer screening trials also are meant to show whether early detection (finding cancer before it causes symptoms) helps a person live longer or decreases a person's chance of dying from the disease. For some types of cancer, the chance of recovery is better if the disease is found and treated at an early stage.

There Is No Standard or Routine Screening Test for Testicular Cancer

There is no standard or routine screening test used for early detection of testicular cancer. Most often, testicular cancer is first found by men themselves, either by chance or during self-exam. Sometimes the cancer is found by a doctor during a routine physical exam.

No studies have been done to find out if testicular self-exams, regular exams by a doctor, or other screening tests in men with no symptoms would decrease the risk of dying from this disease. However, routine screening probably would not decrease the risk of dying from testicular cancer. This is partly because testicular cancer can usually be cured at any stage. Finding testicular cancer early may make it easier to treat. Patients who are diagnosed with testicular cancer that has not spread to other parts of the body may need less chemotherapy and surgery, resulting in fewer side effects.

If a lump is found in the testicle by the patient or during a routine physical exam, tests may be done to check for cancer. Some tests have risks, and may cause anxiety.

Section 48.12 | **Tumor Markers**

This section includes text excerpted from "Tumor Markers," National Cancer Institute (NCI), May 11, 2021.

WHAT ARE TUMOR MARKERS?

A tumor marker is anything present in or produced by cancer cells or other cells of the body in response to cancer or certain benign (noncancerous) conditions that provides information about a cancer, such as how aggressive it is, what kind of treatment it may respond to, or whether it is responding to treatment.

Tumor markers have traditionally been proteins or other substances that are made at higher amounts by cancer cells than normal cells. These can be found in the blood, urine, stool, tumors, or other tissues or bodily fluids of some patients with cancer. Increasingly, however, genomic markers (such as tumor gene mutations, patterns of tumor gene expression, and nongenetic changes in tumor DNA) that are found in tumors themselves and in tumor fragments shed into bodily fluids are being used.

Many different tumor markers have been characterized and are in clinical use. Some are associated with only one type of cancer, whereas others are associated with multiple different cancer types.

HOW ARE TUMOR MARKERS USED IN CANCER CARE?

There are two main types of tumor markers: circulating tumor markers and tumor tissue markers.

Circulating tumor markers can be found in the blood, urine, stool, or other bodily fluids of some patients with cancer. Circulating tumor markers are used to:

- Estimate prognosis
- Determine the stage of cancer
- Detect cancer that remains after treatment (residual disease) or that has returned after treatment
- Assess how well a treatment is working
- Monitor whether the treatment has stopped working

Although an elevated level of a circulating tumor marker may suggest the presence of cancer and can sometimes help to diagnose cancer, this alone is not enough to diagnose cancer. For example, noncancerous conditions can sometimes cause the levels of certain tumor markers to increase. In addition, not everyone with a particular type of cancer will have a higher level of a tumor marker associated with that cancer. Therefore, measurements of circulating tumor markers are usually combined with the results of other tests, such as biopsies or imaging, to diagnose cancer.

Tumor markers may also be measured periodically during cancer therapy. Such "serial measurements," which show how the level of a marker is changing over time, are usually more meaningful than a single measurement. For example, a decrease in the level of a circulating tumor marker may indicate that the cancer is responding to treatment, whereas an increasing or unchanged level may indicate that the cancer is not responding.

Circulating tumor markers may also be measured periodically after treatment has ended to check for recurrence (the return of cancer).

Examples of commonly used circulating tumor markers include calcitonin (measured in blood), which is used to assess treatment response, screen for recurrence, and estimate prognosis in medullary thyroid cancer; CA-125 (measured in blood), to monitor how well cancer treatments are working and if cancer has come back in ovarian cancer; and beta-2-microglobulin (measured in blood, urine, or cerebrospinal fluid), to estimate prognosis and follow response to treatment for multiple myeloma, chronic lymphocytic leukemia, and some lymphomas. Additional circulating tumor markers are described in the list of tumor markers in common use.

Tumor tissue (or cell) markers are found in the actual tumors themselves, typically in a sample of the tumor that is removed during a biopsy. Tumor tissue markers are used to:

- Diagnose, stage, and/or classify cancer
- Estimate prognosis
- Select an appropriate treatment (e.g., treatment with a targeted therapy)

Tumor tissue markers that indicate whether someone is a candidate for a particular targeted therapy are sometimes referred to as biomarkers for cancer treatment. Tests for these biomarkers are usually genetic tests that look for changes in genes that affect cancer growth.

Examples of tumor tissue markers that are used as biomarkers for cancer treatment include estrogen receptor and progesterone receptor, which are tested for to determine whether someone with breast cancer should get treatment with hormone therapy; *FGFR3* gene mutation analysis, to help determine treatment for patients with bladder cancer; and PD-L1, to see if people with any of a number of cancer types are candidates for treatment with an immune checkpoint inhibitor.

Because some tumors shed cells and genetic material into blood, it is sometimes possible to examine biomarkers in blood samples. Although these "liquid biopsies" are not yet routinely used, they have several potential advantages. Because they do not involve surgery, they can be done more frequently than standard biopsies. They can also be performed when surgical biopsies cannot, such as when tumors are difficult to reach or patients cannot tolerate surgery.

Liquid biopsy tests can often detect multiple cancer-associated biomarkers. For example, the Foundation One Liquid CDx test is approved for the detection of genetic mutations in 324 genes and two genomic signatures in any solid tumor type. The test can also identify which patients with nonsmall cell lung cancer, melanoma, breast cancer, colorectal cancer, or ovarian cancer may benefit from 15 different U.S. Food and Drug Administration (FDA)-approved targeted treatment options.

DOES THE NCI HAVE GUIDELINES FOR THE USE OF TUMOR MARKERS?

The National Cancer Institute (NCI) does not have guidelines for the use of tumor markers. However, some national and international organizations have guidelines for the use of tumor markers for some types of cancer:

- The American Society of Clinical Oncology (ASCO) has developed and published *Clinical Practice Guidelines* on a variety of topics, including tumor markers for breast cancer, colorectal cancer, lung cancer, and others.
- The National Academy of Clinical Biochemistry publishes *Laboratory Medicine Practice Guidelines*, including Use of Tumor Markers in Clinical Practice: Quality Requirements, which focuses on the appropriate use of tumor markers for specific cancers.

Because tumor markers are detected using biospecimens (tissue and blood samples), the National Cancer Institute publishes best practices for biospecimen collection, processing, and storage.

CAN TUMOR MARKERS BE USED IN CANCER SCREENING?

Because tumor markers can be used to predict the response of a tumor to treatment and for prognosis, researchers have hoped that they might also be useful in screening tests that aim to detect cancer early, before there are any symptoms.

However, studies to see whether circulating tumor markers can be used to screen for cancer have generally found that these markers do not identify everyone with the disease (they are not sensitive enough) or that they indicate the possible presence of cancer in people who do not have it (they are not specific enough). When a test has low specificity, people have to have further testing to determine whether cancer is present. And some screening tests based on tumor markers have been shown to lead to overdiagnosis, which happens when people are diagnosed with cancers that would never have affected them during their lifetimes.

For example, the prostate-specific antigen (PSA) test was used routinely in the past to screen men for prostate cancer. However, as more was learned about the limitations of the test (including relatively low specificity), medical groups began to recommend against using it for routine population screening.

Several liquid biopsy–based assays that test for multiple tumor markers to detect cancer early, in people without symptoms, are in development:

- PapSEEK identifies ovarian and endometrial cancer–related alterations in DNA obtained from fluids collected during a routine Pap test. In a study that included women already diagnosed with cancer, the test was able to detect some endometrial and ovarian cancers at early, more treatable stages.
- CancerSEEK is a blood test that detects DNA mutations and protein biomarkers linked to multiple types of cancer. In a large trial of women with no history of cancer that combined the blood test with whole-body PET imaging, 65 percent of cancers that were detected were at an early stage.
- UroSEEK is a urine-based test that detects the most common alterations in 11 genes linked to bladder and upper tract urothelial cancers. In a study that included patients not yet diagnosed with bladder cancer, but at high risk of the disease because of symptoms, UroSEEK identified 83 percent of those who developed bladder cancer.

Although these tests are able to detect early cancers, it is not yet known whether treating those cancers would actually reduce deaths from these cancers.

Chapter 49 | Sleep Disorder Tests

A variety of conditions plague the sleep of Americans. These sleep disorders include:

- Sleep deficiency (irregular sleep schedules that result in not getting enough sleep)
- Sleep apnea (a condition that causes pauses in breathing, shallow breaths, and occasionally snoring during sleep)
- Insomnia (trouble falling or staying asleep)
- Restless legs syndrome (also called "Willis-Ekbom disease")
- Narcolepsy (vivid dreams, daytime sleepiness, brief periods of deep sleep, sleep paralysis, muscle weakness)
- Parasomnias (abnormal sleep behaviors)

The challenge with sleep disorders is that unlike many other medical conditions, your health-care provider depends on you to explain the problem, which occurs in the privacy of your bedroom while you are sleeping. There is no pain associated with sleep disorders. Instead, people often have daytime symptoms, such as a morning headache or daytime sleepiness. There is no blood test to help diagnose a sleep disorder. Instead, successful diagnosis depends on the patient. It is important to discuss your symptoms with your physician so she or he can help you determine if you have sleep apnea or another sleep disorder.

This chapter includes text excerpted from "Sports and Concussion," MedlinePlus, National Institutes of Health (NIH), 2015. Reviewed October 2021.

DIAGNOSING SLEEP DISORDERS

Depending on your symptoms, it may help you to gather information on your sleep behaviors. Your health-care provider will review this information and consider several possible tests when trying to diagnose a sleep disorder:

Sleep History and Sleep Log

If you believe you have a sleep problem, consider keeping a sleep diary and bringing it to your next medical appointment. Your physician will ask you how many hours you sleep each night, how often you awaken during the night and for how long, how long it takes you to fall asleep, how well rested you feel upon awakening, and how sleepy you feel during the day. If you do not already keep a sleep diary, your health professional may ask you to keep one for a few weeks. Your provider also may ask you whether you have any symptoms of a sleep disorder, such as loud snoring, snorting or gasping, morning headaches, tingling or unpleasant sensations in the limbs that are relieved by moving them, and jerking of the limbs during sleep. You may want to ask your sleeping partner if you have these symptoms, since you may not be aware of them yourself.

Sleep Recording in a Sleep Laboratory

A sleep recording or polysomnogram (PSG) may be done while you stay overnight at a sleep center or at home. Your doctor will suggest the appropriate location for the PSG based on your symptoms and health. Electrodes and other monitors are placed on your scalp, face, chest, limbs, and finger. While you sleep, these devices measure your brain activity, eye movements, muscle activity, heart rate and rhythm, blood pressure, and how much air moves in and out of your lungs. This test also checks the amount of oxygen in your blood. A PSG test is painless. In certain circumstances, the PSG can be done at home. A home monitor can be used to record heart rate, how air moves in and out of your lungs, the amount of oxygen in your blood, and your breathing effort.

Multiple Sleep Latency Test

This daytime sleep study measures how sleepy you are and is particularly useful for diagnosing problems staying awake during the day. The multiple sleep latency test (MSLT) is conducted in a sleep laboratory and typically done after an overnight sleep recording (PSG). In this test, monitoring devices for sleep stage are placed on your scalp and face. You are asked to nap four or five times for 20 minutes every two hours during the day. Technicians note how quickly you fall asleep and how long it takes you to reach various stages of sleep, especially REM (rapid eye movement) sleep, during your naps. Normal individuals either do not fall asleep during these short, designated naptimes or take a long time to fall asleep. People who fall asleep in less than five minutes are likely to require treatment for a sleep disorder, as are those who quickly reach REM sleep during their naps.

Chapter 50 | **Orthopedic/ Musculoskeletal Examinations**

The muscles, bones, joints, and connective tissues constitute the human musculoskeletal system. An orthopedic/musculoskeletal examination is performed to evaluate the musculoskeletal system and is conducted based on a patient's complaint. It comprises a series of clinical assessments performed by a trained examiner. There are three types of examinations that include:

- A screening examination – A brief assessment of the musculoskeletal system.
- A comprehensive examination – A more detailed examination performed by certified rheumatologists.
- A regional examination – A focused evaluation of a joint or any other structure.

Prior to an orthopedic examination, the examiner must consider factors such as:

- Movement limitations
- Affected joint or joints
- Degree and progression of pain
- Manner of injury, if injured
- History of pain in the same area

A routine orthopedic/musculoskeletal examination comprises procedures such as:

- Inspection
- Palpation
- Determining the range of motion (ROM)
- Neurological examination
- Special tests to evaluate a particular disorder

The examination also includes assessments of muscle strength and movements. In addition, the surrounding tissues, skin changes, lesions in the skin, muscle atrophy, and inflammation are evaluated.

PROCEDURE OF AN ORTHOPEDIC/MUSCULOSKELETAL EXAMINATION

Inspection. It is primarily a visual inspection where any abnormalities on the skin or the musculoskeletal system are detected by visually comparing structures on both sides of the body for any differences.

Palpation. It is the process of feeling or checking an object on the body with one's hands. The patient is examined for temperature changes on the skin of the joint or joints caused by perfusion or infections. Any bony protrusions are also evaluated for tenderness. If lumps are present, their mobility, fluctuation, and texture are also assessed.

Determining the range of motion (ROM). It is an assessment where the maximum range of movement in a joint is measured in degrees and is mediated through:

- Active ROM, where the patient moves the joint voluntarily
- Passive ROM, where the examiner moves the patient's joint

If any pain is noticed during measurement, it is recorded for further diagnosis. A goniometer and inclinometer are used to measure the angles of motion in a joint.

Conducting neurological examinations. A neurological examination of the affected joint is undertaken with a neuropathy impairment score (NIS). The scale uses stimuli such as touch-pressure, pinprick, and vibration, and the scoring system is categorized as:

- 0 – Normal
- 1 – Decreased
- 2 – Absent

Special tests. Other tests are prescribed for patients with complaints in their joints and includes:

- **Spine.** Schober test, neck compression tests, straight leg raise tests, and Mennell sign.
- **Arm and hand.** Mill test, Cozen test, Tinel sign, hand elevation test, and Finkelstein test.
- **Hip joint.** Trendelenburg test, FABER test, and Thomas test.
- **Knee joint.** Anterior drawer test, Lachman test, patellar tap test, and knee bulge test.

Strength evaluation. Joint and muscle strength are evaluated with the help of a muscle strength scale developed by the Medical Research Council (MRC) that categorizes muscle strength from 0–5.

An orthopedic/musculoskeletal examination is crucial in formulating early interventions for musculoskeletal disorders as it helps identify the functional anatomy of specific clinical conditions. In addition, these interventions can help effectively treat chronic musculoskeletal conditions.

References

1. Villela, Renato C; Anil Kumar Reddy Reddivari. "Musculoskeletal Examination," StatPearls, September 8, 2021.
2. Dai, Lei; Zeng, Rui. "Physical Examination of the Musculoskeletal System," *Handbook of Clinical Diagnostics*, August 27, 2019.
3. Goldberg, Charlie. "Musculo-Skeletal Examination," University of California San Diego (UCSD) School of Medicine, February 5, 2006.
4. "Orthopedic Examination Findings," AMBOSS, May 28, 2021.

Chapter 51 | Sports Assessments

All athletes, professional or amateur, are required to undergo a preparticipation physical evaluation (PPE) before participating in any sport. The assessment comprises a series of exercises that help to evaluate an athlete's overall health. Although PPEs cannot prevent mortality during sports, they help detect serious conditions and provide strategies to prevent injuries. A wide range of standardized tests are used for these exams, some intended for medical purposes and some to determine if an athlete is qualified to participate.

PURPOSE OF PREPARTICIPATION PHYSICAL EVALUATION

- Prevent injury
- Collect baseline data such as blood tests
- Ensure optimal medical and musculoskeletal health
- Optimize performance
- Review medications and vaccinations

MEDICAL SCREENING

- **History.** The medical history helps shed light on any underlying medical conditions and covers areas such as asthma, neurological disorders, concussion, musculoskeletal problems, hematologic disorders, etc. For athletes under the age of 18, a parent or guardian should provide full history.

- **Neurological screening.** It provides a history of spinal cord injury, seizure disorder, concussion, or cervical spine disorder.
- **Musculoskeletal screening.** It helps assess the range of motion, muscle strength, muscle asymmetry and identifying significant injuries. It also helps determine recovery from any previous injuries.
- **Cardiovascular screening.** Along with the initial auscultation of the heart with the patient in various positions, a series of specific questions related to cardiovascular risk factors are asked. Cardiac testing such as electrocardiography (ECG) and echocardiography are not required unless patient history suggests it.
- **General medical screening.** This includes full blood count, glucose levels, lipid profile, etc. It helps to find out if the athlete is anemic and reviews medications taken by the athlete.

BENEFITS OF TESTING

The results from tests can help determine:

- Weakness, if any
- Future performance
- Improvement in current performance
- The success of the training program
- The correct training group for the athlete

Factors that influence test results:

- The ambiance (temperature, humidity, noise level, etc.)
- Inappropriate warm-up
- Presence of other people
- The amount of sleep the athlete got the previous night
- Any medications that the athlete is taking
- The emotional state of the athlete
- Athlete's caffeine intake
- Athlete's last meal

- The surface of the test environment (gym, track, grass, road)
- Athletes attire (shoes and clothes)
- Environmental conditions such as wind and rain
- Athlete's knowledge of the test before the experience

COMMON FITNESS TESTS

General Health Evaluation

Before starting a fitness program, it is advisable to get the necessary approval from the doctor and share the medical history with the trainer. Then, the trainer will use one or more screening tools to determine baseline health. This includes basic health information such as an individual's height, weight, resting blood pressure (RBP), and resting heart rate (RHR). The trainer may also ask to fill the Physical Activity Readiness Questionnaire (PAR-Q) to understand the athlete's general health.

Body Composition Testing

Body composition testing is a way to measure the different components that make up the total body weight (muscles, bones, and fat). The most common methods to measure body composition include:

- **Skinfold measurements.** With the help of calipers, the estimated amount of fat present in the skinfold is measured.
- **Body mass index (BMI).** This is calculated based on the person's height and weight.
- **Bioelectrical impedance analysis (BIA).** Electrodes placed on the soles of feet send electrical signals to the abdomen and provide an estimated body composition.

Cardiovascular Endurance Testing

This is also known as "stress testing" and helps measure how effectively the heart and lungs work to supply oxygen and energy to the body during physical activity. The most common tests used are:

- **Exercise stress.** Performed on a stationary bike or treadmill to measure vital signs via a heart monitor and blood pressure cuff.
- **12-minute run test.** This is used to measure the preexercise heart and respiration rate with the postexercise heart and respiration rate. It is performed on a treadmill.
- **VO2 max testing.** This is used to measure the rate of oxygen intake during an activity. It is performed on a stationary bike or treadmill.

Strength and Endurance Testing

Strength testing measures the amount of force a muscle group can exert at a point. Endurance testing is used to measure the time taken for a muscle group to contract and release before it gets tired. This test helps the trainer identify muscle groups that are strong and the ones that need to be strengthened.

Flexibility Testing

It is vital to measure flexibility of the joints to help determine postural imbalances, limitations in range of motion, and foot stability. Three common tests to measure flexibility are:

- **Sit-and-reach testing.** Used to measure the tightness of the lower back and hamstring muscles, this test is performed while sitting on the floor with the legs fully extended. Flexibility is calculated by the number of inches the hands are from the feet while reaching forward to touch the toes.
- **Shoulder flexibility testing.** It is also called the "zipper test" and tests the flexibility of the shoulder joints. It is performed by using one hand to reach behind the neck, between the shoulders, and the other reaching behind the back towards the shoulder.
- **Trunk lift testing.** This is performed while lying face-down on the floor with the arms at the side. You would have to lift your upper body with just your back

muscles. The number of inches one can lift off the ground measures flexibility.

Performance Evaluation Tests

How well a task is performed is based on performance. Meeting performance aims helps to identify how well a training program is working. Testing and measuring are the two means of collecting information. The performance evaluation decisions are based on these. The evaluation process is a recurrent six-step process that includes:

- Selecting characteristics to be measured
- Selecting a suitable method of measuring
- Collecting the data
- Analyzing the collected data
- Making decisions
- Implementing those decisions

Sport Specific Tests

Table 51.1. List of Sport Specific Tests

AFL	Running vertical jump, reaction time, sprint recovery test, agility
Boxing	Quick strike, punching speed and punching power
Baseball	Sprint test from home to first base
Basketball	Lane agility, sprint 3/4 court, max touch, reactive shuttle
Cricket	Run-a-three, 17.68 sprint
Cycling	40-m cycle sprint, 2-km time trial, cycling VO2 max
Ice hockey	Shuttle cross pickup, on-ice beep test
Rowing	Rowing beep test, 500-m rowing ergometer test, 2-km rowing ergo test, 5-K rowing ergo
Rugby union	J.A.M. intermittent test
Football/Soccer	Loughborough intermittent shuttle test, yo-yo intermittent tests, balsom agility, FIFA interval test 1 and test 2, FIFA CODA test, FIT interval test, ARIET, footeval, futsal intermittent endurance test

Table 51.1. Continued

Swimming	Swimming beep test, swimming step test, critical swim speed, swimming beep (Williams), SWOLF, VO2 max swimming test, 12-minute swimming test
Water polo	Vertical jump in the water, shuttle swim test and the intermittent shuttle test
Triathlon	1-km swim, 100-m swim
Skiing (Alpine)	Hexagonal obstacle

Drug Testing in Sport

Drug or antidoping testing is done in sports to ensure that athletes are not using illegal and banned substances such as performance-enhancing drugs to gain an advantage over their competition. A sample of the athlete's urine, blood, and saliva are collected and tested for:

- Cocaine
- Stimulants (caffeine, amphetamines, or ephedra)
- Marijuana
- Alcohol
- Human growth hormone (HGH)
- Steroids

These drug assessments are done to prevent cheating at sports and protect athletes' health and identify athletes who may have substance abuse problems. The athlete submits their blood, urine, or saliva sample in the presence of a testing official who ensures that procedure for submission is followed, the sample belongs to the athlete, and that the sample is not tampered with.

References

1. "Screening in Sport," *Physiopedia*, June 6, 2016.
2. "Performance Evaluation Tests," BrianMAC Sports Coach, January 2, 2012.
3. Quinn, Elizabeth. "How a Fitness Test Is Performed," Verywell Fit, April 18, 2020.
4. "Drug Testing in Sports," Tufts Medical Center Community Care, n.d.
5. "Sport Specific Testing," Topend Sports, August 9, 2021.

Part 6 | **Home and Self-Ordered Tests**

Chapter 52 | An Introduction to Home-Use Medical Tests

Home-use tests allow you to test for some diseases or conditions at home. These tests are cost-effective, quick, and confidential. Home-use tests can help:

- Detect possible health conditions when you have no symptoms, so that you can get early treatment and lower your chance of developing later complications (i.e., cholesterol testing, hepatitis testing).
- Detect specific conditions when there are no signs so that you can take immediate action (i.e., pregnancy testing).
- Monitor conditions to allow frequent changes in treatment (i.e., glucose testing to monitor blood sugar levels in diabetes).

Despite the benefits of home testing, you should take precautions when using home-use tests.

- **See your health-care provider regularly.** Home-use tests are intended to help you with your healthcare, but they should not replace periodic visits to your doctor.
    - Most tests are best evaluated together with your medical history, a physical exam, and other testing.

This chapter contains text excerpted from the following sources: Text in this chapter begins with excerpts from "Home Use Tests," U.S. Food and Drug Administration (FDA), April 4, 2019; Text under the heading "How You Can Get the Best Results with Home Use Tests" is excerpted from "How You Can Get the Best Results with Home Use Tests," U.S. Food and Drug Administration (FDA), December 28, 2017. Reviewed October 2021.

- Always see your doctor if you are feeling sick, are worried about a possible medical condition, or if the test instructions recommend you do so.
- **Always use new test strips that are authorized for sale in the United States.** The U.S. Food and Drug Administration (FDA) has issued a safety communication warning about the risks of using previously owned test strips or test strips that are not authorized for sale in the U.S.

HOW YOU CAN GET THE BEST RESULTS WITH HOME-USE TESTS

Follow the tips listed here to use home-use tests as safely and effectively as possible.

- **Read the label and instructions carefully.** Review all instructions and pictures carefully to make sure you understand how to perform the test. Be sure you know:
  - What the test is for and what it is not for
  - How to store the test before you use it
  - How to collect and store the sample
  - When and how to run the test, including timing instructions
  - How to interpret the test
  - What might interfere with the test
  - The manufacturer's phone number if you have questions
- **Use only tests regulated by FDA.** There are several ways to find out if FDA regulates a home-use test. You can ask your pharmacist or the vendor selling the test. If FDA does not regulate the test, the U.S. government has not determined that the test is reasonably safe or effective, or substantially equivalent to another legally marketed device.
- **Follow all instructions.** You must follow all test instructions to get an accurate result. Most home tests require specific timing, materials, and sample amounts. You should also check the expiration dates and storage conditions before performing a test to make sure the components still work correctly.

- Keep good records of your testing.
- Call the "800" telephone number listed on your home-use test if you have any questions.
- **When in doubt, contact your doctor.** All tests can give false results. You should see your doctor if you believe your test results are wrong.
- Do not change medications or dosages based on a home-use test without talking to your doctor.

Chapter 53 | **Gynecological-Related Home Tests**

Chapter Contents

Section 53.1 | Ovulation (Saliva Test)

This section includes text excerpted from "Ovulation (Saliva Test)," U.S. Food and Drug Administration (FDA), February 4, 2018. Reviewed October 2021.

WHAT DOES THIS TEST DO?

This is a home-use test kit to predict ovulation by looking at patterns formed by your saliva. When your estrogen increases near your time of ovulation, your dried saliva may form a fern-shaped pattern.

WHAT TYPE OF TEST IS THIS?

This is a qualitative test – you find out whether or not you may be near your ovulation time, not if you will definitely become pregnant.

WHY SHOULD YOU DO THIS TEST?

You should do this test if you want to know when you expect to ovulate and be in the most fertile part of your menstrual cycle. This test can be used to help you plan to become pregnant. You should not use this test to help prevent pregnancy, because it is not reliable for that purpose.

HOW ACCURATE IS THIS TEST?

This test may not work well for you. Some of the reasons are:

- Not all women fern
- You may not be able to see the fern
- Women who fern on some days of their fertile period, do not necessarily fern on all of their fertile days
- Ferning may be disrupted by:
    - Smoking
    - Eating
    - Drinking
    - Brushing your teeth
    - How you put your saliva on the slide
    - Where you were when you did the test

HOW DO YOU DO THIS TEST?

In this test, you get a small microscope with built-in or removable slides. You put some of your saliva on a glass slide, allow it to dry, and look at the pattern it makes. You will see dots and circles, a fern (full or partial), or a combination depending on where you are in your monthly cycle.

You will get your best results when you use the test within the 5-day period around your expected ovulation. This period includes the 2 days before and the 2 days after your expected day of ovulation. The test is not perfect, though, and you might fern outside of this time period or when you are pregnant. Even some men will fern.

IS THIS TEST SIMILAR TO THE ONE YOUR DOCTOR USES?

The fertility tests your doctor uses are automated, and they may give more consistent results. Your doctor may use other tests that are not yet available for home-use (i.e., blood and urine laboratory tests) and information about your history to get a better view of your fertility status.

DOES A POSITIVE TEST MEAN YOU ARE OVULATING?

A positive test indicates that you may be near ovulation. It does not mean that you will definitely become pregnant.

DO NEGATIVE TEST RESULTS MEAN THAT YOU ARE NOT OVULATING?

No, there may be many reasons why you did not detect your time of ovulation. You should not use this test to help prevent pregnancy, because it is not reliable for that purpose.

Section 53.2 | **Ovulation (Urine Test)**

This section includes text excerpted from "Ovulation (Urine Test)," U.S. Food and Drug Administration (FDA), February 4, 2018. Reviewed October 2021.

WHAT DOES THIS TEST DO?

This is a home-use test kit to measure luteinizing hormone (LH) in your urine. This helps detect the LH surge that happens in the middle of your menstrual cycle, about 1-1½ days before ovulation. Some tests also measure another hormone – estrone-3-glucuronide (E_3G).

WHAT IS LUTEINIZING HORMONE?

Luteinizing hormone (LH) is a hormone produced by your pituitary gland. Your body always makes a small amount of LH, but just before you ovulate, you make much more LH. This test can detect this LH surge, which usually happens 1-1½ days before you ovulate.

WHAT IS ESTRONE-3-GLUCURONIDE?

E_3G is produced when estrogen breaks down in your body. It accumulates in your urine around the time of ovulation and causes your cervical mucus to become thin and slippery. Sperm may swim more easily in your thin and slippery cervical mucus, increasing your chances of getting pregnant.

WHAT TYPE OF TEST IS THIS?

This is a qualitative test – you find out whether or not you have elevated LH or E_3G levels, not if you will definitely become pregnant.

WHY SHOULD YOU DO THIS TEST?

You should do this test if you want to know when you expect to ovulate and be in the most fertile part of your menstrual cycle. This test can be used to help you plan to become pregnant. You should not use this test to help prevent pregnancy, because it is not reliable for that purpose.

HOW ACCURATE IS THIS TEST?

How well this test will predict your fertile period depends on how well you follow the instructions. These tests can detect LH and E_3G reliably about 9 times out of 10, but you must do the test carefully.

HOW DO YOU DO THIS TEST?

You add a few drops of your urine to the test, hold the tip of the test in your urine stream, or dip the test in a cup of your urine. You either read the test by looking for colored lines on the test or you put the test device into a monitor. You can get results in about 5 minutes. The details of what the color looks like, or how to use the monitor varies among the different brands.

Most kits come with multiple tests to allow you to take measurements over several days. This can help you find your most fertile period, the time during your cycle when you can expect to ovulate based on your hormone levels. Follow the instructions carefully to get good results. You will need to start your testing at the proper time during your cycle, otherwise the test will be unreliable, and you will not find your hormonal surges or your fertile period.

IS THIS TEST SIMILAR TO THE ONE YOUR DOCTOR USES?

The fertility tests your doctor uses are automated, and they may give more consistent results. Your doctor may use other tests that are not yet available for home-use (i.e., blood and urine laboratory tests) and information about your history to get a better view of your fertility status.

Section 53.3 | **Home Pregnancy Test**

This section includes text excerpted from "Pregnancy," U.S. Food and Drug Administration (FDA), April 29, 2019.

WHAT DOES THIS TEST DO?

This is a home-use test kit to measure human chorionic gonadotropin (hCG) in your urine. You produce this hormone only when you are pregnant.

WHAT IS HUMAN CHORIONIC GONADOTROPIN?

hCG is a hormone produced by your placenta when you are pregnant. It appears shortly after the embryo attaches to the wall of the uterus. If you are pregnant, this hormone increases very rapidly. If you have a 28 day menstrual cycle, you can detect hCG in your urine 12-15 days after ovulation.

WHAT TYPE OF TEST IS THIS?

This is a qualitative test – you find out whether or not you have elevated hCG levels indicating that you are pregnant.

WHY SHOULD YOU DO THIS TEST?

You should use this test to find out if you are pregnant.

HOW ACCURATE IS THIS TEST?

The accuracy of this test depends on how well you follow the instructions and interpret the results. If you mishandle or misunderstand the test kit, you may get poor results.

Most pregnancy tests have about the same ability to detect hCG, but their ability to show whether or not you are pregnant depends on how much hCG you are producing. If you test too early in your cycle or too close to the time you became pregnant, your placenta may not have had enough time to produce hCG. This would mean that you are pregnant, but you got a negative test result.

Because many women have irregular periods, and women may miscalculate when their period is due, 10 to 20 pregnant women out of every 100 will not detect their pregnancy on the first day of their missed period.

HOW DO YOU DO THIS TEST?

For most home pregnancy tests, you either hold a test strip in your urine stream or you collect your urine in a cup and dip your test strip into the cup. If you are pregnant, most test strips produce a colored line, but this will depend on the brand you purchased. Read the instructions for the test you bought and follow them carefully. Make sure you know how to get good results. The test usually takes only about 5 minutes.

The different tests for sale vary in their abilities to detect low levels of hCG. For the most reliable results, test 1-2 weeks after you miss your period. There are some tests for sale that are sensitive enough to show you are pregnant before you miss your period.

You can improve your chances for an accurate result by using your first morning urine for the test. If you are pregnant, it will have more hCG in it than later urines. If you think you are pregnant, but your first test was negative, you can take the test again after several days. Since the amount of hCG increases rapidly when you are pregnant, you may get a positive test on later days. Some test kits come with more than one test in them to allow you to repeat the test.

IS THIS TEST SIMILAR TO THE ONE YOUR DOCTOR USES?

The home pregnancy test and the test your doctor uses are similar in their abilities to detect hCG, however your doctor is probably more experienced in running the test. If you produce only a small amount of hCG, your doctor may not be able to detect it any better than you could. Your doctor may also use a blood test to see if you are pregnant. Finally, your doctor may have more information about you from your history, physical exam, and other tests that may give a more reliable result.

DOES A POSITIVE TEST MEAN YOU ARE PREGNANT?

Usually, yes, but you must be sure to read and interpret the results correctly.

DO NEGATIVE TEST RESULTS MEAN THAT YOU ARE NOT PREGNANT?

No, there are several reasons why you could receive false negative test results. If you tested too early in your cycle, your placenta may not have had time to produce enough hCG for the test to detect. Or, you may not have waited long enough before you took this test.

If you have a negative result, you would be wise to consider this a tentative finding. You should not use medications and should consider avoiding potentially harmful behaviors, such as smoking or drinking alcohol, until you have greater certainty that you are not pregnant.

You will probably recognize incorrect results with the passage of time. You may detect false negatives by the unexpected onset of menses (regular vaginal bleeding associated with "periods"). Repeat testing and/or other investigations such as ultrasound may provide corrected results.

Section 53.4 | **Home Vaginal pH Test**

This section includes text excerpted from "Vaginal pH," U.S. Food and Drug Administration (FDA), September 27, 2018. Reviewed October 2021.

WHAT DOES THIS TEST DO?

This is a home-use test kit to measure the pH of your vaginal secretions.

WHAT IS PH?

pH is a way to describe how acidic a substance is. It is given by a number on a scale of 1–14. The lower the number, the more acidic the substance.

WHAT TYPE OF TEST IS THIS?

This is a quantitative test – you find out how acidic your vaginal secretions are.

WHY SHOULD YOU DO THIS TEST?

You should do this test to help evaluate if your vaginal symptoms (i.e., itching, burning, unpleasant odor, or unusual discharge) are likely caused by an infection that needs medical treatment. The test is not intended for human immunodeficiency virus (HIV), chlamydia, herpes, gonorrhea, syphilis, or group B streptococcus.

HOW ACCURATE IS THIS TEST?

Home vaginal pH tests showed good agreement with a doctor's diagnosis. However, just because you find changes in your vaginal pH, does not always mean that you have a vaginal infection. pH changes also do not help or differentiate one type of infection from another. Your doctor diagnoses a vaginal infection by using a combination of: pH, microscopic examination of the vaginal discharge, amine odor, culture, wet preparation, and Gram stain.

DOES A POSITIVE TEST MEAN YOU HAVE A VAGINAL INFECTION?

No, a positive test (elevated pH) could occur for other reasons. If you detect elevated pH, you should see your doctor for further testing and treatment. There are no over-the-counter medications for treatment of an elevated vaginal pH.

If test results are negative, can you be sure that you do not have a vaginal infection? No, you may have an infection that does not show up in these tests. If you have no symptoms, your negative test could suggest the possibility of chemical, allergic, or other noninfectious irritation of the vagina. Or, a negative test could indicate the possibility of a yeast infection. You should see your doctor if you find changes in your vaginal pH or if you continue to have symptoms.

HOW DO YOU DO THIS TEST?

You hold a piece of pH paper against the wall of your vagina for a few seconds, then compare the color of the pH paper to the color on the chart provided with the test kit. The number on the chart for the color that best matches the color on the pH paper is the vaginal pH number.

IS THE HOME TEST SIMILAR TO YOUR DOCTOR'S TEST?

Yes. The home vaginal pH tests are practically identical to the ones sold to doctors. But your doctor can provide a more thorough assessment of your vaginal status through your history, physical exam, and other laboratory tests than you can using a single pH test in your home.

Section 53.5 | **Menopause Home Test**

This section includes text excerpted from "Menopause," U.S. Food and Drug Administration (FDA), September 27, 2018. Reviewed October 2021.

WHAT IS MENOPAUSE?

Menopause is the stage in your life when menstruation stops for at least 12 months. The time before this is called "perimenopause" and could last for several years. You may reach menopause in your early 40's or as late as your 60's.

WHAT DOES THIS TEST DO?

This is a home-use test kit to measure follicle stimulating hormone (FSH) in your urine. This may help indicate if you are in menopause or perimenopause. FSH is produced by your pituitary gland. FSH levels increase temporarily each month to stimulate your ovaries to produce eggs. When you enter menopause and your ovaries stop working, your FSH levels also increase.

WHAT TYPE OF TEST IS THIS?

This is a qualitative test – you find out whether or not you have elevated FSH levels, not if you definitely are in menopause or perimenopause.

WHY SHOULD YOU DO THIS TEST?

You should use this test if you want to know if your symptoms, such as irregular periods, hot flashes, vaginal dryness, or sleep problems are part of menopause. While many women may have little or no trouble when going through the stages of menopause, others may have moderate-to-severe discomfort and may want treatment to alleviate their symptoms. This test may help you be better informed about your current condition when you see your doctor.

HOW ACCURATE IS THIS TEST?

These tests will accurately detect FSH about 9 out of 10 times. This test does not detect menopause or perimenopause. As you grow older, your FSH levels may rise and fall during your menstrual cycle. While your hormone levels are changing, your ovaries continue to release eggs and you can still become pregnant.

Your test will depend on whether you:

- Used your first morning urine,
- Drank large amounts of water before the test,
- Use, or recently stopped using, oral or patch contraceptives, hormone replacement therapy, or estrogen supplements.

HOW DO YOU DO THIS TEST?

In this test, you put a few drops of your urine on a test device, put the end of the testing device in your urine stream, or dip the test device into a cup of urine. Chemicals in the test device react with FSH and produce a color. Read the instructions with the test you buy to learn exactly what to look for in this test.

ARE THE HOME MENOPAUSE TESTS SIMILAR TO THE ONES YOUR DOCTOR USES?

Some home menopause tests are identical to the one your doctor uses. However, doctors would not use this test by itself. Your doctor would use your medical history, physical exam, and other laboratory tests to get a more thorough assessment of your condition.

DOES A POSITIVE TEST MEAN YOU ARE IN MENOPAUSE?

A positive test indicates that you may be in a stage of menopause. If you have a positive test, or if you have any symptoms of menopause, you should see your doctor. Do not stop taking contraceptives based on the results of these tests because they are not foolproof and you could become pregnant.

DO NEGATIVE TEST RESULTS INDICATE THAT YOU ARE NOT IN MENOPAUSE?

If you have a negative test result, but you have symptoms of menopause, you may be in perimenopause or menopause. You should not assume that a negative test means you have not reached menopause, there could be other reasons for the negative result. You should always discuss your symptoms and your test results with your doctor. Do not use these tests to determine if you are fertile or can become pregnant. These tests will not give you a reliable answer on your ability to become pregnant.

Chapter 54 | **Cholesterol Home-Use Test**

WHAT DOES THIS TEST DO?

This is a home-use test kit to measure total cholesterol.

WHAT IS CHOLESTEROL?

Cholesterol is a fat (lipid) in your blood. High-density lipoprotein (HDL) ("good" cholesterol) helps protect your heart, but low-density lipoprotein (LDL) ("bad" cholesterol) can clog the arteries of your heart. Some cholesterol tests also measure triglycerides, another type of fat in the blood.

WHAT TYPE OF TEST IS THIS?

This is a quantitative test – you find out the amount of total cholesterol present in your sample.

HOW OFTEN YOU SHOULD DO THIS TEST?

If you are more than 20 years old, you should test your cholesterol about every 5 years. If your doctor has you on a special diet or drugs to control your cholesterol, you may need to check your cholesterol more frequently. Follow your doctor's recommendations about how often you test your cholesterol.

This chapter includes text excerpted from "Cholesterol," U.S. Food and Drug Administration (FDA), February 4, 2018. Reviewed October 2021.

WHAT YOUR CHOLESTEROL LEVELS SHOULD BE?

Your total cholesterol level should be 200mg/dL or less, according to recommendations in the National Cholesterol Education Program (NCEP) Third Adult Treatment Panel (ATP III). You should try to keep your LDL values less than 100 mg/dL, your HDL values greater or equal to 40 mg/dL, and your triglyceride values less than 150 mg/dL.

HOW ACCURATE IS THIS TEST?

This test is about as accurate as the test your doctor uses, but you must follow the directions carefully.

Total cholesterol tests vary in accuracy from brand to brand. Information about the test's accuracy is printed on its package. Tests that say they are "traceable" to a program of the Centers for Disease Control and Prevention (CDC) may be more accurate than others.

WHAT SHOULD YOU DO IF YOUR TEST SHOWS HIGH CHOLESTEROL?

Talk to your doctor if your test shows that your cholesterol is higher than 200 mg/dL. Many things can cause high cholesterol levels including diet, exercise, and other factors. Your doctor may want you to test your cholesterol again.

HOW DO YOU DO THIS TEST?

You prick your finger with a lancet to get a drop of blood. Then put the drop of blood on a piece paper that contains special chemicals. The paper will change color depending on how much cholesterol is in your blood. Some testing kits use a small machine to tell you how much cholesterol there is in the sample.

Chapter 55 | Diabetes Home Test

Chapter Contents

Section 55.1 | Monitoring Blood Sugar

This section includes text excerpted from "Blood Glucose Monitoring Devices," U.S. Food and Drug Administration (FDA), April 4, 2019.

WHAT IS GLUCOSE?

Glucose is a sugar that your body uses as a source of energy. Unless you have diabetes, your body regulates the amount of glucose in your blood. People with diabetes may need special diets and medications to control blood glucose.

WHAT SHOULD YOUR GLUCOSE LEVELS BE?

According to the American Diabetes Association (ADA), the blood glucose levels for an adult without diabetes are below 100 mg/dL before meals and fasting and are less than 140 mg/dL two hours after meals.

People with diabetes should consult their doctor or health-care provider to set appropriate blood glucose goals. You should treat your low or high blood glucose as recommended by your health-care provider.

WHAT DOES THIS TEST DO?

This is a test system for use at home or in health-care settings to measure the amount of sugar (glucose) in your blood.

WHAT TYPE OF TEST IS THIS?

This is a quantitative test, which means that you will find out the amount of glucose present in your blood sample.

WHY SHOULD YOU TAKE THIS TEST?

You should take this test if you have diabetes and you need to monitor your blood sugar (glucose) levels. You and your doctor can use the results to:

- Determine your daily adjustments in treatment
- Know if you have dangerously high or low levels of glucose

- Understand how your diet and exercise change your glucose levels

The Diabetes Control and Complications Trial (1993) showed that good glucose control using home monitors led to fewer disease complications.

HOW OFTEN SHOULD YOU TEST YOUR GLUCOSE?

Follow your doctor's recommendations about how often you test your glucose. You may need to test yourself several times each day to determine adjustments in your diet or treatment.

HOW ACCURATE IS THIS TEST?

The accuracy of this test depends on many factors including:

- The quality of your meter
- The quality of your test strips
    - Always use new test strips that are authorized for sale in the United States. The U.S. Food and Drug Administration (FDA) has issued a safety communication warning about the risks of using previously owned test strips or test strips that are not authorized for sale in the United States
- How well you perform the test. For example, you should wash and dry your hands before testing and closely follow the instructions for operating your meter.
- Your hematocrit (the amount of red blood cells in the blood). If you are severely dehydrated or anemic, your test results may be less accurate. Your health-care provider can tell you if your hematocrit is low or high, and can discuss with you how it may affect your glucose testing.
- Interfering substances. (Some substances, such as vitamin C, Tylenol, and uric acid, may interfere with your glucose testing.) Check the instructions for your meter and test strips to find out what substances may affect the testing accuracy.

- Altitude, temperature, and humidity. (High altitude, low and high temperatures, and humidity can cause unpredictable effects on glucose results.) Check the meter manual and test strip package insert for more information.
- Store and handle the meter and strips according to manufacturer's instructions. It is important to store test strip vials closed.

HOW DO YOU TAKE THIS TEST?

Before you test your blood glucose, you must read and understand the instructions for your meter. In general, you prick your finger with a lancet to get a drop of blood. Then you place the blood on a disposable "test strip" that is inserted in your meter. The test strip contains chemicals that react with glucose. Some meters measure the amount of electricity that passes through the test strip. Others measure how much light reflects from it. In the U.S., meters report results in milligrams of glucose per deciliter of blood, or mg/dl.

You can get information about your meter and test strips from several different sources, including the toll-free number in the manual that comes with your meter or on the manufacturer's website. If you have an urgent problem, always contact your health-care provider or a local emergency room for advice.

HOW DO YOU CHOOSE A GLUCOSE METER?

There are many different types of meters available for purchase that differ in several ways, including:

- Accuracy
- Amount of blood needed for each test
- How easy it is to use
- Pain associated with using the product
- Testing speed
- Overall size
- Ability to store test results in memory
- Likelihood of interferences
- Ability to transmit data to a computer

- Cost of the meter
- Cost of the test strips used
- Doctor's recommendation
- Technical support provided by the manufacturer
- Special features such as automatic timing, error codes, large display screen, or spoken instructions or results

Talk to your health-care provider about the right glucose meter for you, and how to use it.

HOW CAN YOU CHECK YOUR METER'S PERFORMANCE?

There are three ways to make sure your meter works properly:

- To test a liquid control solution, you test a drop of these solutions just like you test a drop of your blood. The value you get should match the value written on the test strip vial label. Use liquid control solutions:
  - Every time you open a new container of test strips
  - Occasionally as you use the container of test strips
  - If you drop the meter
  - Whenever you get unusual results
- **Use electronic checks.** Every time you turn on your meter, it does an electronic check. If it detects a problem it will give you an error code. Look in your meter's manual to see what the error codes mean and how to fix the problem. If you are unsure if your meter is working properly, call the toll-free number in your meter's manual, or contact your health-care provider.
- **Compare your meter with a blood glucose test performed in a laboratory.** Take your meter with you to your next appointment with your health-care provider. Ask your provider to watch your testing technique to make sure you are using the meter correctly. Ask your health-care provider to have your blood tested with a laboratory method. If the values you obtain on your glucose meter match the laboratory values, then your meter is working well and you are using good technique.

WHAT SHOULD YOU DO IF YOUR METER MALFUNCTIONS?

If your meter malfunctions, you should tell your health-care provider and contact the company that made your meter and strips.

CAN YOU TEST BLOOD GLUCOSE FROM SITES OTHER THAN YOUR FINGERS?

Some meters allow you to test blood from sites other than the fingertip. Examples of such alternative sampling sites are your palm, upper arm, forearm, thigh, or calf. Alternative site testing (AST) should not be performed at times when your blood glucose may be changing rapidly, as these alternative sampling sites may provide inaccurate results at those times. You should use only blood from your fingertip to test if any of the following applies:

- You have just taken insulin
- You think your blood sugar is low
- You are not aware of symptoms when you become hypoglycemic
- The results do not agree with the way you feel
- You have just eaten
- You have just exercised
- You are ill
- You are under stress

Also, you should never use results from an alternative sampling site to calibrate a continuous glucose monitor (CGM), or in insulin dosing calculations.

Section 55.2 | **Continuous Glucose Monitoring**

This section includes text excerpted from "Continuous Glucose Monitoring," National Institute of Diabetes and Digestive and Kidney Diseases (NIDDK), June 2017. Reviewed October 2021.

WHAT IS CONTINUOUS GLUCOSE MONITORING?

Continuous glucose monitoring (CGM) automatically tracks blood glucose levels, also called "blood sugar," throughout the day and night. You can see your glucose level anytime at a glance. You can also review how your glucose changes over a few hours or days to see trends. Seeing glucose levels in real time can help you make more informed decisions throughout the day about how to balance your food, physical activity, and medicines.

HOW DOES A CONTINUOUS GLUCOSE MONITOR WORK?

A CGM works through a tiny sensor inserted under your skin, usually on your belly or arm. The sensor measures your interstitial glucose level, which is the glucose found in the fluid between the cells. The sensor tests glucose every few minutes. A transmitter wirelessly sends the information to a monitor.

The monitor may be part of an insulin pump or a separate device, which you might carry in a pocket or purse. Some CGMs send information directly to a smartphone or tablet. Several models are available and are listed in the American Diabetes Association's (ADA) product guide.

Special Features of a Continuous Glucose Monitoring

Continuous glucose monitors are always on and recording glucose levels – whether you are showering, working, exercising, or sleeping. Many CGMs have special features that work with information from your glucose readings:

- An alarm can sound when your glucose level goes too low or too high.
- You can note your meals, physical activity, and medicines in a CGM device, too, alongside your glucose levels.
- You can download data to a computer or smart device to more easily see your glucose trends.

Some models can send information right away to a second person's smartphone – perhaps a parent, partner, or caregiver. For example, if a child's glucose drops dangerously low overnight, the CGM could be set to wake a parent in the next room.

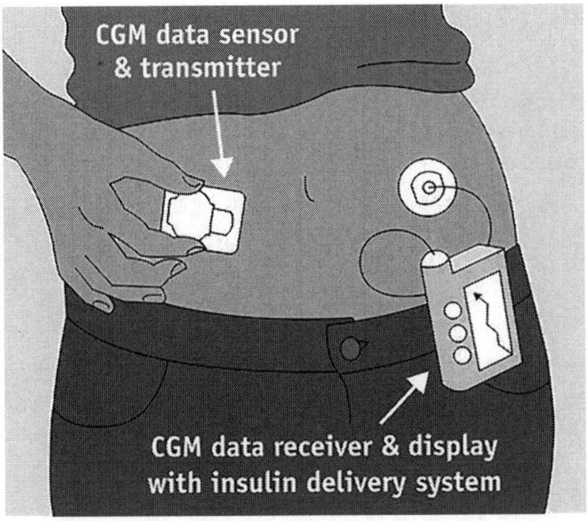

Figure 55.1. Continuous Glucose Monitoring System

A tiny CGM sensor under the skin checks glucose. A transmitter sends data to a receiver. The CGM receiver may be part of an insulin pump, as shown here, or a separate device.

Currently, one CGM model is approved for treatment decisions, the Dexcom G5 Mobile. That means you can make changes to your diabetes care plan based on CGM results alone. With other models, you must first confirm a CGM reading with a fingerstick blood glucose test before you take insulin or treat hypoglycemia.

Special Requirements Needed to Use a Continuous Glucose Monitoring

Twice a day, you may need to check the CGM itself. You will test a drop of blood on a standard glucose meter. The glucose reading should be similar on both devices.

You will also need to replace the CGM sensor every 3 to 7 days, depending on the model.

For safety it is important to take action when a CGM alarm sounds about high or low blood glucose. You should follow your treatment plan to bring your glucose into the target range, or get help.

WHO CAN USE A CONTINUOUS GLUCOSE MONITORING?

Most people who use CGMs have type 1 diabetes. Research is underway to learn how CGMs might help people with type 2 diabetes.

CGMs are approved for use by adults and children with a doctor's prescription. Some models may be used for children as young as age 2. Your doctor may recommend a CGM if you or your child:

- Are on intensive insulin therapy, also called "tight blood sugar control"
- Have hypoglycemia unawareness
- Often have high or low blood glucose

Your doctor may suggest using a CGM system all the time or only for a few days to help adjust your diabetes care plan.

WHAT ARE THE BENEFITS OF A CONTINUOUS GLUCOSE MONITORING?

Compared with a standard blood glucose meter, using a CGM system can help you:

- Better manage your glucose levels every day
- Have fewer low blood glucose emergencies
- Need fewer finger sticks

A graphic on the CGM screen shows whether your glucose is rising or dropping – and how quickly – so you can choose the best way to reach your target glucose level.

Over time, good management of glucose greatly helps people with diabetes stay healthy and prevent complications of the disease. People who gain the largest benefit from a CGM are those who use it every day or nearly every day.

WHAT ARE THE LIMITS OF A CONTINUOUS GLUCOSE MONITORING?

Researchers are working to make CGMs more accurate and easier to use. But, you still need a fingerstick glucose test twice a day to check the accuracy of your CGM against a standard blood glucose meter.

With most CGM models, you cannot yet rely on the CGM alone to make treatment decisions. For example, before changing your insulin dose, you must first confirm a CGM reading by doing a fingerstick glucose test.

A CGM system is more expensive than using a standard glucose meter. Check with your health insurance plan or Medicare to see whether the costs will be covered.

Chapter 56 | HIV Home Test

WHAT DOES THIS TEST DO?

This is a home-use collection kit to detect whether or not you have antibodies to HIV (human immunodeficiency virus). HIV is the virus that causes AIDS (acquired immunodeficiency syndrome).

WHAT TYPE OF TEST IS THIS?

This is a qualitative test – you find out whether or not you have this infection, not how advanced your disease is.

WHY SHOULD YOU DO THIS TEST?

You should do this test to find out if you have an HIV infection. If you know that you have an HIV infection:

- You can obtain medical treatment that helps slow the course of the disease, and
- You can take precautions to keep from infecting others.

Untreated, HIV destroys your immune system. The most advanced stage of HIV infection is AIDS, an often – fatal disease.

WHEN SHOULD YOU DO THIS TEST?

You should do this test if you believe there is a chance you may have an HIV infection. You are at greatest risk for HIV if you:

- Have ever shared injection drug needles and syringes or "works."
- Have ever had sex without a condom with someone who had HIV.

This chapter includes text excerpted from "Human Immunodeficiency Virus (HIV)," U.S. Food and Drug Administration (FDA), September 27, 2018. Reviewed October 2021.

- Have ever had a sexually transmitted disease (STD), like chlamydia or gonorrhea.
- Received a blood transfusion or a blood-clotting factor between 1978 and 1985.
- Have ever had sex with someone who has done any of those things

If you use this test, no one, but you will know you were tested for HIV or what the results showed.

HOW ACCURATE IS THIS TEST?

This test is similar to the test your doctor would use. Researchers have found that about 90 of 100 home-users were able to obtain acceptable samples for sending to the laboratory. After the laboratory got these 90 samples, they could get results for about 81 of 100 of them. Of these 81 samples, the laboratory almost always shows whether or not the person tested had HIV infection.

DOES A POSITIVE TEST MEAN YOU HAVE HIV?

If you test positive in this test, you are infected with the HIV virus. You should take precautions so you do not spread this infection to your sexual partners or others who might be at risk. You should not donate blood because this infection could spread to others. Having HIV infection does not necessarily mean you have AIDS. You should see your doctor so you can learn the status of your disease and decide what therapy, if any, you need.

IF YOUR RESULTS ARE NEGATIVE, CAN YOU BE SURE THAT YOU DO NOT HAVE HIV INFECTION?

If you test negative for HIV, it means you did not have antibodies to HIV at the time of the test. However, if you are newly infected, it will take time for you to make antibodies. It is uncertain how long it may take you to develop antibodies – it may take more than 3 months. So, although you may be infected, the results of your testing will not verify that you are infected for several months.

If you think you were exposed to the virus and might be infected, you should test yourself again in a few months.

HOW DO YOU DO THIS TEST?

The test comes with sterile lancets, an alcohol pad, gauze pads, a blood specimen collection card, a bandage, a lancet disposal container, a shipping pouch, and instructions. To do the test, you:

- Call a specified telephone number,
- Register a code number that is included with the specimen collection kit,
- Prick your finger with a lancet to get a drop of blood,
- Place drops of blood on the card,
- Send the shipping pouch by express courier service to the central testing laboratory,
- Receive results by phone after 3 to 7 business days later, and
- If you test positive for HIV, you get counseling on what to do about your infection.

Chapter 57 | Prothrombin Home Test

WHAT DOES THIS TEST DO?

This is a home-use test kit to measure how long it takes for your blood to clot.

WHAT TYPE OF TEST IS THIS?

This is a quantitative test – you find out the length of time it takes your blood to clot.

WHY SHOULD YOU DO THIS TEST?

If you take blood-thinning drugs such as coumadin or warfarin, you may need to test you blood regularly to make sure it clots properly. Doctors often prescribe these drugs to prevent blood clots in patients who have artificial heart valves, irregular heartbeats or inherited clotting tendencies. Your doctor will prescribe this test for you if you need to do it.

HOW OFTEN SHOULD YOU DO THIS TEST?

You should follow your doctor's instructions about how often you do this test. Your doctor may ask you to use the results to adjust the amount of drugs you to take to control your blood clotting. Never change the drugs you take without your doctor's permission.

This chapter includes text excerpted from "Prothrombin," U.S. Food and Drug Administration (FDA), September 27, 2018. Reviewed October 2021.

HOW DO YOU DO THIS TEST?

You prick your finger with a lancet to get a drop of blood. Place the drop of blood on a test strip or cartridge, and insert it into your test meter. Your meter will measure how long it takes for the blood to form a clot and how much anticoagulant effect there is.

HOW CAN YOU MAKE SURE YOUR METER WORKS PROPERLY?

Your meter has some built-in features that allow it to test itself and detect problems in its operation. Your meter comes with sample solutions to use instead of your blood to assure that it is working properly. Look in your meter's operator manual to see how to check on its accuracy.

Take your meter with you to your doctor's office. Have your doctor watch you do your testing. Your doctor may want to take a sample of your blood and compare the clotting time of that sample with the time your meter gives. If the value you get matches your doctor's value, that you will know your meter is working well and that you are doing the test correctly.

Chapter 58 | Drugs of Abuse Home Tests

WHAT DO THESE TESTS DO?

These tests indicate if one or more prescription or illegal drugs are present in urine. These tests detect the presence of drugs such as marijuana, cocaine, opiates, methamphetamine, amphetamines, phencyclidine (PCP), benzodiazepine, barbiturates, methadone, tricyclic antidepressants, ecstasy, and oxycodone.

The testing is done in two steps. First, you do a quick at-home test. Second, if the test suggests that drugs may be present, you send the sample to a laboratory for additional testing.

WHAT ARE DRUGS OF ABUSE?

Drugs of abuse are illegal or prescription medicines (e.g., oxycodone or Valium) that are taken for a nonmedical purpose. Nonmedical purposes for a prescription drug include taking the medication for longer than your doctor prescribed it for or for a purpose other than what the doctor prescribed it for. Medications are not drugs of abuse if they are taken according to your doctor's instructions.

WHAT TYPE OF TEST ARE THESE?

They are qualitative tests – you find out if a particular drug may be in the urine, but not how much is present.

This chapter includes text excerpted from "Drugs of Abuse Home Use Test," U.S. Food and Drug Administration (FDA), September 27, 2018. Reviewed October 2021.

WHEN SHOULD YOU DO THESE TESTS?

You should use these tests when you think someone might be abusing prescription or illegal drugs. If you are worried about a specific drug, make sure to check the label to confirm that this test is designed to detect the drug you are looking for.

HOW ACCURATE ARE THESE TESTS?

The at-home testing part of this test is fairly sensitive to the presence of drugs in the urine. This means that if drugs are present, you will usually get a preliminary (or presumptive) positive test result. If you get a preliminary positive result, you should send the urine sample to the laboratory for a second test.

It is very important to send the urine sample to the laboratory to confirm a positive at-home result because certain foods, food supplements, beverages, or medicines can affect the results of at-home tests. Laboratory tests are the most reliable way to confirm drugs of abuse.

Many things can affect the accuracy of these tests, including (but not limited to):

- The way you did the test
- The way you stored the test or urine
- What the person ate or drank before taking the test
- Any other prescription or over-the-counter drugs the person may have taken before the test

Note that a result showing the presence of an amphetamine should be considered carefully, even when this result is confirmed in the laboratory testing. Some over-the-counter medications will produce the same test results as illegally-abused amphetamines.

DOES A POSITIVE TEST MEAN THAT YOU FOUND DRUGS OF ABUSE?

No. Take no serious actions until you get the laboratory's result. Remember that many factors may cause a false positive result in the home test.

Remember that a positive test for a prescription drug does not mean that a person is abusing the drug, because there is no way for the test to indicate acceptable levels compared to abusive levels of prescribed drugs.

IF THE TEST RESULTS ARE NEGATIVE, CAN YOU BE SURE THAT THE PERSON YOU TESTED DID NOT ABUSE DRUGS?

No. No drug test of this type is 100 percent accurate. There are several factors that can make the test results negative even though the person is abusing drugs. First, you may have tested for the wrong drugs. Or, you may not have tested the urine when it contained drugs. It takes time for drugs to appear in the urine after a person takes them, and they do not stay in the urine indefinitely; you may have collected the urine too late or too soon. It is also possible that the chemicals in the test went bad because they were stored incorrectly or they passed their expiration date.

If you get a negative test result, but still suspect that someone is abusing drugs, you can test again at a later time. Talk to your doctor if you need more help deciding what steps to take next.

HOW SOON AFTER A PERSON TAKES DRUGS, WILL THEY SHOW UP IN A DRUG TEST? AND HOW LONG AFTER A PERSON TAKES DRUGS, WILL THEY CONTINUE TO SHOW UP IN A DRUG TEST?

The drug clearance rate tells how soon a person may have a positive test after taking a particular drug. It also tells how long the person may continue to test positive after the last time she or he took the drug. Clearance rates for common drugs of abuse are given below. These are only guidelines, however, and the times can vary significantly from these estimates based on how long the person has been taking the drug, the amount of drug they use, or the person's metabolism.

HOW DO YOU DO A DRUGS OF ABUSE TEST?

These tests usually contain a sample collection cup, the drug test (it may be test strips, a test card, a test cassette, or other method for

Table 58.1. Drug Clearance Rates for Common Drugs of Abuse

Drug	How Soon after Taking Drug Will There Be a Positive Drug Test?	How Long after Taking Drug Will There Continue to Be a Positive Drug Test?
Marijuana/Pot	1–3 hours	1–7 days
Crack (Cocaine)	2–6 hours	2–3 days
Heroin (Opiates)	2–6 hours	1–3 days
Speed/Uppers (Amphetamine, methamphetamine)	4–6 hours	2–3 days
Angel Dust/PCP	4–6 hours	7–14 days
Ecstasy	2–7 hours	2–4 days
Benzodiazepine	2–7 hours	1–4 days
Barbiturates	2–4 hours	1–3 weeks
Methadone	3–8 hours	1–3 days
Tricyclic antidepressants	8–12 hours	2–7 days
Oxycodone	1–3 hours	1–2 days

testing the urine), and an instruction leaflet or booklet. It is very important that the person doing the test reads and understands the instructions first, before even collecting the sample. This is important because with most test kits, the result must be visually read within a certain number of minutes after the test is started.

You collect urine in the sample collection cup and test it according to the instructions. If the test indicates the preliminary presence of one or more drugs, the sample should be sent to a laboratory where a more specific chemical test will be used order to obtain a final result. Some home-use kits have a shipping container and preaddressed mailer in them. If you have questions about using these tests, or the results that you are getting, you should contact your health-care provider.

Chapter 59 | Direct-to-Consumer Genetic Testing

WHAT IS DIRECT-TO-CONSUMER GENETIC TESTING?

Most of the time, genetic testing is done through health-care providers such as physicians, nurse practitioners, and genetic counselors. Health-care providers determine which test is needed, order the test from a laboratory, collect and send the deoxyribonucleic acid (DNA) sample, interpret the test results, and share the results with the patient. Often, a health insurance company covers part or all of the cost of testing.

Direct-to-consumer genetic testing is different: these genetic tests are marketed directly to customers via television, print advertisements, or the Internet, and the tests can be bought online or in stores. Customers send the company a DNA sample and receive their results directly from a secure website or in a written report. Direct to consumer genetic testing provides people access to their genetic information without necessarily involving a health-care provider or health insurance company in the process.

Dozens of companies currently offer direct-to-consumer genetic tests for a variety of purposes. The most popular tests use genetic variations to make predictions about health, provide information about common traits, and offer clues about a person's ancestry. The number of companies providing direct-to-consumer genetic testing is growing, along with the range of health conditions and traits covered by these tests. Because there is currently little regulation of direct-to-consumer genetic testing services, it is important to assess the quality of available services before pursuing any testing.

This chapter includes text excerpted from "Direct-to-Consumer Genetic Testing," MedlinePlus, National Institutes of Health (NIH), September 10, 2020.

Other names for direct-to-consumer genetic testing include DTC genetic testing, direct-access genetic testing, at-home genetic testing, and home DNA testing. Ancestry testing (also called "genealogy testing") is also considered a form of direct-to-consumer genetic testing.

WHAT KINDS OF DIRECT-TO-CONSUMER GENETIC TESTS ARE AVAILABLE?

With so many companies offering direct-to-consumer genetic testing, it can be challenging to determine which tests will be most informative and helpful to you. When considering testing, think about what you hope to get out of the test. Some direct-to-consumer genetic tests are very specific (such as paternity tests), while other services provide a broad range of health, ancestry, and lifestyle information.

Major types of direct-to-consumer genetic tests include:

Disease Risk and Health

The results of these tests estimate your genetic risk of developing several common diseases, such as celiac disease, Parkinson disease, and Alzheimer disease. Some companies also include a person's carrier status for less common conditions, including cystic fibrosis and sickle cell disease. A carrier is someone who has one copy of a gene mutation that, when present in two copies, causes a genetic disorder. The tests may also look for genetic variations related to other health-related traits, such as weight and metabolism (how a person's body converts the nutrients from food into energy).

Ancestry or Genealogy

The results of these tests provide clues about where a person's ancestors might have come from, their ethnicity, and genetic connections between families.

Kinship

The results of these tests can indicate whether tested individuals are biologically related to one another. For example, kinship testing can establish whether one person is the biological father of another (paternity testing). The results of direct-to-consumer kinship tests, including paternity tests, are usually not admissible in a court of law.

Lifestyle

The results of these tests claim to provide information about lifestyle factors, such as nutrition, fitness, weight loss, skincare, sleep, and even your wine preferences, based on variations in your DNA. Many of the companies that offer this kind of testing also sell services, products, or programs that they customize on the basis of your test results.

Before choosing a direct-to-consumer genetic test, find out what kinds of health, ancestry, or other information will be reported to you. Think about whether there is any information you would rather not know. In some cases, you can decline to find out specific information if you tell the company before it delivers your results.

WHAT ARE THE BENEFITS AND RISKS OF DIRECT-TO-CONSUMER GENETIC TESTING?

Direct-to-consumer genetic testing has both benefits and limitations, although they are somewhat different than those of genetic testing ordered by a health-care provider.

Benefits

- Direct-to-consumer genetic testing promotes awareness of genetic diseases.
- It provides personalized information about your health, disease risk, and other traits.
- It may help you be more proactive about your health.
- It does not require approval from a health-care provider or health insurance company.
- It is often less expensive than genetic testing obtained through a health-care provider.
- DNA sample collection is usually simple and noninvasive, and results are available quickly.

- Your data is added to a large database that can be used to further medical research. Depending on the company, the database may represent up to several million participants.

Risks and Limitations

- Tests may not be available for the health conditions or traits that interest you.
- This type of testing cannot tell definitively whether you will or will not get a particular disease.
- Unexpected information that you receive about your health, family relationships, or ancestry may be stressful or upsetting.
- People may make important decisions about disease treatment or prevention based on inaccurate, incomplete, or misunderstood information from their test results.
- There is currently little oversight or regulation of testing companies.
- Unproven or invalid tests can be misleading. There may not be enough scientific evidence to link a particular genetic variation with a given disease or trait.
- Genetic privacy may be compromised if testing companies use your genetic information in an unauthorized way or if your data is stolen.
- The results of genetic testing may impact your ability to obtain life, disability, or long-term care insurance.

Direct-to-consumer genetic testing provides only partial information about your health. Other genetic and environmental factors, lifestyle choices, and family medical history also affect the likelihood of developing many disorders. These factors would be discussed during a consultation with a doctor or genetic counselor, but in many cases they are not addressed when using at-home genetic tests.

HOW IS DIRECT-TO-CONSUMER GENETIC TESTING DONE?

For most types of direct-to-consumer genetic testing, the process involves:

Purchasing a Test

Test kits can be purchased online (and are shipped to your home) or at a store. The price of some test kits includes the analysis and interpretation, while in other cases this information is purchased separately.

Collecting the Sample

Collection of the DNA sample usually involves spitting saliva into a tube or swabbing the inside of your cheek. You then mail the sample as directed by the company. In some cases, you will need to visit a health clinic to have blood drawn.

Analyzing the Sample

A laboratory will analyze the sample to look for particular genetic variations. The variations included in the test depend on the purpose of the test.

Receiving Results

In most cases, you will be able to access your results on a secure website. Other test companies share results in the mail or over the phone. The results usually include interpretation of what specific genetic variations may mean for your health or ancestry. In some cases, a genetic counselor or other health-care provider is available to explain the results and answer questions.

The test kit will include step-by-step instructions, so be sure you understand them before you begin. If you have questions, contact the company before collecting your sample.

WHAT DO THE RESULTS OF DIRECT-TO-CONSUMER GENETIC TESTING MEAN?

Direct-to-consumer genetic testing can provide interesting information about your health, traits, and ancestry. However, the results may not be as clear-cut as many people assume. Companies that provide these tests often tell their customers that the results are for information, education, and research purposes only – they are not meant to diagnose, prevent, or treat any disease or health condition. It is useful to keep this distinction in mind when interpreting your own test results.

Health and Disease Risk

The results of these genetic tests provide information about your chance of developing certain diseases and the likelihood that you have particular traits (such as dimples or lactose intolerance). These results are usually based on an analysis of one or more genetic variations that are known or suspected to be associated with the disease or trait.

The results of tests to predict disease risk do not provide a "yes or no" answer about whether a person will develop a given disease. Other factors, including genetic variations that were not tested, environmental factors, and lifestyle choices (such as diet and exercise) also contribute to disease risk in ways that may not be fully understood. Therefore, a result showing an increased risk does not mean you will definitely develop the disease, and a result showing a reduced risk does not mean you will never develop the disease.

Ancestry

The results of these tests give clues about major geographic areas that are your family's origins. These results are calculated on the basis of genetic variations that are more common in people from certain areas of the world than in others. You may also choose to receive information about individuals who are likely related to you. (These individuals have also undergone testing, and the predictions are based on similarities among DNA sequences.)

Sometimes the results of ancestry testing are unexpected or inconsistent with what a person understands about her or his family history. These tests can uncover previously unknown information about biological relationships among people (such as paternity). People who are closely related, such as siblings, may receive slightly different information about their ancestry because results are limited by the number and diversity of people who have submitted DNA samples to a given direct-to-consumer genetic testing company. It is important to be aware that receiving unexpected or ambiguous information about your background or family is a potential risk with this type of testing.

Lifestyle

In most cases, direct-to-consumer lifestyle tests assess genetic variations related to very specific traits, such as how your body converts the nutrients from food into energy (metabolism), day/night (circadian) rhythm, or the senses of taste and smell. The company may recommend specific diet or fitness programs, dietary supplements, skincare products, or other products and services on the basis of your results. However, in most cases the link between a given genetic variation and a complex trait like weight, athletic performance, or sleep is indirect or unknown. Therefore, the results of these tests can be challenging to interpret, and it can be difficult to predict whether a recommended product or service will be helpful to you.

If you have questions about the meaning of your test results, professional support (such as guidance from a genetic counselor) may be available from the company that provided the test. You can also share questions about your results with your own health-care provider. Talk to your doctor before making any major changes in managing your health, diet, or fitness after you receive results of a direct-to-consumer genetic test.

Chapter 60 | COVID-19 Self-Testing

Testing is critically important to help reduce the spread of coronavirus disease (COVID-19).

If you need to be tested for COVID-19 and cannot get tested by a health-care provider, you can consider using either a self-collection kit or a self-test that can be performed at home or anywhere else. Sometimes a self-test is also called a "home test" or an "at-home test." The U.S. Food and Drug Administration (FDA) provides information on which self-tests are authorized for use.

These self-collection kits and tests are available either by prescription or over the counter (OTC), without a prescription, in a pharmacy or retail store. At present, self-collection kits and tests are used for the detection of current infection.

TYPES OF SPECIMENS

- Some tests require a nasal specimen that can be collected using an anterior nasal swab or a nasal mid-turbinate swab.
- Other tests require a saliva specimen.

PREPARE TO COLLECT A SPECIMEN

- Wash your hands with soap.
- Open the box and follow the manufacturer's instructions included with the specimen collection or test kit to collect your own nasal or saliva specimen.

This chapter includes text excerpted from "Self-Testing," Centers for Disease Control and Prevention (CDC), October 4, 2021.

- If you do not collect the specimens as directed, your test results may be incorrect.

Once collected, send the specimen to a testing facility or use the specimen, as described in the manufacturer's instructions, to complete the self-test.

PERFORMING THE TEST

Follow the manufacturer's instructions exactly and perform the steps in the order that they are listed. The manufacturer may also provide other resources, such as quick reference guides or instructional videos, to help you perform the test correctly.

Tips

- Store all test components according to the manufacturer's instructions until ready for use.
- Check the expiration date. Do not use expired tests or test components that are damaged or appear discolored based on the manufacturer's instructions.
- Clean the countertop, table, or other surfaces where you will do the test.
- Do not open test devices or other test components until you are ready to start the testing process.
- Read and record test results only within the amount of time specified in the manufacturer's instructions. A result read before or after the specified timeframe may be incorrect.
- Do not reuse test devices or other components.

After you have the results, discard the specimen collection swab and test kit in the trash, clean all surfaces that the specimen may have touched, and wash your hands.

REPORTING RESULTS

Give your results to your health-care provider or, if you do not have a health-care provider, to your local or state health department.

Some self-tests have an app that will automatically report your results to the appropriate public-health authorities.

IF YOUR TEST IS POSITIVE

Tell a health-care provider about your positive test result and stay in contact with them during your illness. If your illness becomes severe, seek medical attention. To avoid spreading the virus to others, follow the Centers for Disease Control and Prevention (CDC) recommendations.

As much as possible, stay in a specific room and away from other people and pets in your home or place of residence. If possible, you should use a separate bathroom. If you need to be around other people or animals in or outside of the home or place of residence, wear a mask. Do not share personal household items, like cups, towels, and utensils. Monitor your symptoms. If you have an emergency warning sign (including trouble breathing), seek emergency medical care immediately.

Tell your close contacts that they may have been exposed to SARS-CoV-2, the virus that causes COVID-19. An infected person can spread COVID-19 starting 48 (or 2 days) before the person has any symptoms or tests positive. By letting your close contacts know they may have been exposed to COVID-19, you are helping to protect everyone.

IF YOUR TEST IS NEGATIVE

A negative test result means that SARS-CoV-2, the virus that causes COVID-19, was not found in your specimen. If you took the test while you had symptoms and followed all instructions carefully, a negative result means your current illness is probably not COVID-19.

However, it is possible for a test to give a negative result in some people who have COVID-19. This is called a "false negative." You could also test negative if the specimen was collected too early in your infection. In this case, you could test positive later during your illness.

Some self-tests are designed to be used in a series. Serial testing is when a person tests themselves multiple times for COVID-19 on a routine basis, such as every few days. By testing more frequently, you might detect COVID-19 more quickly and could reduce the spread of infection. Some self-administered tests come with more than one test and instructions for performing serial testing.

If your self-test is negative, you should follow the manufacturer's instructions for serial testing that are included within the kit during purchase, or you can find the instructions for your test (molecular or antigen) on the FDA website. They will likely recommend you test again within 2 or 3 days. Contact a health-care provider if you have any questions about your test results or serial testing. You may also use the COVID-19 Viral Testing Tool to help you determine the next steps after testing. If you have COVID-19 symptoms, especially if you have been exposed to someone who has COVID-19, you should quarantine according to CDC recommendations.

IF YOUR RESULT SHOWS INVALID OR ERROR

Sometimes the results are inconclusive or not clear, and the test cannot tell you if your results are positive or negative.

If the display on the self-test shows an invalid result or a test error, the test did not work properly. If this happens, refer to the instructions for use in the package insert and contact the manufacturer for assistance.

Invalid results can occur for many reasons. Your specimen may not have been collected correctly, or the testing instrument may have malfunctioned. Invalid test results are rare, but can occur.

Regardless of what your test results are, you should always review the results with a health-care provider. The health-care provider will consider the test result together with your symptoms and possible exposure in deciding how to care for you.

Part 7 | Additional Help and Information

Chapter 61 | Glossary of Terms Related to Medical Tests

anesthesia: A drug that is used to make you sleepy or to numb a part of your body before surgery so that you do not feel pain during the procedure.

angiography: A procedure to x-ray blood vessels. The blood vessels can be seen because of an injection of a dye that shows up in the x-ray.

A1c: A test that measures a person's average blood glucose level over the past two to three months.

arrhythmia: An abnormal heart rhythm. The heartbeats may be too slow, too rapid, too irregular, or too early.

assessment: In healthcare, a process used to learn about a patient's condition. This may include a complete medical history, medical tests, a physical exam, a test of learning skills, tests to find out if the patient is able to carry out the tasks of daily living, a mental-health evaluation, and a review of social support and community resources available to the patient.

biopsy: The removal of cells or tissues for examination by a pathologist. The pathologist may study the tissue under a microscope or perform other tests on the cells or tissue.

bronchoscopy: A procedure that uses a bronchoscope to examine the inside of the trachea, bronchi, and lungs. A bronchoscope is a thin, tube-like instrument with a light and a lens for viewing. It may also have a tool to remove tissue to be checked under a microscope for signs of disease.

chemotherapy: Treatment with drugs that kill cancer cells.

This glossary contains terms excerpted from documents produced by several sources deemed reliable.

colonoscopy: Examination of the inside of the colon using a colonoscope, inserted into the rectum. A colonoscope is a thin, tube-like instrument with a light and a lens for viewing. It may also have a tool to remove tissue to be checked under a microscope for signs of disease.

complete blood count (CBC): A test to check the number of red blood cells (RBCs), white blood cells (WBCs), and platelets in a sample of blood.

computed tomography (CT) scan: A series of detailed pictures of areas inside the body taken from different angles. The pictures are created by a computer linked to an x-ray machine.

contrast material: A dye or other substance that helps show abnormal areas inside the body. It is given by injection into a vein, by enema, or by mouth. Contrast material may be used with x-rays, CT scans, magnetic resonance imaging (MRI), or other imaging tests.

cystoscopy: Examination of the bladder and urethra using a cystoscope, inserted into the urethra. A cystoscope is a thin, tube-like instrument with a light and a lens for viewing. It may also have a tool to remove tissue to be checked under a microscope for signs of disease.

DEXA scan: An imaging test that measures bone density by passing x-rays with two different energy levels through the bone. It is used to diagnose osteoporosis.

dialysis: The process of filtering wastes from the blood artificially in a person with end-stage kidney disease.

elastography: A medical imaging technique that measures the elasticity or stiffness of a tissue. The technique captures snapshots of shear waves, a special type of sound wave, as they move through the tissue.

electrocardiogram (EKG): A line graph that shows changes in the electrical activity of the heart over time. It is made by an instrument called an "electrocardiograph" (ECG or EKG). The graph can show that there are abnormal conditions, such as blocked arteries, changes in electrolytes, and changes in the way electrical currents pass through the heart tissue.

electromagnetic radiation (EMR): Radiation that has both electric and magnetic fields and travels in waves. It comes from natural and human-made sources. Electromagnetic radiation can vary in strength from low energy to high energy. It includes radio waves, microwaves, infrared light, visible light, ultraviolet light, x-rays, and gamma rays.

endoscopic retrograde cholangiopancreatography (ERCP): A procedure that uses an endoscope to examine and x-ray the pancreatic duct, hepatic duct, common bile duct, duodenal papilla, and gallbladder. An endoscope is a thin, tube-like instrument with a light and a lens for viewing.

endoscopy: A procedure that uses an endoscope to examine the inside of the body. An endoscope is a thin, tube-like instrument with a light and a lens for viewing. It may also have a tool to remove tissue to be checked under a microscope for signs of disease.

false-positive test result: A test result that indicates that a person has a specific disease or condition when the person actually does not have the disease or condition.

fine-needle aspiration (FNA) biopsy: The removal of tissue or fluid with a thin needle for examination under a microscope.

fluoroscopy: An x-ray procedure that makes it possible to see internal organs in motion.

genetic testing: Analyzing deoxyribonucleic acid (DNA) to look for a genetic alteration that may indicate an increased risk for developing a specific disease or disorder.

histology: The study of tissues and cells under a microscope.

imaging: In medicine, a process that makes pictures of areas inside the body. Imaging uses methods such as x-rays and radio waves.

in vitro: A laboratory experiment or process performed in a test tube, culture dish, or elsewhere outside a living animal.

laboratory test: A medical procedure that involves testing a sample of blood, urine, or other substance from the body. Tests can help determine a diagnosis, plan treatment, check to see if treatment is working, or monitor the disease over time.

lower gastrointestinal (GI) series: X-rays of the colon and rectum that are taken after a person is given a barium enema.

lumbar puncture: A procedure in which a thin needle called a "spinal needle" is injected into the lower part of the spinal column to collect cerebrospinal fluid (CSF) or to give drugs.

magnetic resonance imaging (MRI): A procedure in which radio waves and a powerful magnet linked to a computer are used to create detailed pictures of areas inside the body. These pictures can show the difference between normal and diseased tissue. MRI makes better images of organs and soft tissue than other scanning techniques, such as computed tomography (CT) or x-ray. MRI is especially useful for imaging the brain, the spine, the soft tissue of joints, and the inside of bones.

mammogram: A mammogram is an x-ray picture of the breast. Doctors use a mammogram to look for early signs of breast cancer. Regular mammograms are the best tests doctors have to find breast cancer early, sometimes up to three years before it can be felt.

microscopy: Using microscopes to view samples and objects that cannot be seen with the unaided eye.

minimally invasive surgery: A surgical procedure typically utilizing one or more small incisions through which laparoscopic surgical tools are inserted and manipulated by a surgeon. Minimally invasive surgery can reduce damage to surrounding healthy tissue, decrease the need for pain medication, and reduce patient recovery time.

monitor: In healthcare, to regularly watch and check a person or condition to see if there is any change. Also refers to a device that records and/or displays patient data, such as for an electrocardiogram (EKG).

myelogram: An x-ray of the spinal cord after an injection of dye into the space between the lining of the spinal cord and brain.

newborn screening: The examination of blood samples from a newborn to detect disease-related abnormalities or deficiencies in gene products.

optical coherence tomography (OCT): A technique for obtaining subsurface images such as diseased tissue just below the skin. For example, ophthalmologists use OCT to obtain detailed images from within the retina. Cardiologists also use it to help diagnose coronary artery disease (CAD).

optical imaging: A technique for noninvasively looking inside the body, as is done with x-rays. Unlike x-rays, which use ionizing radiation, optical imaging uses visible light and the special properties of photons to obtain detailed images of organs and tissues as well as smaller structures including cells and molecules.

oral glucose tolerance test (OGTT): A test to diagnose prediabetes and diabetes, given after an overnight fast. Test results show how the body uses glucose over time.

Pap test: A test that finds changes in the cells of the cervix. The test can find cancer or cells that can turn into cancer. To perform a Pap test, a health-care provider uses a small brush to gently scrape cells from the cervix for examination under a microscope.

pelvic exam: A physical examination in which the health-care professional will feel for lumps or changes in the shape of the vagina, cervix, uterus, fallopian tubes, ovaries, and rectum. The health-care professional will also use a speculum to open the vagina to look at the cervix and take samples for a Pap test.

personal health record (PHR): An electronic application through which individuals can maintain and manage their health information (and that of others for whom they are authorized) in a private, secure, and confidential environment.

physical examination: An exam of the body to check for general signs of disease.
positive test result: A test result that reveals the presence of a specific disease or condition for which the test is being done.

positron emission tomography (PET) scan: A procedure in which a small amount of radioactive glucose is injected into a vein, and a scanner is used to make detailed, computerized pictures of areas inside the body where the glucose is used. Because cancer cells often use more glucose than normal cells, the pictures can be used to find cancer cells in the body.

radiation therapy: The use of high-energy radiation from x-rays, gamma rays, neutrons, protons, and other sources to kill cancer cells and shrink tumors. Radiation may come from a machine outside the body (external-beam radiation therapy), or it may come from radioactive material placed in the body near cancer cells (internal radiation therapy).

radiology: The use of radiation (such as x-rays) or other imaging technologies to diagnose or treat disease.

randomized clinical trial (RCT): A study in which the participants are assigned by chance to separate groups that compare different treatments and the treatments they receive can be compared objectively. At the time of the trial, it is not known which treatment is best. It is the patient's choice to be in a randomized trial.

screening: Checking for disease when there are no symptoms. Since screening may find diseases at an early stage, there may be a better chance of curing the disease. Screening can also include checking for a person's risk of developing an inherited disease by doing a genetic test.

sensors: In medicine and biotechnology, sensors are tools that detect specific biological, chemical, or physical processes and then transmit or report this data. Some sensors work outside the body while others are designed to be implanted within the body. Sensors help health-care providers and patients monitor health conditions.

sentinel lymph node biopsy (SLNB): Removal and examination of the sentinel nodes (the first lymph nodes to which cancer cells are likely to spread from a primary tumor).

sigmoidoscopy: Examination of the lower colon using a sigmoidoscope, inserted into the rectum. A sigmoidoscope is a thin, tube-like instrument with a light and a lens for viewing. It may also have a tool to remove tissue to be checked under a microscope for signs of disease.

single photon emission computed tomography (SPECT): A special type of computed tomography (CT) scan in which a small amount of a radioactive drug is injected into a vein and a scanner is used to make detailed images of areas inside the body where the radioactive material is taken up by the cells. SPECT can give information about blood flow to tissues and chemical reactions in the body.

skin test: A test for an immune response to a compound by placing it on or under the skin.

spinal fusion: A procedure where the entire disc is removed and replaced with a bone graft. In a spinal fusion, the two vertebrae are then fused together. Although the operation can cause the spine to stiffen, resulting in lost flexibility, the procedure serves one critical purpose: protection of the spinal cord.

telehealth: The use of communication technologies to provide and support healthcare at a distance.

ultrasound: A procedure in which high-energy sound waves are bounced off internal tissues or organs and make echoes. The echo patterns are shown on the screen of an ultrasound machine, forming a picture of body tissues called a "sonogram."

upper endoscopy: Examination of the inside of the stomach using an endoscope, passed through the mouth and esophagus. An endoscope is a thin, tube-like instrument with a light and a lens for viewing. It may also have a tool to remove tissue to be checked under a microscope for signs of disease.

upper gastrointestinal (GI) series: A series of x-ray pictures of the esophagus, stomach, and duodenum. The x-ray pictures are taken after the patient drinks a liquid containing barium sulfate. The barium sulfate coats and outlines the inner walls of the upper gastrointestinal tract so that they can be seen on the x-ray pictures.

ureteroscopy: Examination of the inside of the kidney and ureter, using a ureteroscope. A ureteroscope is a thin, tube-like instrument with a light and a lens for viewing. It may also have a tool to remove tissue to be checked under a microscope for signs of disease. The ureteroscope is passed through the urethra into the bladder, ureter, and renal pelvis.

urinalysis: A test that determines the content of the urine.

vaccine: A substance or an agent that provides active immunity to a particular infectious disease.

virtual colonoscopy (VC): A method to examine the inside of the colon by taking a series of x-rays. A computer is used to make two-dimensional and three-dimensional pictures of the colon from these x-rays. The pictures can be saved, changed to give better viewing angles, and reviewed after the procedure, even years later.

x-ray: A type of high-energy radiation. In low doses, x-rays are used to diagnose diseases by making pictures of the inside of the body. In high doses, x-rays are used to treat cancer.

Chapter 62 | **Organizations with Resources for People Undergoing Medical Tests**

GOVERNMENT ORGANIZATIONS THAT PROVIDE INFORMATION ABOUT MEDICAL TESTS

Agency for Healthcare Research and Quality (AHRQ)

5600 Fishers Ln.
7th Fl.
Rockville, MD 20857
Phone: 301-427-1364
Website: www.ahrq.gov
E-mail: AHRQPubs@ahrq.hhs.gov

Centers for Disease Control and Prevention (CDC)

1600 Clifton Rd.
Atlanta, GA 30329-4027
Toll-Free: 800-CDC-INFO (800-232-4636)
Phone: 404-639-3311
Toll-Free TTY: 888-232-6348
Website: www.cdc.gov
E-mail: cdcinfo@cdc.gov

Centers for Medicare & Medicaid Services (CMS)

7500 Security Blvd.
Baltimore, MD 21244
Toll-Free: 877-267-2323
Phone: 410-786-3000
TTY: 410-786-0727
Toll-Free TTY: 866-226-1819
Website: www.cms.gov
E-mail: CMSHealthInformaticsOffice@cms.hhs.gov

Federal Trade Commission (FTC)

600 Pennsylvania Ave., N.W.
Washington, DC 20580
Toll-Free: 877-FTC-HELP (877-382-4357)
Phone: 202-326-2222
Website: www.ftc.gov

Resources in this chapter were compiled from several sources deemed reliable; all contact information was verified and updated in October 2021.

National Cancer Institute (NCI)
9609 Medical Center Dr.
BG 9609, MSC 9760
Bethesda, MD 20892-9760
Toll-Free: 800-4-CANCER
(800-422-6237)
Website: www.cancer.gov
E-mail: NCIinfo@nih.gov

National Eye Institute (NEI)
31 Center Dr., MSC 2510
Bethesda, MD 20892-2510
Phone: 301-496-5248
Website: www.nei.nih.gov
E-mail: 2020@nei.nih.gov

National Institute of Diabetes and Digestive and Kidney Diseases (NIDDK)
9000 Rockville Pike
Bethesda, MD 20892
Toll-Free: 800-860-8747
Toll-Free TTY: 866-569-1162
Website: www.niddk.nih.gov
E-mail: healthinfo@niddk.nih.gov

National Institute of Mental Health (NIMH)
6001 Executive Blvd.
Rm. 6200, MSC 9663
Bethesda, MD 20892-9663
Toll-Free: 866-615-6464
Phone: 301-443-4536
TTY: 301-443-8431
Toll-Free TTY: 866-415-8051
Fax: 301-443-4279
Website: www.nimh.nih .gov
E-mail: nimhinfo@nih.gov

National Institute of Neurological Disorders and Stroke (NINDS)
P.O. Box 5801
Bethesda, MD 20824
Toll-Free: 800-352-9424
Website: www.ninds.nih.gov
E-mail: braininfo@ninds.nih.gov

National Institute on Aging (NIA)
31 Center Dr., MSC 2292
Bldg. 31, Rm. 5C27
Bethesda, MD 20892
Toll-Free: 800-222-2225
Toll-Free TTY: 800-222-4225
Website: www.nia.nih.gov
E-mail: niaic@nia.nih.gov

National Institute on Deafness and Other Communication Disorders (NIDCD)
31 Center Dr., MSC 2320
Bldg. 31, Rm. 5C27
Bethesda, MD 20892-2320
Toll-Free: 800-241-1044
Phone: 301-827-8183
Toll-Free TTY: 800-241-1055
Fax: 301-402-0018
Website: www.nidcd.nih.gov
E-mail: nidcdinfo@nidcd.nih.gov

Substance Abuse and Mental Health Services Administration (SAMHSA)
5600 Fishers Ln.
Rockville, MD 20857
Toll-Free: 877-SAMHSA-7
(877-726-4727)
Toll-Free TTY: 800-487-4889
Fax: 240-221-4292
Website: www.samhsa.gov
E-mail: SAMHSAinfo@samhsa.hhs.gov

U.S. Department of Health and Human Services (HHS)
200 Independence Ave., S.W.
Hubert H. Humphrey Bldg.
Washington, DC 20201
Toll-Free: 877-696-6775
Website: www.hhs.gov
E-mail: media@hhs.gov

U.S. Food and Drug Administration (FDA)
10903 New Hampshire Ave.
Silver Spring, MD 20993-0002
Toll-Free: 888-INFO-FDA
(888-463-6332)
Website: www.fda.gov
E-mail: FDAOMA@fda.hhs.gov

U.S. National Library of Medicine (NLM)
8600 Rockville Pike
Bethesda, MD 20894
Toll-Free: 888-FIND-NLM
(888-346-3656)
Phone: 301-594-5983
Website: www.nlm.nih.gov
E-mail: NLMCommunications@nih.gov

PRIVATE ORGANIZATIONS THAT PROVIDE INFORMATION ABOUT MEDICAL TESTS

American Academy of Allergy, Asthma, and Immunology (AAAAI)
555 E. Wells St., Ste. 1100
Milwaukee, WI 53202-3823
Phone: 414-272-6071
Website: www.aaaai.org
E-mail: info@aaaai.org

American Academy of Family Physicians (AAFP)
11400 Tomahawk Creek Pkwy.
Leawood, KS 66211-2680
Toll-Free: 800-274-2237
Phone: 913-906-6000
Fax: 913-906-6075
Website: www.nf.aafp.org
E-mail: aafp@aafp.org

The American Academy of Pediatrics (AAP)
345 Park Blvd.
Itasca, IL 60143
Toll-Free: 800-433-9016
Fax: 847-434-8000
Website: www.aap.org
E-mail: mcc@aap.org

American Association of Neurological Surgeons (AANS)
5550 Meadowbrook Dr.
Rolling Meadows, IL 60008-3852
Toll-Free: 888-566-AANS (888-556-2267)
Phone: 847-378-0500
Fax: 847-378-0600
Website: www.aans.org
E-mail: info@aans.org

American Cancer Society (ACS)
250 Williams St., N.W.
Atlanta, GA 30303
Toll-Free: 800-227-2345
Website: www.cancer.org

American College of Physicians (ACP)
190 N. Independence Mall W.
Philadelphia, PA 19106-1572
Toll-Free: 800-523-1546
Phone: 215-351-2400
Website: www.acponline.org
E-mail: custserv@acponline.org

American College of Radiology® (ACR)
1891 Preston White Dr.
Reston, VA 20191
Toll-Free: 800-227-5463
Phone: 703-648-8900
Website: www.acr.org
E-mail: info@acr.org

American Diabetes Association® (ADA)
2451 Crystal Dr., Ste. 900
Arlington, VA 22202
Toll-Free: 800-DIABETES (800-342-2383)
Website: www.diabetes.org
E-mail: askada@diabetes.org

American Gastroenterological Association (AGA)
4930 Del Ray Ave.
Bethesda, MD 20814
Phone: 301-654-2055
Fax: 301-654-5920
Website: www.gastro.org
E-mail: member@gastro.org

American Heart Association (AHA)
7272 Greenville Ave.
Dallas, TX 75231
Toll-Free: 800-AHA-USA-1 (800-242-8721)
Phone: 214-570-5978
Website: www.heart.org
E-mail: inquiries@heart.org

American Kidney Fund (AKF)
11921 Rockville Pike, Ste. 300
Rockville, MD 20852
Toll-Free: 800-638-8299
Website: www.kidneyfund.org
E-mail: info@kidneyfund.org

American Society of Echocardiography (ASE)
2530 Meridian Pkwy., Ste. 450
Durham, NC 27713
Phone: 919-861-5574
Fax: 919-882-9900
Website: asecho.org
E-mail: ase@asecho.org

American Society of Radiologic Technologists (ASRT)
15000 Central Ave., S.E.
Albuquerque, NM 87123-3909
Toll-Free: 800-444-2778
Phone: 505-298-4500
Fax: 505-298-5063
Website: www.asrt.org
E-mail: memberservices@asrt.org

American Speech-Language-Hearing Association (ASHA)
2200 Research Blvd.
Rockville, MD 20850-3289
Toll-Free: 800-638-8255
Phone: 301-296-5700
TTY: 301-296-5650
Fax: 301-296-8580
Website: www.asha.org
E-mail: actioncenter@asha.org

American Stroke Association
7272 Greenville Ave.
Dallas, TX 75231
Toll-Free: 888-4-STROKE
(888-478-7653)
Website: www.stroke.org

Glaucoma Research Foundation (GRF)
251 Post St., Ste. 600
San Francisco, CA 94108
Toll-Free: 800-826-6693
Phone: 415-986-3162
Fax: 415-986-3763
Website: www.glaucoma.org
E-mail: grf@glaucoma.org

Health Physics Society (HPS)
950 Herndon Pkwy., Ste. 450
Herndon, VA 20170
Phone: 703-790-1745
Fax: 703-790-2672
Website: www.hps.org
E-mail: hps@BurkInc.com

Healthline Media, Inc.
660 3rd St.
San Francisco, CA 94107
Phone: 415-281-3100
Website: www.healthline.com
E-mail: info@healthline.com

International Foundation for Gastrointestinal Disorders (IFFGD)
3015 Dunes W. Blvd., Ste. 512
Mount Pleasant, SC 29466
Phone: 414-964-1799
Website: www.iffgd.org
E-mail: iffgd@iffgd.org

The Joint Commission
701 Pennsylvania Ave., N.W.
Ste. 700
Washington, DC 20004
Phone: 630-792-5800
Fax: 630-792-5005
Website: www.jointcommission.org
E-mail: customerservice@joint-commission.org

Juvenile Diabetes Research Foundation (JDRF)
26 Bdwy., 14th Fl.
New York, NY 10004
Toll-Free: 800-533-CURE (800-533-2873)
Fax: 212-785-9595
Website: www.jdrf.org
E-mail: info@jdrf.org

March of Dimes (MOD)
1550 Crystal Dr., Ste. 1300
Arlington, VA 22202
Toll-Free: 888-663-4637
Website: www.marchofdimes.org
E-mail: donorservice@marchofdimes.org

Mental Health America (MHA)
500 Montgomery St., Ste. 820
Alexandria, VA 22314
Toll-Free: 800-969-6642
Phone: 703-684-7722
Fax: 703-684-5968
Website: www.mentalhealthamerica.net
E-mail: info@mhanational.org

National Kidney Foundation® (NKF)
30 E. 33rd St.
New York, NY 10016
Toll-Free: 800-622-9010
Phone: 212-689-9261
Website: www.kidney.org
E-mail: info@kidney.org

National Sleep Foundation (NSF)
1414 N.E., 42nd St., Ste. 400
Seattle, WA 98105
Website: sleepfoundation.org
E-mail: contact@sleepfoundation.org

National Stroke Association (NSA)
9707 E. Easter Ln., Ste. B
Centennial, CO 80112
Toll-Free: 800-STROKES (800-787-6537)
Phone: 303-649-9299
Fax: 303-649-1328
Website: www.stroke.org
E-mail: info@stroke.org

The Nemours Foundation/ KidsHealth®
10140 Centurion Pkwy., N.
Jacksonville, FL 32256
Phone: 904-697-4100
Website: www.nemours.org
E-mail: media@nemours.org

Radiological Society of North America (RSNA)
820 Jorie Blvd., Ste. 200
Oak Brook, IL 60523-2251
Toll-Free: 800-381-6660
Phone: 630-571-2670
Fax: 630-571-7837
Website: www.rsna.org
E-mail: customerservice@rsna.org

RESOLVE: The National Infertility Association
7918 Jones Branch Dr., Ste. 300
McLean, VA 22102
Phone: 703-556-7172
Fax: 703-506-3266
Website: www.resolve.org
E-mail: info@resolve.org

Susan G. Komen
5005 LBJ Fwy., Ste. 526
Dallas, TX 75244
Toll-Free: 877-GO-KOMEN
(877-465-6636)
Website: ww5.komen.org
E-mail: info@komen.org

University of Maryland Medical Center (UMMC)
22 S. Greene St.
Baltimore, MD 21201-1595
Toll-Free: 800-492-5538
Phone: 410-328-8667
Website: www.umms.org
E-mail: media@umm.edu

WebMD, LLC.
1201 Peachtree St., N.E., 400
Colony Sq., Ste. 2100
Atlanta, GA 30361
Toll-Free: 866-788-3097
Website: www.webmd.com

INDEX

INDEX

Page numbers followed by 'n' indicate a footnote. Page numbers in *italics* indicate a table or illustration.

A

B

C

Index

D

E

F

G

N

O

P

Q

R

S

V

W

X

Y